Head and Neck Surgery: Latest Findings

Head and Neck Surgery: Latest Findings

Edited by Adrien Butler

hayle
medical

New York

Hayle Medical,
750 Third Avenue, 9th Floor,
New York, NY 10017, USA

Visit us on the World Wide Web at:
www.haylemedical.com

ISBN: 978-1-63241-724-4

Cataloging-in-Publication Data

Head and neck surgery : latest findings / edited by Adrien Butler.
      p. cm.
Includes bibliographical references and index.
ISBN 978-1-63241-724-4
1. Head--Surgery. 2. Neck--Surgery. 3. Otolaryngology, Operative.
4. Otolaryngology. I. Butler, Adrien.
RD521 .H43 2019
617.51--dc23

Table of Contents

Preface

This book was inspired by the evolution of our times; to answer the curiosity of inquisitive minds. Many developments have occurred across the globe in the recent past which has transformed the progress in the field.

Head and neck surgery is a surgical sub-field of medicine which is concerned with the structures of the head, neck, ear, nose and throat (ENT). Specialist doctors in this field are called head and neck surgeons. Some of the common surgical procedures performed by head and neck surgeons include thyrotomy, thyroplasty and tracheotomy. The procedure involving an incision of the larynx through the thyroid cartilage is known as thyrotomy. Thyroplasty is a procedure used to improve one's voice by altering the thyroid cartilage of the larynx. The procedure involving an incision on the anterior aspect of the neck, which is used to open a direct airway in the trachea, is known as tracheotomy. This book explores all the important aspects of head and neck surgery in the present day scenario. It strives to provide a fair idea about this discipline and to help develop a better understanding of the latest advances within this field. For all readers who are interested in head and neck surgery, the case studies included in this book will serve as an excellent guide to develop a comprehensive understanding.

This book was developed from a mere concept to drafts to chapters and finally compiled together as a complete text to benefit the readers across all nations. To ensure the quality of the content we instilled two significant steps in our procedure. The first was to appoint an editorial team that would verify the data and statistics provided in the book and also select the most appropriate and valuable contributions from the plentiful contributions we received from authors worldwide. The next step was to appoint an expert of the topic as the Editor-in-Chief, who would head the project and finally make the necessary amendments and modifications to make the text reader-friendly. I was then commissioned to examine all the material to present the topics in the most comprehensible and productive format.

I would like to take this opportunity to thank all the contributing authors who were supportive enough to contribute their time and knowledge to this project. I also wish to convey my regards to my family who have been extremely supportive during the entire project.

Editor

Does medical school research productivity predict a resident's research productivity during residency?

Scott Kohlert[1,2]* (iD), Laura Zuccaro[2], Laurie McLean[1,2] and Kristian Macdonald[1,2]

Abstract

Background: Research productivity is an important component of the CanMEDS Scholar role and is an accreditation requirement of Canadian Otolaryngology training programs. Our objective was to determine if an association exists between publication rates before and during Otolaryngology residency.

Methods: We obtained the names for all certified Canadian Otolaryngologists who graduated between 1998 and 2013 inclusive, and conducted a Medline search for all of their publications. Otolaryngologists were subgrouped based on year of residency graduation and the number of articles published pre-residency and during residency (0 or $\geq$1). Chi-squared analyses were used to evaluate whether publications pre-residency and year of graduation were associated with publications during residency.

Results: We obtained data for 312 Canadian Otolaryngologists. Of those 312 graduates, 46 (14.7%) had no identifiable publications on PubMed and were excluded from the final data analysis. Otolaryngology residents had a mean 0.65 (95% CI 0.50-0.80) publications before residency and 3.35 (95% CI 2.90-3.80) publications during residency. Between 1998 and 2013, mean publication rates before and during residency both increased significantly ($R^2 = 0.594$ and $R^2 = 0.759$, respectively), whereas publication rates after residency graduation has stagnated ($R^2 = 0.023$). The odds of publishing during residency was 5.85 times higher (95% CI 2.69-12.71) if a resident published prior to residency ($p < 0.0001$). The Spearman correlation coefficient between publications before and during residency is 0.472 ($p < 0.0001$).

Conclusion: Residents who publish at least one paper before residency are nearly six times as likely to publish during residency than those who did not publish before residency. These findings may help guide Otolaryngology program selection committees in ranking the best CaRMS candidates.

Keywords: Residency, CanMEDS, Publishing, Resident selection, Otolaryngology

Background

Medical students compete each year for approximately 30 Otolaryngology - Head and Neck Surgery (OTOHNS) residency positions country-wide through the Canadian Residency Matching Service (CaRMS). In 2015, 60 Canadian medical graduates applied for the 29 available residency positions, making OTOHNS the third most competitive surgical discipline [1]. Candidates are ranked based on their academic record, letters of recommendations, personal statements, elective experience, publications and research experience, extracurricular talents, personality and interpersonal traits, and overall impression. These factors, combined with their performance during face-to-face interviews, are used to assign an overall final rank for the match process.

There is previous literature that can help program selection committees predict which applicants will be most successful during residency [2, 3]. In 2012, Chole and colleagues found that many of the application factors typically used to select Otolaryngology resident candidates—such as exam performance, letters of recommendation, and performance during internship—might not be predictive of future capabilities as a clinician. In addition, Alpha Omega Alpha

* Correspondence: kohlert@me.com
[1]Department of Otolaryngology, The Ottawa Hospital, 501 Smyth Rd, Ottawa, ON K1H 8L6, Canada
[2]University of Ottawa, Ottawa, ON, Canada

membership and United States Medical Licensing Examination (USMLE) Part 1 examinations were not correlated with physician success [4]. However, rank of the medical school and faculty interview, as well as having excelled in a team sport correlated with higher clinical performance [5]. Previous studies that attempted to demonstrate an association between clinical performance in medical school and residencies in other surgical subspecialties have shown mixed results [6, 7].

Most medical schools and residency programs now support and expect completion of a scholarly project as part of postgraduate training. A recent study by Chen and colleagues showed a significant increase in the number of resident publications in the last few years [8]. While it is generally felt that publishing as a medical student and/or resident helps demonstrate proficiency in the CanMEDS "Scholar" role [9], a study involving general internal medicine residents [10] revealed that having pre-residency publications was not associated with higher evaluations in the scholar category. That said, previous work has demonstrated that publishing as a medical student or resident is significantly associated with subsequent career publications [11–13] and that medical school publications are associated with a higher propensity towards an academic career after completion of residency [14]. Of note, all data in these prior studies comes from medical and surgical specialties other than Otolaryngology.

We theorized that research productivity in medical school was associated with research productivity in OTOHNS residency. A recent study by Gupta and colleagues found that publishing prior to residency is significantly associated with publishing during a Pediatrics residency [15]. While prior research may be valued during the CaRMS selection process for applicants to an OTOHNS residency program, to our knowledge no similar study has examined this link among applicants to competitive surgical specialties. Our objective was to identify whether an association exists between publishing before and during OTOHNS residency. Our secondary outcome was to evaluate the trend of research productivity among medical students, residents and attending physicians over time.

Methods

Participants

This study targeted all practicing otolaryngologists who were certified by the Royal College of Physicians and Surgeons of Canada (RCPSC) between 1998 and 2013, inclusive. We created a database from information contained in the publicly available Royal College Specialist Directory [16] which included each surgeon's last name,

first name, middle names, certification date and current city of practice.

Publication collection

Each otolaryngologist was searched by full name in PubMED and any publications matching to that author were recorded. To increase the sensitivity of our search, multiple permutations were used for each search query (Table 1). In an attempt to reduce the likelihood of false positive identification, we used the following supportive characteristics for each publication collected: publication topic of Otolaryngology, corresponding geographic location of affiliated institution, and matching middle initials between publication and RCPSC database. If multiple authors with the same name were found, publications were only attributed to the target otolaryngologist if at least one of the previously mentioned supporting characteristics was present. To further increase the accuracy of our search, publication lists were cross-referenced with any identifiable publically available external sources including Research Gate, LinkedIn and online curriculum vitaes (CVs). Missed publications were added and false positives were removed from the final list of publications. Data collection was performed on April 1, 2015, and no papers published after this date were captured in this study.

Publication categorization

Otolaryngology – Head and Neck Surgery (OTOHNS) certification in Canada is completed in the summer of each year on June 30, following the final RCPSC examinations. The expected during residency and pre-residency time periods were classified based on the certification date. OTOHNS residency in Canada is five years in duration, thus the five years preceding certification were designated as residency, and prior to this was considered pre-residency. Each period was extended by one year, to capture articles that were likely completed within the pre or during residency period, but not published until afterwards (see Fig. 1). Articles were then categorized based on their date of initial abstract submission.

Table 1 Search permutations used to collect publications from PubMed

Search Permutations
Last, First
Last, First Middle
Last, F
Last, F*
Last, FM

*PubMed truncation symbol

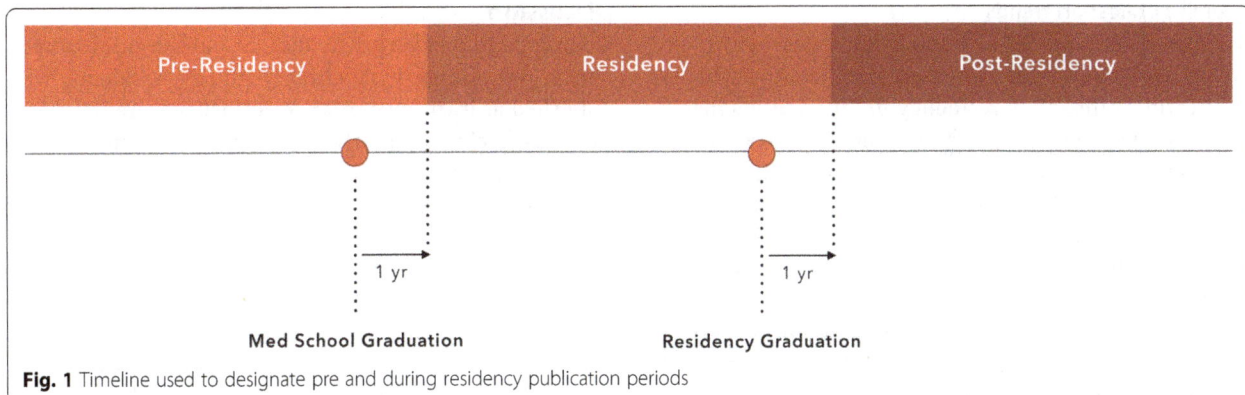

Fig. 1 Timeline used to designate pre and during residency publication periods

Statistical analysis

Each otolaryngologist was categorized as having either 0, 1, 2 or ≥ 3 publications for both of the time periods. Descriptive statistics were performed, including the mean rates of publication in each group, with 95% confidence intervals (95% CI). The data was separated by certification year in order to calculate trends in average publication rates over time using linear regression (Coefficient of Determination, R^2). Chi-squared analyses were used to evaluate whether publications pre-residency and year of graduation were associated with publications during residency. A Mantel-Haenszel calculation was used to measure the combined odds-ratio for the study population. A Spearman correlation coefficient was calculated for the relationship between the number of publications before residency compared to the number during residency.

Validation

To validate whether this method truly identifies a clinician's list of publications, an email was sent to all members of the Canadian Society of Otolaryngology who graduated between the years of 1998 and 2013 asking for a copy of their CV, as it was assumed that the CV could be used as the gold standard list of an author's publications (relying on the assumption that the authors would maintain an accurate list of their publications). This CV was subsequently cross-referenced against the list of publications that had been identified in our search. Any publications meeting the following exclusion criteria outlined in Table 2 were removed from the list.

Table 2 Validation Process - Exclusion Criteria

1. Papers published after April 1, 2015 (the date of data collection)

2. Articles published in non peer-reviewed journals, or in biomedical journals that are not indexed by Pubmed (as this is a basic marker of journal quality) including popular magazines and newspaper articles

3. Textbook chapters

4. Patents

Papers meeting the inclusion criteria were then manually cross-referenced against the publications identified in our search. True positives, false positives and false negatives were tracked and used to determine sensitivity and positive predictive value.

Ethics and permissions

As all data was publically available on PubMed and the Royal College website, research ethics board approval was not necessary for this study.

Results

Publication rates

Using the Royal College database and Medline/PubMed, 3441 publications for 312 residents were identified between 1998 and 2013. 46 (14.7%) of these had no publications during their career. There was an average of 0.65 (95% CI 0.50-0.80) publications before residency and 3.35 (95% CI 2.90-3.80) publications during residency. The number of residents with no publications was 216 (63%) prior to residency compared to 83 (26.6%) during residency. Only 7% (23/312) had ≥3 publications before residency, while 42% (131/312) had ≥3 publications during residency.

Residents who had at least 1 publication prior to residency were nearly six times more likely to publish at least once during residency (OR 5.85; 95% CI 2.7-12.7; $p < 0.0001$). There was a linear correlation between research publications prior to and during residency ($r = 0.472$, $p < 0.0001$). Table 3 shows the mean, median and mode publication rates among residents before and during residency.

Table 3 Overall mean, median and mode publication rates among Otolaryngology residents from 1998-2013

Number of publications	Before residency	During Residency
Mean	0.65	3.35
Median	0	2
Mode	0 (216/312 residents)	0 (83/312 residents)

Overall publication trends

Between 1998 and 2013, publication rates before and during residency both increased significantly, whereas publication rates after residency graduation stagnated. Residents who graduated from residency in 1998 had an average of 0.3 publications prior to residency, compared to 1.2 publications for graduates from 2013 ($R^2 = 0.594$). Individuals completing residency in 1998 published an average of 1.7 publications during residency, compared to 5.5 publications for those finishing in 2013 ($R^2 = 0.758$). This strong trend of increasing research productivity over time did not persist when looking at publication rates after completion of residency. Following graduation from Otolaryngology residency, individuals published an average 0.6 publications/year in 1998 compared to 0.3 publications/year in 2013 ($R^2 = 0.023$). Figures 2, 3, 4, and Table 4 highlight the trends in mean and median publication rates over time.

Validation

Thirty-one authors (10.3% response rate) provided us with either a copy of their CV or a separate up-to-date list of their publications. Each of the 874 publications that met the inclusion criteria were cross-referenced against the list of publications identified in our initial study. We identified 35 missed publications (i.e. false negatives), resulting in a search sensitivity of 96.1%. Based on the validation data, we identified an average of 1.1 missed publications per author.

The validation process initially identified 15 articles (from a total of 5 authors) as false positives as they were not found on the CV provided by the authors. These 5 authors were contacted to verify the accuracy of their CV. Upon further investigation, each of these 15 publications were in fact accurately attributed to the author in question (leaving us with zero false positives, and a positive predictive value of 100%).

Discussion

Compared to residents who did not publish prior to residency, we found that Otolaryngology residents who published at least once prior to residency were nearly six times as likely to publish in postgraduate training. Our results suggest a moderately correlated linear relationship of the number of papers published before residency with the number during residency. These findings indicate that research conducted prior to residency increases the likelihood the resident will publish scholarly work after residency begins.

Despite the demonstrated association between pre-residency publication and publications during residency, other variables are likely also at play and further work is required to identify and account for these confounding factors. Not all residency candidates have research experience, and publishing as a medical student or resident has not been shown to make an individual a better clinician. As previously stated, nearly 15% of Otolaryngologists in our study did not have any identifiable publications. Further, pre-residency publication status is not a definite predictor of a resident's publication potential, as 65% (141/216) of individuals without pre-residency publications did proceed to publish as a resident.

The results from this study could be used to help guide the research curriculum within Otolaryngology residency programs. For example, residents without prior research experience may benefit from early mentorship and formal training in research skills, and residents with prior experience may benefit from an amount of protected research time proportional to their research interests.

Potential limitations

Although a strength of our dataset is that it is a recent comprehensive national population study not affected by response rates, the correct author and publication time

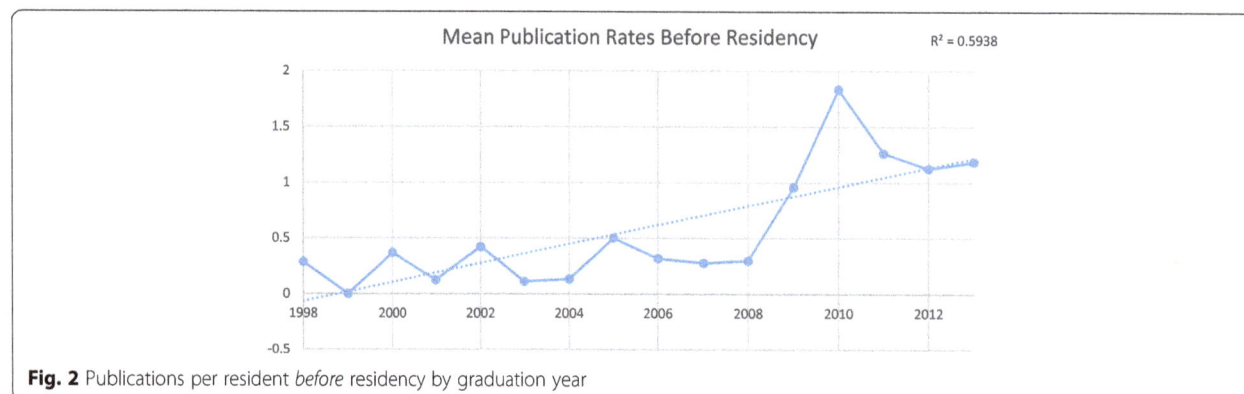

Fig. 2 Publications per resident *before* residency by graduation year

Does medical school research productivity predict a resident's research productivity during...

5

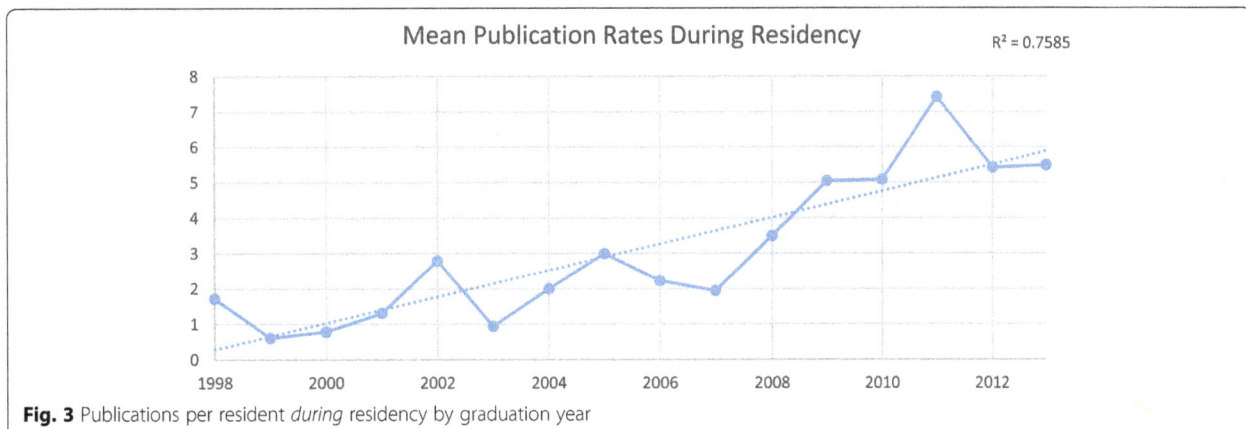

Fig. 3 Publications per resident *during* residency by graduation year

period could not be confirmed on an individual basis. Individuals whose residency periods were extended to greater than five years (e.g. due to completion of masters' degrees, maternity leave, or examination failure) may not be accurately identified in our analysis. This could result in misclassification of publications into the wrong time period (pre vs. during residency) and could skew our results either towards or away from the null hypothesis (that there is no correlation between pre or during residency publications).

Further, PubMed was exclusively used for data collection and any publications not listed on PubMed were not captured in the dataset, potentially underestimating the true number of a researcher's publications. We exclusively used this search method because of the basic scientific rigor associated with the PubMed's abstract listing criteria [17].

Future directions

Future research may include attempting to further stratify candidates based on various personal, program and publication variables.

Personal variables include: an individual's previous graduate degrees held, medical school, and completion of a

fellowship. Another interesting personal variable is the individual's *h-index*, an objective and easily calculable measure to evaluate both the number, as well as the relative importance of an author's scientific contributions. By looking not only at the number of publications but also the number of times each paper has been cited in the literature, the *h-index* is considered to be a more accurate marker of publication quality and academic success [18].

Future studies could also investigate the effect that the research environment (residency program, dedicated research time, support resources, attending physician research productivity, etc) has on the resident's research productivity.

Publication variables that could be examined include type of publication (eg: case report vs. systematic review vs. randomized control trial) and journal impact factor. Furthermore, future studies could also investigate the authorship trends of research in Otolaryngology. Single authorship is becoming increasingly less common in our current academic world, and inappropriate assignment of authorship credit is an increasingly well known phenomenon [19]. For example, a survey of authors in the "basic and medical sciences category" found that 26% of non-first authors admitted to not contributing substantially to the paper [20].

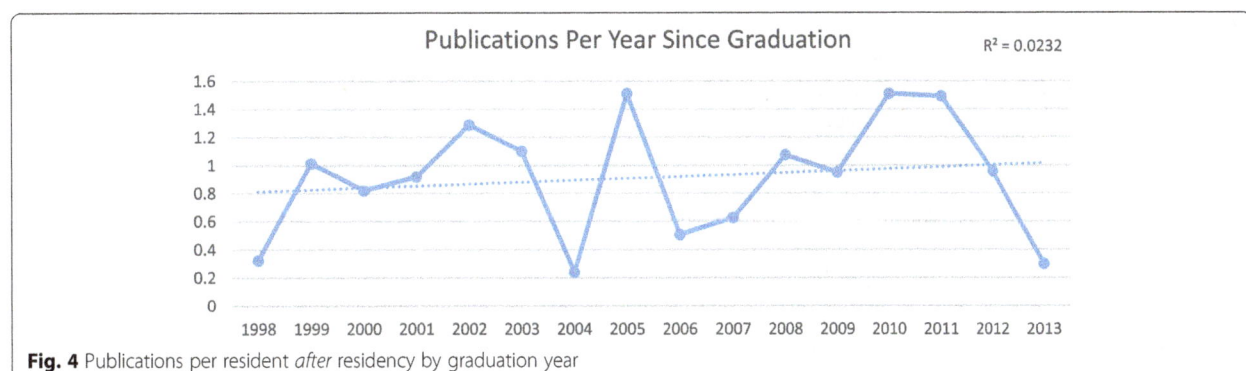

Fig. 4 Publications per resident *after* residency by graduation year

Table 4 Mean and median publication rates by residency graduation year

	Before Residency (total number of publications)		During Residency (total number of publications)		After Residency (number of publications per year)	
Grad Year	Mean	Median	Mean	Median	Mean	Median
1998	0.29	0	1.71	0	0.32	0.00
1999	0.00	0	0.62	0	1.02	0.33
2000	0.37	0	0.79	0	0.82	0.07
2001	0.13	0	1.31	0	0.92	0.31
2002	0.42	0	2.79	1	1.29	0.17
2003	0.11	0	0.94	1	1.10	0.09
2004	0.13	0	2.00	2	0.24	0.10
2005	0.50	0	3.00	2	1.51	0.28
2006	0.32	0	2.23	2	0.51	0.13
2007	0.28	0	1.94	2	0.63	0.36
2008	0.30	0	3.50	2	1.08	0.33
2009	0.96	0	5.04	4	0.95	0.40
2010	1.83	1	5.08	4	1.51	0.75
2011	1.26	0	7.42	5	1.49	0.67
2012	1.13	1	5.42	4	0.96	0.50
2013	1.19	1	5.48	4	0.30	0.00

Otolaryngology may be not immune to this phenomenon, with multiple authors in our study having been credited with publishing at an average rate of ≥1 paper/month over the past 5 years. Further studies looking at research productivity could evaluate author order, degree of author contribution, and total number of co-authors listed per publication.

While our study found that publication rates after residency graduation have not been rising over time, our data was not detailed enough to allow us to separate academic otolaryngologists from community otolaryngologists. A future study could collect this data and perform a subgroup analysis to compare the trends in research productivity over time between these two groups.

Conclusion

In this nation-wide sample of Canadian certified otolaryngologists, we demonstrated that pre-residency publication is significantly associated with subsequent publication during residency. Over the past 16 years, publication rates have steadily increased both before and during residency. During that same timespan, publication rates among practicing otolaryngologists has remained relatively stagnant. Our analysis did not take into account several potential confounding variables.

Pre-residency research productivity is a predictor for research productivity in residency and can act as a helpful marker for residency program selection committees in ranking candidates for the CaRMS match.

Abbreviations
OTOHNS: Otolaryngology - Head and Neck Surgery; CaRMS: Canadian Residency Matching Service; USMLE: United States Medical Licensing Examination; RCPSC: Royal College of Physicians and Surgeons of Canada; CV: Curriculum vitae; R^2: Coefficient of Determination

Acknowledgements
The authors would like to thank Dr. Daniel Corsi and Mr. William Petrcich of the Ottawa Methods Centre for their assistance with the statistical analysis of our dataset.

Funding
No funding was received by any of the authors in relation to this study.

Authors' contributions
SK assisted with the study design, data collection, data analysis, and writing of the manuscript. LZ was involved in data collection and writing of the manuscript. LM critically appraised and made edits leading to the final manuscript. KM assisted with study design, supervised the drafting of the initial manuscript, critically appraised and made edits leading to the final manuscript. All authors have read and approved the final version of the manuscript.

Competing interests
The authors declare that they have no competing interests.

References

1. Canadian Residency Matching Service. R-1 match reports – 2015 - CaRMS. carms. ca. 2015. at <http://www.carms.ca/en/data-and-reports/r-1/reports-2015/>.
2. Bent JP, et al. Otolaryngology resident selection: do rank lists matter? Otolaryngol Head Neck Surg. 2011;144:537–41.
3. Calhoun KH, Hokanson JA, Bailey BJ. Predictors of residency performance: a follow-up study. Otolaryngol Head Neck Surg. 1997;116:647–51.
4. Daly KA, Levine SC, Adams GL. Predictors for resident success in otolaryngology. J Am Coll Surg. 2006;202:649–54.
5. Chole RA, Ogden MA. Predictors of future success in otolaryngology residency applicants. Arch Otolaryngol Head Neck Surg. 2012;138:707–12.
6. Egol KA, Collins J, Zuckerman JD. Success in orthopaedic training: resident selection and predictors of quality performance. J Am Acad Orthop Surg. 2011;19:72–80.
7. Stohl HE, Hueppchen NA, Bienstock JL. Can medical school performance predict residency performance? Resident selection and predictors of successful performance in obstetrics and gynecology. J Grad Med Educ. 2010;2:322–6.
8. Chen JX, et al. Increased Resident Research over an 18-Year Period: A Single Institution's Experience. Otolaryngol Head Neck Surg. 2015;153:350–6.
9. Frank JR, Snell L, Sherbino J. CanMEDS 2015: Physician Competency Framework. 2015. at < http://canmeds.royalcollege.ca/en/framework >.
10. Cavalcanti RB, Detsky AS. Publishing history does not correlate with clinical performance among internal medicine residents. Med Educ. 2010;44:468–74.
11. Dorsey ER, Raphael BA, Balcer LJ, Galetta SL. Predictors of future publication record and academic rank in a cohort of neurology residents. Neurology. 2006;67:1335–7.
12. Rezek I, McDonald RJ, Kallmes DF. Pre-residency publication rate strongly predicts future academic radiology potential. Acad Radiol. 2012;19:632–4.
13. Yang G, et al. Urology resident publication output and its relationship to future academic achievement. J Urol. 2011;185:642–6.
14. Grimm LJ, et al. Predictors of an academic career on radiology residency applications. Acad Radiol. 2014;21:685–90.
15. Gupta R, Norris ML, Writer H. Preresidency publication record and its association with publishing during paediatric residency. Paediatr Child Health. 2016;21(4):187–90.
16. The Royal College of Physicians and Surgeons of Canada. Royal College Specialist Directory. royalcollege.ca. 2015. at <http://www.royalcollege.ca/rcdir/>.
17. National Institutes of Health (NIH),. Fact Sheet: MEDLINE® Journal Selection. nlm.nih.gov. 2015. at <https://www.nlm.nih.gov/pubs/factsheets/jsel.html>.
18. Svider PF, et al. The use of the h-index in academic otolaryngology. Laryngoscope. 2013;123:103–6.
19. Shaffer E. Too many authors spoil the credit. Can J Gastroenterol Hepatol. 2014;28(11):605.
20. Osborne JW, Holland A. What is authorship, and what should it be? A survey of prominent guidelines for determining authorship in scientific publications. Practical Assessment, Research & Evaluation. 2009;14:1–19.

2

An automated A-value measurement tool for accurate cochlear duct length estimation

John E. Iyaniwura[1*], Mai Elfarnawany[2], Hanif M. Ladak[1,2,3,4†] and Sumit K. Agrawal[1,2,4,5†]

Abstract

Background: There has been renewed interest in the cochlear duct length (CDL) for preoperative cochlear implant electrode selection and postoperative generation of patient-specific frequency maps. The CDL can be estimated by measuring the A-value, which is defined as the length between the round window and the furthest point on the basal turn. Unfortunately, there is significant intra- and inter-observer variability when these measurements are made clinically. The objective of this study was to develop an automated A-value measurement algorithm to improve accuracy and eliminate observer variability.

Method: Clinical and micro-CT images of 20 cadaveric cochleae specimens were acquired. The micro-CT of one sample was chosen as the atlas, and A-value fiducials were placed onto that image. Image registration (rigid affine and non-rigid B-spline) was applied between the atlas and the 19 remaining clinical CT images. The registration transform was applied to the A-value fiducials, and the A-value was then automatically calculated for each specimen. High resolution micro-CT images of the same 19 specimens were used to measure the gold standard A-values for comparison against the manual and automated methods.

Results: The registration algorithm had excellent qualitative overlap between the atlas and target images. The automated method eliminated the observer variability and the systematic underestimation by experts. Manual measurement of the A-value on clinical CT had a mean error of $9.5 \pm 4.3\%$ compared to micro-CT, and this improved to an error of $2.7 \pm 2.1\%$ using the automated algorithm. Both the automated and manual methods correlated significantly with the gold standard micro-CT A-values ($r = 0.70$, $p < 0.01$ and $r = 0.69$, $p < 0.01$, respectively).

Conclusion: An automated A-value measurement tool using atlas-based registration methods was successfully developed and validated. The automated method eliminated the observer variability and improved accuracy as compared to manual measurements by experts. This open-source tool has the potential to benefit cochlear implant recipients in the future.

Keywords: Cochlear duct length, A-value, Computer tomography, Atlas-based registration, Cochlear implants

Background

Cochlear implants (CI) are now commonly used worldwide to restore hearing in patients with severe to profound sensorineural hearing loss (SNHL) [1–3]. The literature has described significant variation in the human cochlear duct length (CDL) [4–8], which may have an impact on CI electrode selection for patients [9, 10]. An electrode cannot be too long (which would result in incomplete insertion), or too short (poorer cochlear coverage). Knowledge of the CDL a priori would help with pre-operative electrode selection.

Several studies have examined the benefits of deep insertions and complete cochlear coverage. Roy et al. reported a benefit in musical appreciation with deeper insertions [11] while Qi et al. highlighted similar benefits with tonal language discrimination [12]. Mistrik and Jolly emphasized that low frequency information delivered to the cochlear apex is particularly important for spatial hearing [13]. In addition, they commented that the matching of the electrode array length and cochlear length is the most important factor which directly affects the mapping of CI electrode array to the auditory nerve of the cochlea.

* Correspondence: jiyaniwu@uwo.ca
†Equal contributors
[1]Biomedical Engineering Graduate Program, Western University, 1151 Richmond Street, London, ON N6A 3K7, Canada
Full list of author information is available at the end of the article

Apart from lower frequency information, Hochmair et al. [10] noted that deeper insertions provide the opportunity for: 1) better mapping of tonotopic locations within the cochlea, 2) increase in the coverage of cochlear locations, and 3) the reduction of potential channel overlap due to larger contact divisions per channel.

In addition to the *pre-operative* electrode selection to maximize cochlear coverage, the CDL can be used *post-operatively* to create custom frequency maps for patients, potentially reducing place pitch mismatch, the effect of which has been studied clinically. The greenwood equation is used as a guideline for post-operative frequency mapping of the CI electrode arrays and it is directly dependant on the CDL. Based on this equation, Koch et al. demonstrated a CDL length mismatch of 6 mm would translate to a frequency mismatch of 1100 Hz in the basal region and 400 Hz in the apical region [14–16]. Fu et al. carried out a clinical study that showed a shift of just 2–4 mm affected patients' rehabilitation times [17]. With bilateral CI users, Kan et al. and Stelmach et al. highlighted that a place mismatch can occur between the left and right electrode arrays and that this mismatch can simply be as a result of insertion depth differences [18, 19]. Studies have also shown that such place pitch mismatches can lead to poor speech recognition in noisy environments [20], a shift in the perceive location of sound sources [18], and poor interaural time differences (ITD) [21, 22]. In addition, with regards to cochlear implant users with single sided deafness (SSD), Rader et al. concluded that place dependant stimulation can be expected to improve pitch perception [23]. Other studies have shown conceivable shortcomings in CI performances due to significant levels of place pitch mismatching [15, 24–26]. In order to reduce pitch place mismatch, CDL estimates would be needed to create custom frequency maps.

The complete effects of deep insertions, frequency place pitch mismatch, and the potential benefits of customizable electrode lengths and individualized frequency map fitting, is still an ongoing active area of research, and preliminary results hold significant clinical relevance [4, 27–30].

Currently the CDL can be estimated using the A-value; a measurement defined as the length of the straight line between the middle of the round window, passing through the modiolar axis, and reaching the furthest point on the basal turn [31]. This measurement was proposed by Escudé et al., who utilized the correlation between the A-value and the CDL [31]. Alexiades et al. [32] proposed an equation to determine CDLs using the A-value, and these equations were further modified using high resolution imaging by Koch et al. [14]. However, despite the simplicity of this method and its relevance, there is significant inter-observer and intra-observer variability associated with the A-value measurement on clinical CT scans [33, 34]. The development of an automated tool to measure the A-value could alleviate this user variability.

The primary objective of this study is to develop an automated algorithm using atlas-based registration techniques on an open-source platform. The secondary objective is to compare the accuracy of the automated tool against manual measurements by experts. A set of micro-CT (μCT) images of the same sample set was used as the gold standard for measurement.

Methods
Image acquisition
Twenty fixed cadaveric temporal bone specimens were obtained for the study. Ethics approval was acquired through the Department of Anatomy at the Schulich School of Medicine and Dentistry at Western University, Ontario Canada.

Clinical CT images
All 20 specimens were scanned at a clinical resolution of 600 μm using the Discovery CT750 HD Clinical Scanner (GE Healthcare, Chicago, IL), equipped with GE's Gemstone CT detector. The Scanner was set to a slice thickness of 0.625 mm and an x-ray voltage of 120 kV. The acquisition time for each of the 20 specimens was approximately 20 s.

Micro-CT images
High resolution micro-CT (μCT) images were acquired for all 20 specimens. The temporal bone specimens where trimmed using a cylindrical drill bit, with a diameter of 40 mm and a height of 60 mm. Special care was taken to ensure the region of interest was preserved. The trimmed specimens could then be imaged with the eXplore Locus μCT scanner (GE Healthcare, Chicago, IL), which was set at 80 kV and 0.45 mA. Using an incremental angle of 0.4 degrees, approximately 900 views could be captured. A modified cone beam algorithm [35] was used to reconstruct a 3D image with a voxel size of 20μm.

Gold standard values
A fellowship trained neurotologist (SKA) measured the A-value on a set of 20 high resolution μCT images. These images were reconstructed at an oblique angle that enabled the full basal turn of the cochlea to be visualized. The reconstructed views were subsequently displayed with an appropriate minimum-intensity projection (MinIP) as described by Escudé et al. [31]. The A-value for all 20 specimens served as the gold standard reference values [33]. As a note, intra- and inter-observer variation was insignificant on these high-resolution μCT scans as the round window membrane

and outer cochlear wall were clearly visible on the MinIP projections.

Atlas generation

The μCT image of the specimen with the median gold standard A-value was selected to be used as the single atlas for the automated algorithm. The atlas was mirrored to ensure that models were available for both right and left cochleae. To facilitate accurate registration, the atlas was cropped to only contain the region of interest in 3D Slicer [36]. Two fiducials were then placed; one on the centre of the round window and the other on furthest point on the basal turn as shown in Fig. 1.

Registration algorithm

The registration algorithm was developed on an open source software platform, 3D Slicer [36, 37]. The algorithm components are illustrated in the flowchart (Fig. 2). The atlas (source image) was loaded along with the clinical CT (target) image. Fiducials were placed on the following landmarks: the cochlear apex, modiolus, round window and oval window. Landmark registration was then used to ensure the source and target images were in the same spatial region. Finally, the target image was cropped to extract the region of interest (i.e., the cochlea and immediate surrounding structures).

Affine registration

Affine image registration is a form of linear registration that incorporates translation, rotation, scaling, and shearing. The dimension of the image determines the degrees of freedom in the registration [38]. The CT images were 3-dimensional, which resulted in a total of 12 degrees of freedom (DOF) (translation, rotation, scaling, and shearing were performed in each of the x, y, and z axis). Affine registration is restricted in that it only captures global differences between images, therefore, it is typically used as a technique to align a set of images before non-linear registration techniques are applied [38, 39]. To capture global differences alone, only 0.1% of the clinical CT (target image) was considered by the algorithm. Normalized cross correlation (NCC) was used as the image similarity comparison metric, which defined the registration's objective function. Table 1 outlines the complete set of parameters used.

B-Spline registration

A free-form deformation (FFD) model based on b-splines, was used to address local differences between the images. FFDs allows for local deformation of an image through the manipulation of a mesh of control points [39]. After the movement of the control points, a b-spline function is used to interpolate the corresponding movement in the image and the degrees of freedom for b-spline registration is determined by the number of control points [40]. After the affine registration addressed global differences, b-spline registration was then used to address local differences between the images. The parameters used for the b-spline registration in Table 1 were based on Elfarnawany et al. [41]. A 3D mesh of control points (4 x 4 x 4) allowed for a total of 64 DOF and NCC again was used as the image similarity metric used to define the objective function. The whole clinical sample (100%) was used in the registration process in an attempt to capture all the local differences between the clinical CT and atlas images. The generated b-spline transform matrix was applied to the atlas and its corresponding A-value fiducials, and the new distance between the fiducials was computed as the A-value of the target image.

Evaluation of automated method

The registration algorithm was implemented on 19 specimens, as the atlas was excluded from the analysis. Depending on whether the target image was a right or left cochlea, the registration algorithm was applied using the corresponding atlas. The results of the automated

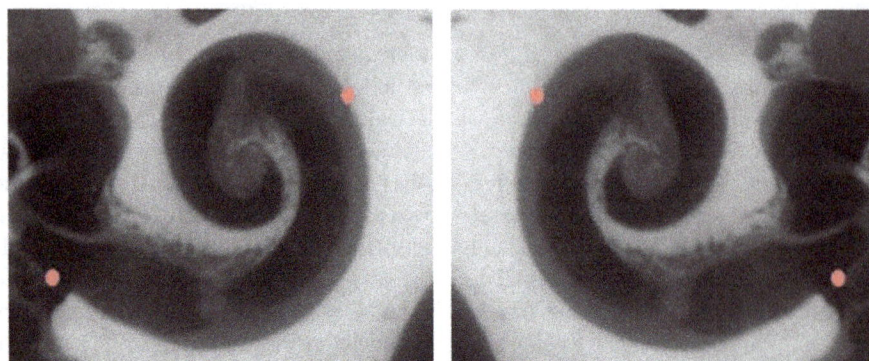

Fig. 1 Atlas with two fiducials on the right and left cochleae

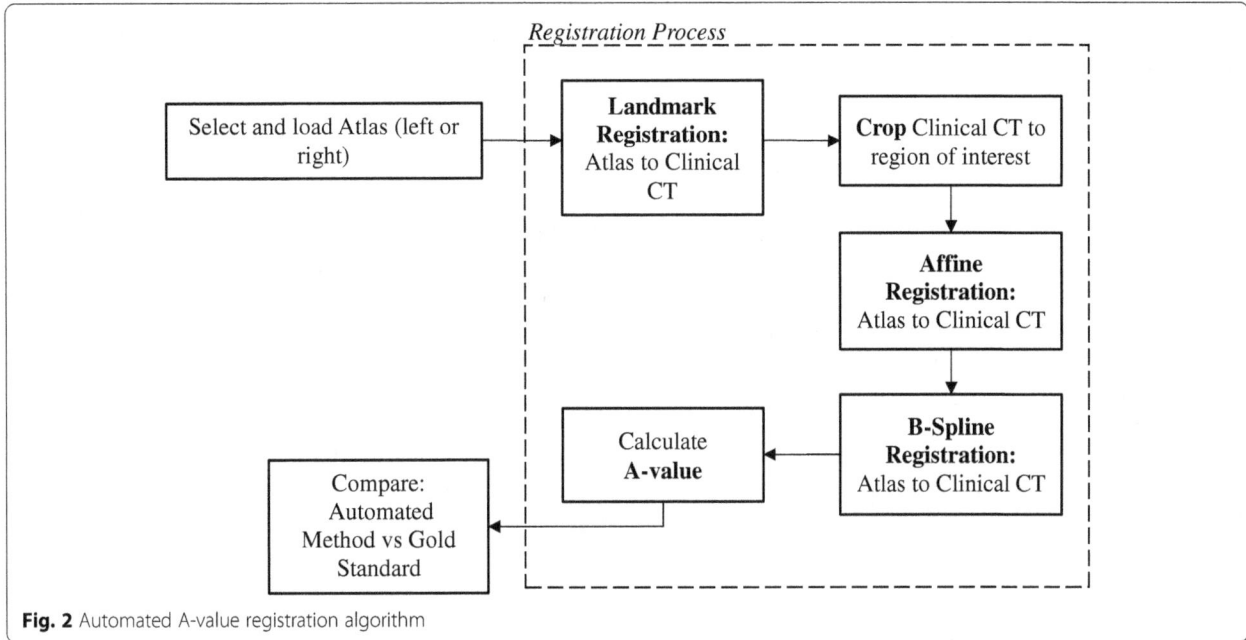

Fig. 2 Automated A-value registration algorithm

method applied on the clinical CT images were compared to the gold standard A-values from the μCT images of the same samples. Additionally, the automated method results were compared to the A-values manually acquired by experts on the same set of clinical CT images in a previous study [33].

Qualitative evaluation

3D models of the atlas and a clinical CT image sample were created. The overlap of the models and the A-value fiducials were qualitatively evaluated before and after the registration algorithm. The deformation grids of the atlas, before and after each registration step, were also generated and visualized.

Quantitative evaluation

A-values obtained using the automated registration-based method were compared to the gold standard reference values by calculating the absolute percentage difference. The mean percentage difference of the automated method from the gold standard was compared to the difference of the manual method reported in Iyaniwura et al. [33]. The automated and manually measured A-values were tested for normality using the Shapiro-Wilk test. Based on this result, the Wilcoxon

matched pairs test was used to compare these values against the gold standard. The correlation between the two sets (automated and manual) of A-values and the gold standard A-values were evaluated using the Spearman correlation.

Lastly, Bland-Altman plots were used to display the differences between the A-values from clinical CT (automated method and manually measured) and the gold standard A-value measurements. A clinically acceptable A-value error range of ± 1.05 mm was determined based on the revised cochlear length equations published by Koch et al. [18] and is indicated on the derived Bland-Altman plots.

Results
Qualitative results

The cochlear models generated from the μCT (atlas), clinical CT (target), and the corresponding deformation grids were analysed. In all cases, affine registration successfully aligned the atlas and clinical CT images, addressing the majority of the global differences between the two images. Subsequently, the b-spline registration further improved the alignment addressing the local difference between the two images.

Table 1 Automated method parameters for Landmark, Affine, and B-Spline registration

Registration	Initialization	Objective function	Degrees Of Freedom (DOF)	% of Sample
Landmark	Fiducial placements	Least squares	6 DOF	N/A
Affine	Geometric alignment	Normalized Cross Correlation (NCC)	12 DOF	0.1
B-Spline	Affine transform	Normalized Cross Correlation (NCC)	64 DOF	100

Figure 3 provides a specific example where the target image was larger than the atlas. Affine registration globally expanded the atlas as shown by the deformation grid, and this achieved a partial overlap with the target (Fig. 3b). B-spline registration was then able to deal with the local differences, and the individual protrusions can be visualized on the deformation grid (Fig. 3c).

Quantitative results

The absolute percentage difference (mean ± standard deviation), Wilcoxon test, and Spearman correlation were used to analyze manual and automated A-value measurements. Table 2 summarizes these results as compared to the gold standard measurements from μCT. The automated method had a 2.7 ± 2.1% absolute difference from the gold standard compared to a difference of 9.5 ± 4.3% for the manual method reported in Iyaniwura et al. [33]. Using the Wilcoxon test, the automated method was not significantly different from the gold standard ($p = 0.061$, ns), but the manual method was significantly different from the gold standard ($p < 0.0001$). Comparing the automated method against the manual method, the results were significantly different from each other ($p < 0.0001$). Both the automated and manual methods had significant Spearman correlations of $r = 0.70$ ($p < 0.01$) and $r = 0.69$ ($p < 0.01$), respectively, when compared to the gold standard measurements.

Bland-Altman plots were generated as shown in Fig. 4. A comparison of the automated method against the gold standard revealed that all measurements fell within the acceptable range (Fig. 4a). Experts' manual measurements reported by Iyaniwura et al. [33] depicted an

Table 2 Percentage difference, Spearman correlation & Wilcoxon test comparison of manual and automated method

	% Difference	Wilcoxon	Spearman
Manual	9.5 ± 4.3%	$p < 0.0001$	$r = 0.69**$
Automated	2.7 ± 2.1%	$p = 0.061$ (ns)	$r = 0.70**$

$**p < 0.01$

underestimation of true A-values. A second Bland-Altman plot was generated from these previously reported manual measurements and 26% of those measurements were found to be outside of the acceptable range (Fig. 4b).

Discussion

As discussed, there is significant variation in cochlear size and morphology described in the literature [4–8, 42]. To develop a robust algorithm, 50 cochleae were initially scanned and a subset of 20 cochleae were chosen to represent a wide range of A-values. An additional strength of the study was the availability of corresponding μCT images of the clinical CT images, which allowed for a gold standard validation of the algorithm.

Overall, the quantitative results revealed a statistically significant 6.8 ± 4.8% improvement in accuracy using the automated method. This algorithm also corrected the 26% of values that fell outside the clinically acceptable range using the manual method as observed on the Bland-Altman plots. The type of error on these plots was also different between the automated and manual methods. The automated algorithm had a random error centred on the origin, whereas the manual measurements consistently underestimated the true A-value (Fig. 4). The error observed in Fig. 4b can be described as a systematic error in the manual measurements. This error is most likely

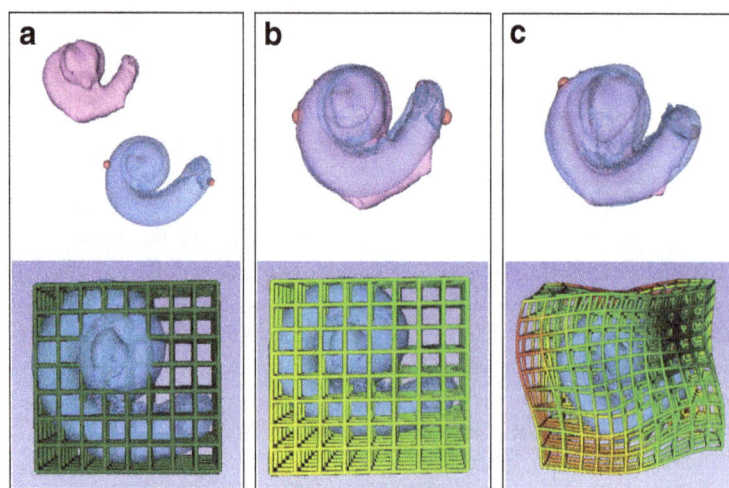

Fig. 3 Micro-CT Atlas (blue) and Clinical CT Target (pink) before registration. **a** Original deformation grid around atlas shown. **b** Atlas and Target overlapped after affine registration with associated deformation grid. **c** Atlas and Target overlapped after B-Spline registration with associated deformation grid

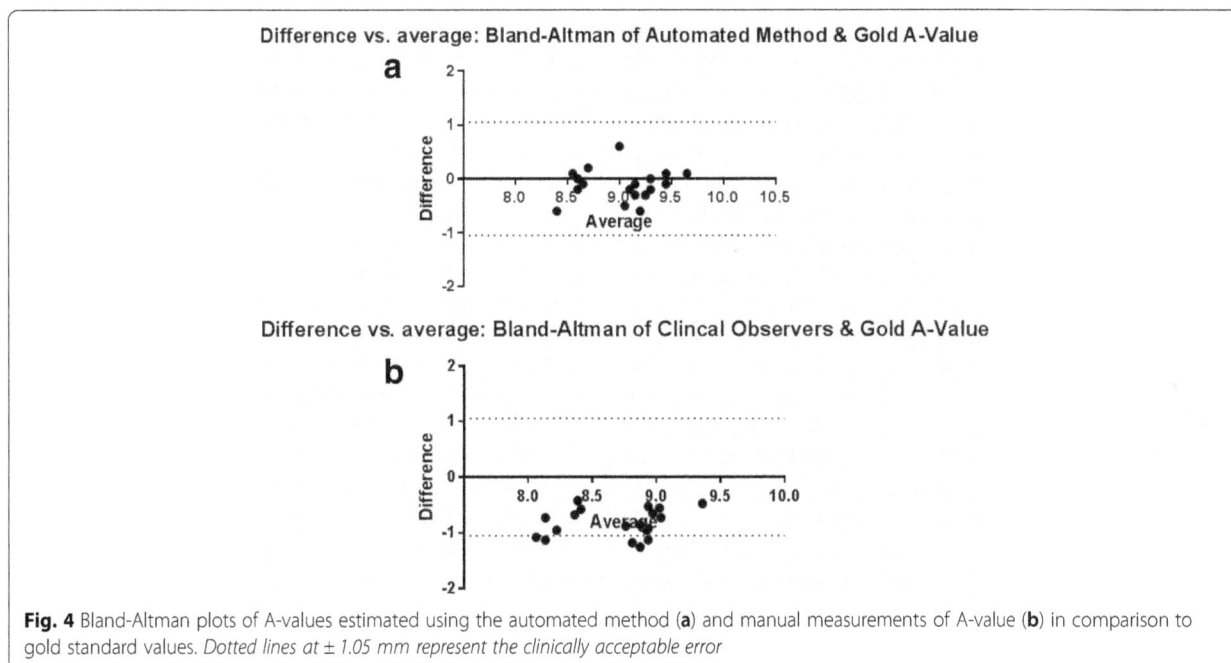

Fig. 4 Bland-Altman plots of A-values estimated using the automated method (**a**) and manual measurements of A-value (**b**) in comparison to gold standard values. *Dotted lines at ± 1.05 mm represent the clinically acceptable error*

attributed to both the poor visibility of the round window in clinical CT images, and the variability associated with the selection of an oblique plane for the multiplanar reconstruction of each clinical CT image; however, a similar study with a larger n (participants would need to be conducted [33]. Furthermore the clinical CT images used in this study were of relatively low resolution (625um); however, other commonly used clinical CT scanning modalities such as cone beam computed tomography (CBCT), typically exhibit higher resolutions [43, 44]. As such an improvement in the algorithm's performance would be hypothesized if utilized on CBCT images, for example.

Intra- and inter-observer variability between specialists also has been identified as a major source of error when measuring A-values on clinical CT [33, 34]. Iyaniwura et al. [19] reported intraclass correlation (ICC) coefficients for inter-observer variability (ICC = 0.57) and intra-observer variability (ICC range = 0.54 to 0.90). Rivas et al. [20] reported a mean absolute difference as high as 8 mm for CDL estimates calculated from manual A-value measurements. The automated algorithm described eliminates this observer variability.

The clinical significance of improved accuracy and consistency can be assessed by examining its effect on electrode selection and on the frequency mapping of the cochlea via the Greenwood equation. [16, 32, 45]. With regards to electrode selection, Iyaniwura et al. [33], using an average CDL value of 32.9 mm, derived an average CDL variation of ±3.9 mm with the manual method. Cochlear implant manufacturers have off the shelf

implants available in 15, 17, 20, 24, 25, 28 and 31 mm variants, therefore a variation of ±3.9 mm could lead to improper electrode selection preoperatively [13, 46–49]. In terms of customized frequency maps, Koch et al. [14] calculated that a 6 mm error in CDL would result in a frequency-place mismatch of 400 Hz at the apical turn and 1100 Hz along the basal turn of the cochlea. These discrepancies could translate into discernible effects on cochlear implant performance [15, 24].

There have been a number of registration techniques that have been described in the medical imaging literature. In structures with significant variability, FFD (non-linear/non-rigid) registration like b-spline, as well as atlas-based registration techniques, are typically used [39, 41, 50–56]. In this study, a single atlas with b-spline registration was sufficient in improving the accuracy of A-value measurements, which are based upon the basal turn of the cochlea. However, the cochlear apex can exhibit significant additional variation between patients [5, 14, 32, 45] If the apex was to be directly modeled in the future, this could be overcome using multi-atlas registration techniques. [56–58].

Other studies have attempted to register inner ear structures for a variety of purposes. Christensen et al. used a deformable atlas based registration technique to measure shapes within the inner ear [59], however they did not measure the A-value or the CDL. Rivas et al. [34] developed a sophisticated algorithm for measuring the CDL, however no high-resolution μCT images were available to validate their results. The A-value measured by the algorithm can then be used to estimate the CDL at the lateral wall and Organ of Corti by using equations developed by Alexiades et al. [32] and Koch et al. [14]. These equations have been built into the module as part of the output to the end-user.

The implemented automated algorithm will be made available as an open-source software extension to 3D Slicer. This would allow for further development by other groups and validation of the methodology on a wider variety of cochleae.

Conclusion

An automated method to estimate cochlear length based on the A-value was developed using open-source atlas-based registration tools. The automated method produced more accurate results than the manual method, and eliminated the observer variability between experts. This improved accuracy may be clinically important for electrode selection and patient-specific frequency mapping of cochlear implants.

Abbreviations
3D: Three dimensional; CBCT: Cone beam computed tomography; CDL: Cochlear duct length; CI: Cochlear implants; CT: Computed tomography; DOF: Degrees of freedom; FFD: Free-form deformation; ICC: Intraclass correlation; NCC: Normalized cross correlation; SNHL: Sensorineural hearing loss; μCT: Micro-CT

Acknowledgements
Financial support for John Enioluwa Iyaniwura was provided by MITACS Accelerate, Natural Sciences and Engineering Research Council of Canada (NSERC), and the Otolaryngology Graduate Research Scholarship (Department of Otolaryngology - Head and Neck Surgery, Western University, Canada).

Funding
This study was funded by an Otolaryngology Graduate Research Scholarship (The Department of Otolaryngology – Head and Neck Surgery, Schulich Medicine & Dentistry, Western University, Canada), a MITACS Accelerate Internship (Canada) and an Engineering Research Council of Canada (NSERC) Discovery Grant.

Authors' contributions
JEI developed the algorithm under the guidance of ME and HML. JEI, ME and SKA wrote the manuscript. HML and SKA were primary supervisors for JEI. All authors read and approved the final manuscript.

Authors' information
HML and SKA were co-senior authors on this study.

Competing interests
The authors declare that they have no competing interests.

Author details
[1]Biomedical Engineering Graduate Program, Western University, 1151 Richmond Street, London, ON N6A 3K7, Canada. [2]Department of Otolaryngology-Head and Neck Surgery, Western University, London, ON, Canada. [3]Department of Medical Biophysics, Western University, London, ON, Canada. [4]Department of Electrical and Computer Engineering, Western University, London, ON, Canada. [5]London Health Science Centre, Room B1-333, University Hospital, 339 Windermere Rd., London, ON, Canada.

References
1. Peterson NR, Pisoni DB, Miyamoto RT. Cochlear implants and spoken language processing abilities: review and assessment of the literature. Restor Neurol Neurosci. 2010;28:237–50.
2. Montes F, Peñaranda A, Correa S, Peñaranda D, García J-M, Aparicio ML, et al. Cochlear implants versus hearing aids in a middle-income country: costs, productivity, and quality of life. Otol Neurotol Off Publ Am Otol Soc Am Neurotol Soc Eur Acad Otol Neurotol. 2017;
3. Biller A, Bartsch A, Knaus C, Müller J, Solymosi L, Bendszus M. Neuroradiological imaging in patients with sensorineural hearing loss prior to cochlear implantation. ROFO Fortschr Geb Rontgenstr Nuklearmed. 2007;179:901–13.
4. Meng J, Li S, Zhang F, Li Q, Qin Z. Cochlear size and shape variability and implications in Cochlear implantation surgery. Otol Neurotol. 2016;37:1307–13.
5. Erixon E, Hogstorp H, Wadin K, Rask-Andersen H. Variational anatomy of the human cochlea: implications for Cochlear implantation. Otol Neurotol. 2009; 30:14–22.
6. Miller JD. Sex diffferences in the length of the organ of Corti in humans. J Acoust Soc Am. 2007;121:EL151–5.
7. Ketten DR, Vannier MW, Skinner MW, Gates GA, Wang G, Neely JG. In vivo measures of cochlear length and insertion depth of nucleus cochlear implant electrode arrays. Ann Otol Rhinol Laryngol. 1998;107:1–16.
8. Ulehlova L, Voldrich L, Janisch R. Correlative study of sensory cell-density and Cochlear length in humans. Hear Res. 1987;28:149–51.
9. Landsberger DM, Mertens G, Punte AK, Van De Heyning P. Perceptual changes in place of stimulation with long cochlear implant electrode arrays. J Acoust Soc Am. 2014;135:EL75–81.
10. Hochmair I, Hochmair E, Nopp P, Waller M, Jolly C. Deep electrode insertion and sound coding in cochlear implants. Hear Res. 2015;322:14–23.
11. Roy AT, Penninger RT, Pearl MS, Wuerfel W, Jiradejvong P, Carver C, et al. Deeper Cochlear implant electrode insertion angle improves detection of musical sound quality deterioration related to bass frequency removal. Otol Neurotol. 2016;37:146–51.
12. Qi B, Liu B, Krenmayr A, Liu S, Gong S, Liu H, et al. The contribution of apical stimulation to mandarin speech perception in users of the MED-EL COMBI 40+ cochlear implant. Acta Otolaryngol (Stockh). 2011;131:52–8.
13. Mistrík P, Jolly C. Optimal electrode length to match patient specific cochlear anatomy. Eur Ann Otorhinolaryngol Head Neck Dis. 2016;133(Suppl 1):S68–71.
14. Koch RW, Elfarnawany M, Zhu N, Ladak HM, Agrawal SK. Evaluation of Cochlear duct length computations using synchrotron radiation phase-contrast imaging. Otol Neurotol.
15. Jiam NT, Pearl MS, Carver C, Limb CJ. Flat-panel CT imaging for individualized pitch mapping in Cochlear implant users. Otol Neurotol. 2016;37:672–9.
16. Greenwood DD. A cochlear frequency-position function for several species–29 years later. J Acoust Soc Am. 1990;87:2592–605.
17. Fu Q-J, Shannon RV, Galvin JJ. Perceptual learning following changes in the frequency-to-electrode assignment with the Nucleus-22 cochlear implant. J Acoust Soc Am. 2002;112:1664–74.
18. Kan A, Stoelb C, Litovsky RY, Goupell MJ. Effect of mismatched place-of-stimulation on binaural fusion and lateralization in bilateral cochlear-implant users. J Acoust Soc Am. 2013;134:2923–36.
19. Stelmach J, Landsberger DM, Padilla M, Aronoff JM. Determining the minimum number of electrodes that need to be pitch matched to accurately estimate pitch matches across the array. Int J Audiol. 2017;56:1–6.
20. Li T, Fu Q-J. Effects of spectral shifting on speech perception in noise. Hear Res. 2010;270:81–8.

21. Long CJ, Eddington DK, Colburn HS, Rabinowitz WM. Binaural sensitivity as a function of interaural electrode position with a bilateral cochlear implant user. J Acoust Soc Am. 2003;114:1565–74.

22. Poon BB, Eddington DK, Noel V, Colburn HS. Sensitivity to interaural time difference with bilateral cochlear implants: development over time and effect of interaural electrode spacing. J Acoust Soc Am. 2009;126:806–15.

23. Rader T, Döge J, Adel Y, Weissgerber T, Baumann U. Place dependent stimulation rates improve pitch perception in cochlear implantees with single-sided deafness. Hear Res. 2016;339:94–103.

24. Ali H, Noble JH, Gifford RH, Labadie RF, Dawant BM, Hansen JHL, et al. Image-guided customization of frequency-place mapping in cochlear implants. In: 2015 IEEE international conference on acoustics, speech and signal processing (ICASSP), 19–24 April 2015: IEEE; 2015. p. 5843–7.http://ieeexplore.ieee.org/document/7179092/

25. Ma N, Morris S, Kitterick PT. Benefits to speech perception in noise from the binaural integration of electric and acoustic signals in simulated unilateral deafness. Ear Hear. 2016;37:248–59.

26. Goupell MJ. Interaural envelope correlation change discrimination in bilateral cochlear implantees: effects of mismatch, centering, and onset of deafness. J Acoust Soc Am. 2015;137:1282–97.

27. Noble JH, Hedley-Williams AJ, Sunderhaus L, Dawant BM, Labadie RF, Camarata SM, et al. Initial results with image-guided Cochlear implant programming in children. Otol Neurotol. 2016;37:e63–9.

28. Venail F, Mathiolon C, Menjot de champfleur S, Piron JP, Sicard M, Villemus F, et al. Effects of electrode array length on frequency-place mismatch and speech perception with cochlear implants. Audiol Neurootol. 2015;20:102–11.

29. Hochmair I, Arnold W, Nopp P, Jolly C, Müller J, Roland P. Deep electrode insertion in cochlear implants: apical morphology, electrodes and speech perception results. Acta Otolaryngol (Stockh). 2003;123:612–7.

30. Di Nardo W, Scorpecci A, Giannantonio S, Cianfrone F, Paludetti G. Improving melody recognition in cochlear implant recipients through individualized frequency map fitting. Eur Arch Oto-Rhino-Laryngol Off J Eur Fed Oto-Rhino-Laryngol Soc EUFOS Affil Ger Soc Oto-Rhino-Laryngol - Head Neck Surg. 2011;268:27–39.

31. Escudé B, James C, Deguine O, Cochard N, Eter E, Fraysse B. The size of the cochlea and predictions of insertion depth angles for Cochlear implant electrodes. Audiol Neurotol. 2006;11:27–33.

32. Alexiades G, Dhanasingh A, Jolly C. Method to estimate the complete and two-turn cochlear duct length. Otol Neurotol. 2015;36:904–7.

33. Iyaniwura JE, Elfarnawany M, Riyahi-Alam S, Sharma M, Kassam Z, Bureau Y, et al. Intra- and Interobserver Variability of Cochlear Length Measurements in Clinical CT. Otol Neurotol. 2017;38:828–32.

34. Rivas A, Cakir A, Hunter JB, Labadie RF, Zuniga MG, Wanna GB, et al. Automatic Cochlear duct length estimation for selection of Cochlear implant electrode arrays. Otol Neurotol. 2017;38:339–46.

35. Feldkamp LA, Davis LC, Kress JW. Practical cone-beam algorithm. JOSA A. 1984;1:612–9.

36. 3D. Slicer. https://www.slicer.org/. Accessed 28 Mar 2016.

37. Fedorov A, Beichel R, Kalpathy-Cramer J, Finet J, Fillion-Robin J-C, Pujol S, et al. 3D slicer as an image computing platform for the quantitative imaging network. Magn Reson Imaging. 2012;30:1323–41. `

38. Peters TM, Cleary K, editors. Image-guided interventions: technology and applications. First: Springer; 2008. http://www.springer.com/gp/book/9780387738567

39. Rueckert D, Sonoda LI, Hayes C, Hill DLG, Leach MO, Hawkes DJ. Nonrigid registration using free-form deformations: application to breast MR images. IEEE Trans Med Imaging. 1999;18:712–21.

40. Lee S, Wolberg G, Shin SY. Scattered data interpolation with multilevel B-splines. IEEE Trans Vis Comput Graph. 1997;3:228–44.

41. Elfarnawany M, Alam SR, Agrawal SK, Ladak HM. Evaluation of non-rigid registration parameters for atlas-based segmentation of CT images of human cochlea. In: Styner MA, Angelini ED, editors. ; 2017. p. 101330Z. https://doi.org/10.1117/12.2254040.

42. Hardy M. The length of the organ of Corti in man. Am J Anat. 1938;62:291–311.

43. De Seta D, Mancini P, Russo FY, Torres R, Mosnier I, Bensimon JL, et al. 3D curved multiplanar cone beam CT reconstruction for intracochlear position assessment of straight electrodes array. A temporal bone and clinical study. Acta Otorhinolaryngol Ital. 2016;36:499–505.

44. Gerber N, Reyes M, Barazzetti L, Kjer HM, Vera S, Stauber M, et al. A multiscale imaging and modelling dataset of the human inner ear. Sci Data. 2017;4:170132.

45. Koch RW, Ladak HM, Elfarnawany M, Agrawal SK. Measuring Cochlear duct length – a historical analysis of methods and results. J Otolaryngol - Head Neck Surg. 2017;46 https://doi.org/10.1186/s40463-017-0194-2.

46. Finley CC, Holden TA, Holden LK, Whiting BR, Chole RA, Neely GJ, et al. Role of electrode placement as a contributor to variability in Cochlear implant outcomes. Otol Neurotol. 2008;29:920–8.

47. MED-EL | Cochlear Implants for Hearing Loss. http://www.medel.com/ca/. Accessed 29 May 2017.

48. Advanced Bionics | The Cochlear Implant Technology Innovation Leader - Cochlear Implants for Children and Adults. https://www.advancedbionics.com/. Accessed 1 June 2017.

49. Cochlear Hearing Implants | Official Website | Cochlear. http://www.cochlear.com/wps/wcm/connect/us/home. Accessed 1 June 2017.

50. Huang X, Ren J, Abdalbari A, Green M. Deformable image registration for tissues with large displacements. J Med Imaging Bellingham Wash. 2017;4:14001.

51. Liao YL, Chen HB, Zhou LH, Zhen X. Construction of an anthropopathic abdominal phantom for accuracy validation of deformable image registration. Technol Health Care Off J Eur Soc Eng Med. 2016;24(Suppl 2):S717–23.

52. Fukumitsu N, Nitta K, Terunuma T, Okumura T, Numajiri H, Oshiro Y, et al. Registration error of the liver CT using deformable image registration of MIM maestro and velocity AI. BMC Med Imaging. 2017;17 https://doi.org/10.1186/s12880-017-0202-z.

53. Khalvati F, Salmanpour A, Rahnamayan S, Haider MA, Tizhoosh HR. Sequential registration-based segmentation of the prostate gland in MR image volumes. J Digit Imaging. 2016;29:254–63.

54. Ehrhardt J, Handels H, Plötz W, Pöppl SJ. Atlas-based recognition of anatomical structures and landmarks and the automatic computation of orthopedic parameters. Methods Inf Med. 2004;43:391–7.

55. Taghizadeh E, Reyes M, Zysset P, Latypova A, Terrier A, Büchler P. Biomechanical role of bone anisotropy estimated on clinical CT scans by image registration. Ann Biomed Eng. 2016;44:2505–17.

56. Farjam R, Tyagi N, Veeraraghavan H, Apte A, Zakian K, Hunt MA, et al. Multi-atlas approach with local registration goodness weighting for MRI-based electron density mapping of head and neck anatomy. Med Phys. 2017. doi: https://doi.org/10.1002/mp.12303. ISSN: 2473-4209.

57. Tian Z, Liu L, Fei B. A fully automatic multi-atlas based segmentation method for prostate MR images. Proc SPIE Int Soc Opt Eng. 2015;9413 https://doi.org/10.1117/12.2082229.

58. Ren S, Hara W, Wang L, Buyyounouski MK, Le Q-T, Xing L, et al. Robust estimation of electron density from anatomic magnetic resonance imaging of the brain using a unifying multi-atlas approach. Int J Radiat Oncol. 2017; 97:849–57.

59. Christensen GE, He J, Dill JA, Rubinstein JT, Vannier MW, Wang G. Automatic measurement of the labyrinth using image registration and a deformable inner ear atlas. Acad Radiol. 2003;10:988–99.

3

Management delays in patients with squamous cell cancer of neck node(s) and unknown primary site

Kevin Martell[1,2]* , Joanna Mackenzie[3], Warren Kerney[4] and Harold Yeehau Lau[1,2]

Abstract

Background: We aim to characterize the workup received by and identify any delays to diagnosis or treatment in patients referred to a tertiary cancer centre with the diagnosis of squamous cell carcinoma in neck node(s) and no identifiable primary (SCCNIP).

Methods: Over 1 year, 68 patients were initially referred to the Head and Neck clinic with a label of "primary unknown". After extensive workup, 29 of the 68 patients were found to have pathologically confirmed SCCNIP. For these 29 patients, imaging tests, biopsies, examinations and times to treatment were reviewed and compared to 145 patients referred for known primaries.

Results: In 21/29 (72%) patients, ultrasound was ordered prior to biopsy or referral. After referral, the first imaging test used was CT neck in 28 patients and PET/CT in 1 patient.
Median time from referral to primary identification ($n = 23$) or workup completion ($n = 6$) were 16 (range: 0-48) and 36 (17-82) days respectively. Median time from referral to treatment was 55 (27-90; $n = 26$) days and was longer than those referred for known primaries (48 days; 20-162; $p < 0.001$). Across all patients, median time between first diagnostic imaging test and pathologic diagnosis were 20.5 and -8.0 days ($p < 0.0001$) in patients receiving ultrasound and CT, respectively.

Conclusions: In our cohort, delays to management were linked to community use of ultrasound and scheduling of both CT and PET/CT after thorough head and neck examination in patients with SCCNIP.

Keywords: Unknown primary, Neck node, Squamous cell carcinoma, Head and neck, Diagnostic workup, Treatment delay, Diagnostics

Background

Head and neck malignancies of unknown primary are unique malignancies in their workup and treatment [1–6]. These patients often receive unnecessary tests which can delay diagnosis and treatments. There is also additional emotional distress in patients who receive delays in treatment for sequential tests which fail to give additional diagnostic information.

For true unknown primaries, Grau et al. [7] have demonstrated that the addition of bilateral neck irradiation in treatment of these malignancies doubles 5 year control rates. Conversely, in head and neck malignancies with known primaries, bilateral neck irradiation often increases toxicity without increasing disease control. Hence, a diagnosis of "unknown primary" should only be made after an extensive workup [1, 6, 8].

Initial literature reviews showed no other studies analyzing the delays in treatment resulting from workup performed for head and neck malignancies after referral to a tertiary cancer centre. However, several strategies for workup of unknown primaries have been suggested

---

* Correspondence: kevin.martell@albertahealthservices.ca
[1]Division of Radiation Oncology, Tom Baker Cancer Centre, Calgary, AB, Canada
[2]Department of Oncology, University of Calgary, 1331 29 Street Northwest, Calgary, AB T2N 4 N2, Canada
Full list of author information is available at the end of the article

[2, 3, 5, 9]. Unfortunately, these often included restricted tests or specialized invasive procedures such as tonsillectomy which Randall et al. [10] showed can provide diagnosis for up to 20% of these patients. Also, more recently, both Reglink et al. [11] and Rudmik et al. [12] have shown the utility of FDG-PET (Fluorodeoxyglucose positron emission tomography) imaging in these malignancies.

Hence we seek to characterize the workup received by patients with metastatic squamous cell carcinoma (SCC) to neck nodes and unknown primary at our centre, quantify the delay from referral to treatment as compared to known primary patients and identify any potential delays to diagnosis or treatment caused by use of unnecessary tests either before or after referral.

Methods

Setting

The Tom Baker Cancer Centre (TBCC) is the tertiary cancer centre for southern Alberta, Canada and has a catchment population of approximately two million. Head and neck cancer patient referrals to this centre primarily come from family practitioners. Otolaryngologists, and oromaxillofacial surgeons. The main requirement for referral is a pathologic diagnosis of malignancy. After referral, a multidisciplinary team involving otolaryngologists, radiation oncologists and medical oncologists will review the patient in clinic, perform a complete head and neck exam including nasopharyngoscopy and arrange for any required additional investigations and decide on management recommendations.

Study population

Between January 1 and December 31, 2014, a total of 286 patients were referred to the TBCC multidisciplinary head and neck clinic for consideration of head and neck malignancies. For purposes of this study the 68 patients referred with a diagnosis of "head and neck malignancy of unknown primary" were then retrospectively reviewed by two independent physicians. Patients were then excluded from analysis if they were treated elsewhere (3), refused further workup (2), did not have squamous pathology (3), had a non-head and neck primary (5; 3 skin and 2 lung) or a primary lesion was identified through imaging or clinical examination performed prior to referral (26). This left 29 patients with pathologically confirmed squamous cell carcinoma diagnosed on cervical lymph node fine needle aspirate (25) or core/excisional biopsy (4) which forms the cohort of our analysis [Fig. 1]. To quantify the delay to treatment resulting from workup of unknown primaries, an additional, subsequent population consisting of the 145 patients referred to TBCC during the same time period and having known head and neck SCC with identifiable primaries at the time of referral was used to perform a comparative analysis.

Ethical considerations and data collection

This study is a retrospective cohort analysis. It was designed for purposes of quality review and patient outcome enhancement. Ethical review was performed by an independent third party reviewer using the institutionally approved method described by Hagen et al. [13]. A prospectively collected database containing all referrals to the Tom Baker Cancer Centre multidisciplinary head and neck cancer treatment team was then used to identify patients with initial diagnosis of unknown primary. Retrospective chart reviews of both the local electronic medical record and the provincial electronic health record which houses results for all diagnostic tests performed in Alberta was then undertaken for these patients (including those ordered by a primary care provider). All subsequent diagnostic investigations, appointment and treatment dates were then collected for each patient. These tests were then assessed and a test was considered to have given a diagnosis when two independent physician reviewers agreed that sufficient evidence to identify the primary malignancy was acquired.

Statistical methods

The primary study cohort was characterized using descriptive statistics. Times from referral to TBCC to diagnosis, then confirmation of diagnosis for each patient were then calculated. Additionally, days to appointment and treatment were calculated. For calculations of delays caused by inappropriate workup, the time from the inappropriate test (eg ultrasound) to pathologic confirmation of disease were calculated. For comparison, time between pathologic diagnosis and the first imaging test was calculated for patients with only appropriate diagnostic workups was calculated. The Shapiro-Wilks test was employed on all calculated time differences for determination of normality. For comparative analysis with the reference group, the Mann-Whitney test was employed to determine significance between medians for times to treatment. Two tailed p-values of <0.05 were then accepted as representing statistical significance. All data was analyzed using the R-programming language version 3.1.1 (www.r-project.org).

Results

Unknown primary cohort

A total of 29 patients had confirmed unknown primary site of malignancy at the time of diagnosis. All 29 underwent CT scan, 23 received PET scans and 19 required EUAs. As shown in Fig. 2, the first investigation following referral was CT neck in 28 patients and PET/CT in 1 patient. From these investigations, 10 (34%) patients had a primary site of malignancy identified (9 from CT and 1 from PET). Of the remaining 18 patients 2 patients underwent targeted biopsies and were subsequently diagnosed with a salivary gland and a tonsillar primary pathologically;

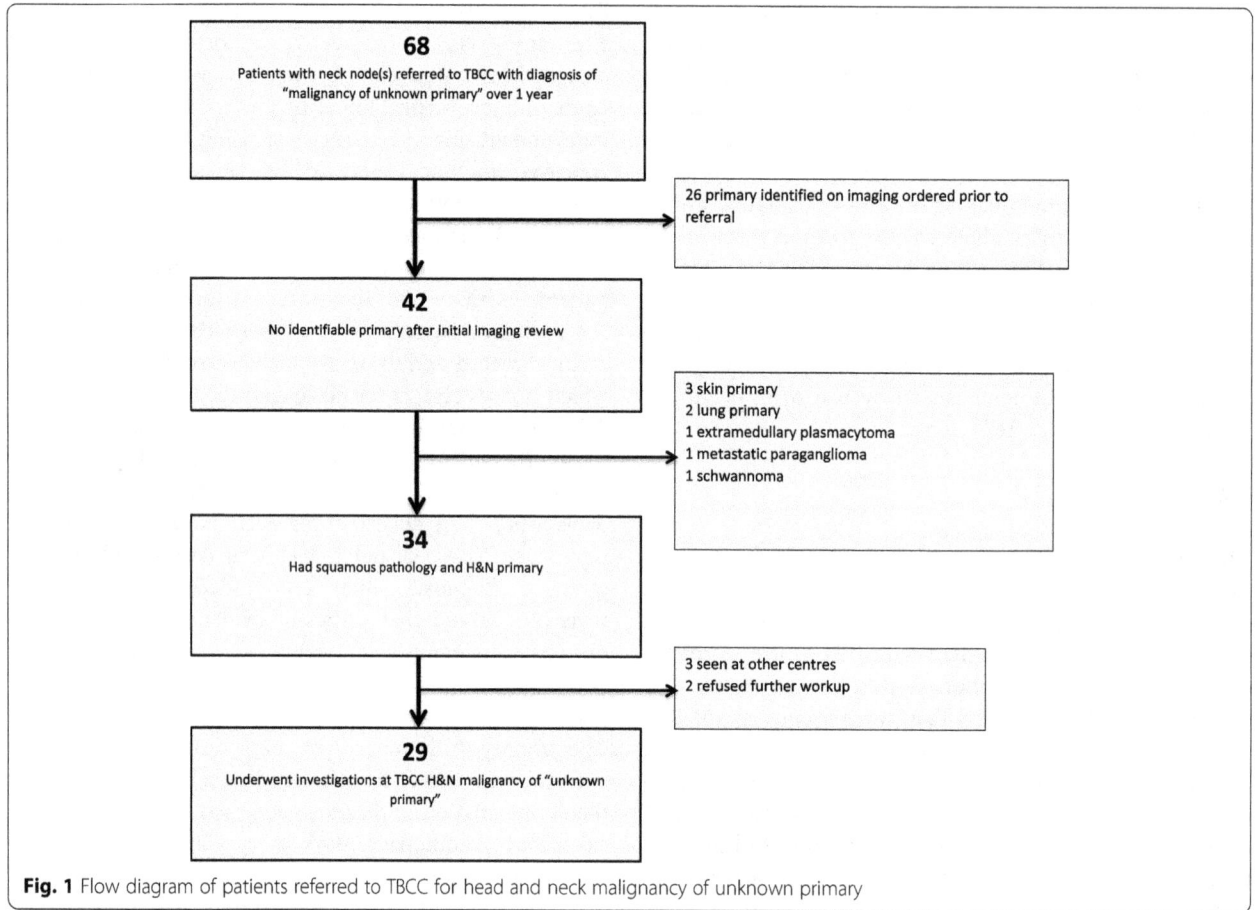

Fig. 1 Flow diagram of patients referred to TBCC for head and neck malignancy of unknown primary

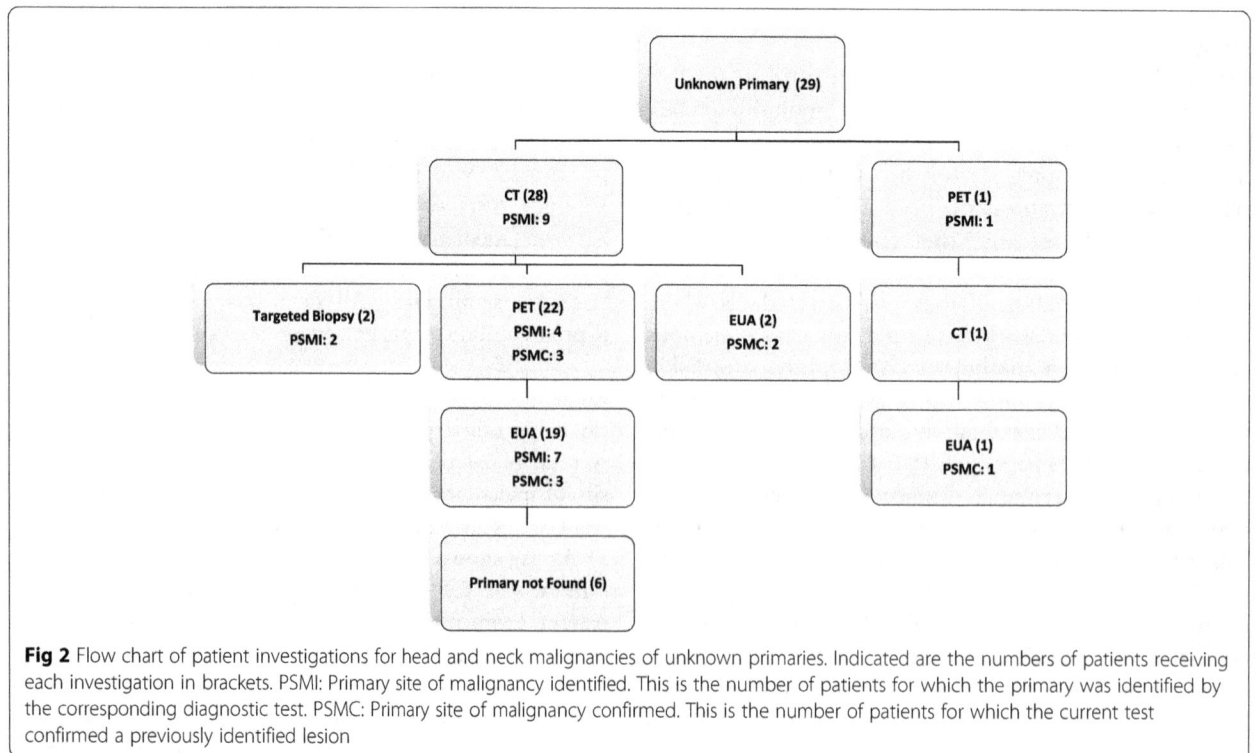

Fig 2 Flow chart of patient investigations for head and neck malignancies of unknown primaries. Indicated are the numbers of patients receiving each investigation in brackets. PSMI: Primary site of malignancy identified. This is the number of patients for which the primary was identified by the corresponding diagnostic test. PSMC: Primary site of malignancy confirmed. This is the number of patients for which the current test confirmed a previously identified lesion

4 patients were diagnosed on subsequent PET scan; and 7 were diagnosed after examination under anesthetic (EUA). This left six patients (21%) where CT, PET and EUA showed no evidence of a primary site. These patients were given a final diagnosis of 'head and neck carcinoma of unknown primary' and represent 2% of referrals to our multi-disciplinary head and neck clinic.

Of the 29 patients, the referring physicians were otolaryngologists (14), general practitioners (14) and 1 was referred by an oncologic surgeon.

Review of the initial community based workup of these patients revealed that 21 patients (72%) had undergone ultrasound (USS) for consideration of neck mass before being diagnosed with a malignancy. For these, median time from USS to FNA (fine needle aspirate) or core biopsy was 20 days (range: 0-51). Initial pathology was via fine needle aspirate and core biopsy in 25 and four patients respectively.

p16 is a cyclin dependent kinase inhibitor and a surrogate marker for HPV related malignancies [14]. Fourteen patients had p16 status reported initially (4/4 core biopsies, 8/25 FNA). Of these 12 were p16 positive and two were p16 -ve. A further 11 went on to have repeat pathology or review and were p16 positive. In four patients p16 testing was not performed because their original biopsy specimens were inadequate and no further positive biopsies were made.

Median time from referral to TBCC to completion of workup and diagnosis of "Head and neck SCC of unknown primary" was 36 days (range: 17-82; $n = 6$). Median time from referral to identification of a primary was 16 days (0-48; $n = 23$). Of the 23 primary sites of malignancies identified, 12 (52.2%), 8 (34.8%) and 2 (8.7%) of these cancers were tonsillar, base of tongue and nasopharyngeal primaries. There was one (4.3%) salivary gland tumor. 9 (39%), 9 (39%), 3 (13%) and 2 (8%) were T1, T2, T4 and TX malignancies. 26 (90%) patients received treatment (1 patient declined and 2 had yet to start before the data were locked). Median time from diagnosis to treatment was 36 (14-84) days. Twenty-five patients (86%) went on to have chemoradiotherapy. Other treatments included 1 (3%) patient having surgery, 1 (3%) with surgery followed by radiotherapy and 1 (3%) with radiotherapy alone.

Comparison

Median number of days between referral to TBCC and treatment was 48 (20-162) vs 55 (27-90); $p < 0.001$ [Fig. 3] and from appointment to treatment was 34 (12-153) vs 42 (20-77); $p < 0.001$ [Fig. 4] for patients with known (145) and unknown primaries (29) at the time of referral respectively.

The largest delays from referral to treatment were noted in the known primary cohort. In explanation of this, 3 patients initially refused treatment resulting in

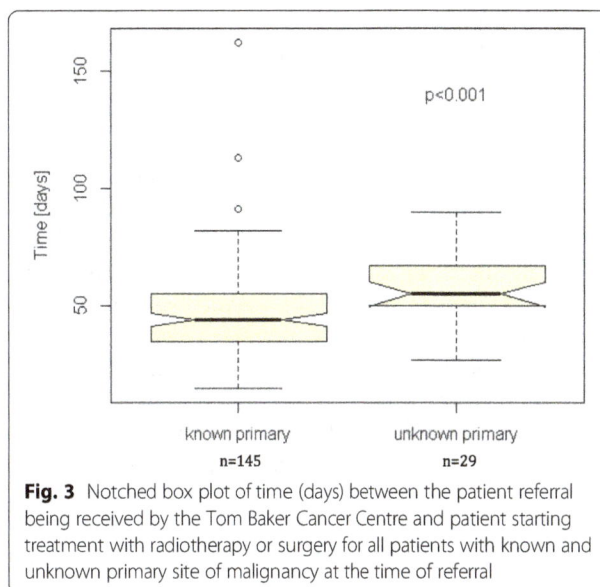

Fig. 3 Notched box plot of time (days) between the patient referral being received by the Tom Baker Cancer Centre and patient starting treatment with radiotherapy or surgery for all patients with known and unknown primary site of malignancy at the time of referral

times from referral to treatment of 162, 113 and 76 days. An additional 7 patients in this cohort required additional workup resulting in times from referral to treatment between 67 and 91 days. Use of ultrasound as a first diagnostic imaging investigation again led to a median of a 20.5 [(-53) to (+359); $n = 62$] day delay to pathologic diagnosis. With patients undergoing CT/MR, pathologic diagnosis was made a median of 8 days before their imaging investigation [-8.0; (-77) to (+202); $n = 80$; $p < 0.0001$].

Discussion

We identified several sources of delay in patients referred to a Canadian tertiary cancer centre for head and neck

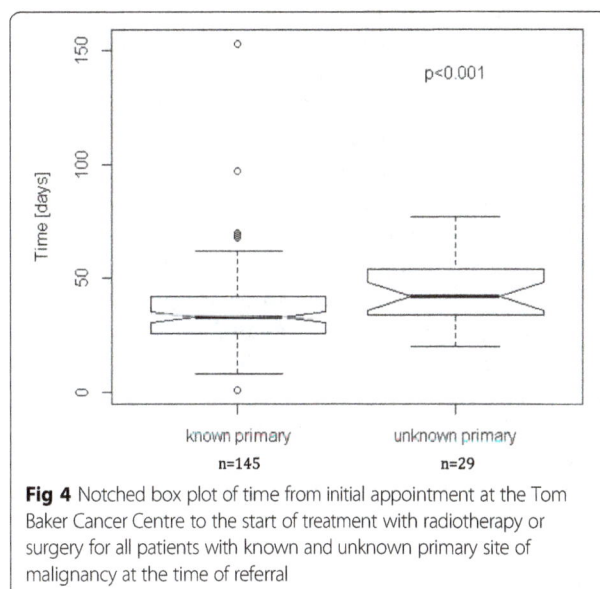

Fig 4 Notched box plot of time from initial appointment at the Tom Baker Cancer Centre to the start of treatment with radiotherapy or surgery for all patients with known and unknown primary site of malignancy at the time of referral

malignancies with unknown primary. Median time to pathologic diagnosis of malignancy was significantly greater (20.5 days vs -8.0) in patients undergoing community requested ultrasound for confirmation of a neck mass when compared to those having only appropriate workup ordered. Additionally, patients referred for unknown primaries undergo many diagnostic tests including PET, CT and EUA after referral which results in a statistically significant increase in time from referral to treatment when compared to patients with identifiable primaries (48 vs 55 days).

All 29 patients went on to have CT scans and 23 had PET scans. In the 3 patients who underwent PET after a diagnosis was made on CT, the PET scan confirmed the diagnosis. There were only 6 patients diagnosed via CT who did not go on to have a PET. Of note, our PET detection rate (35% in those receiving PET) is quite similar to those cited elsewhere [12, 15–17]. Our results are also similar to Regelink et al. [11], who analyzed outcomes in 50 patients who received PET, EUA and CT. They identified 16, 12 and 11 primaries respectively. This implies that, in centres where it is readily available and easily accessible, PET scan should be the first test of choice after thorough head and neck examination for these patients. This could lead to reduction in delays to treatment and an additional cost savings from the unnecessary diagnostic CT scans [11, 18].

Furthermore, 22 patients had EUA examination after referral and 1 out of 2 targeted biopsies was of a site that would normally be sampled during EUA. An additional attempt to reduce time to treatment could be made by scheduling PET scan and EUA at the time of triaging. This is supported by Waltonen et al. [19], however careful review of the patient chart would be necessary as many patients triaged as malignancy of unknown primary did have a diagnosis. Finally, it has been shown that transoral robotic surgery in diagnostic workup of unknown primaries can improve rates of primary site detection to 80-90% [20, 21]. As this procedure becomes more popular it may be beneficial to schedule this early in the diagnostic workup and perhaps at the time of EUA [22].

Delays to *pathologic* diagnosis in this cohort were attributable to ultrasound being utilized as a first investigation after presentation to their primary care provider for a neck mass (median time to pathologic diagnosis of 20.5 days vs -8 days when compared to patients having only appropriate workup). On review of current practice guidelines, ultrasound was not identified as a recommended diagnostic procedure [23–27]. It is important to acknowledge that the number of community ultrasounds interpreted as benign lymphadenopathy is not addressed in this analysis and remains unknown. However, over the last decade there has been a substantial increase in HPV related oropharyngeal cancers which often present as painless neck lymphadenopathy [28]. Furthermore, the clinical presentation of a persistent, painless neck node should arouse suspicion for malignancy [29]. Hence, ordering an ultrasound guided FNA as the initial diagnostic procedure may be preferred as it could reduce time to diagnosis [30]. Additional measures could include the creation of a specialized clinic for expedited workup and diagnosis of a neck mass.

When interpreting the results of this study it is important to acknowledge that this is a retrospective cohort analysis and inherent bias from unknown confounders is possible. As a single centre study it may not be generalizable to other jurisdictions. For example, PET/CT is not readily available in all centres. Additionally, there were fewer patients than anticipated with head and neck squamous cell carcinomas of unknown primary at the time of referral. Hence, these numbers should be interpreted with caution until larger, multicentre studies are conducted. Finally, this study does not address whether the treatment delays seen in this cohort affected survival outcomes.

Conclusions

We present an analysis of the typical workup and delay in time to treatment experienced by patients with squamous cell cancer in a neck node without an identifiable primary. One major source of delay was community delays to diagnosis caused by use of ultrasound. This can be avoided in the future though enhanced primary care education, updating primary care guidelines to specifically address ultrasound as an inappropriate test and suggest ultrasound guided biopsy or introduction of expedited care pathways or creation of dedicated clinics to assist primary care practitioners with assessment. A second source of delay was the waitlist for CT scans. As a large majority of these patients ultimately received PET scans, perhaps if patients referred with biopsy proven malignancy in neck nodes could proceed to expedited PET/CTs, this could shorten delays to diagnosis and treatment but would require additional resources for cancer centres.

Abbreviations
CT: Computed tomography; EUA: Examination under anaesthesia; FNA: Fine needle aspirate; HPV: Human papilloma virus; MRI: Magnetic resonance imaging; PET: Positron emission tomography; SCC: Squamous cell carcinoma; TBCC: Tom Baker Cancer Centre; USS: Ultrasound

Acknowledgements
Not Applicable.

Funding
This research was supported in part by departmental funding through the Tom Baker Cancer Centre. The funding source had no participation in study design, implementation, data analysis, data interpretation or decision to publish.

Authors' contributions

KM aided in the collection of data, performed the primary data analysis and wrote the manuscript. JM aided in the collection of data and was a major contributor to the manuscript. WK held the primary databases through with patients applicable for the study were identified. HL is the senior investigator on this study and provided advice on its design and implementation. He also was a major contributor to writing the manuscript. All authors reviewed and approved the final manuscript.

Competing interests

The authors declare that they have no competing interests.

Author details

[1]Division of Radiation Oncology, Tom Baker Cancer Centre, Calgary, AB, Canada. [2]Department of Oncology, University of Calgary, 1331 29 Street Northwest, Calgary, AB T2N 4 N2, Canada. [3]Edinburgh Cancer Centre, Western General Hospital, Edinburgh, Scotland, UK. [4]Calgary Zone, Alberta Health Services, Calgary, AB, Canada.

References

1. Eisbruch A, Foote RL, O'Sullivan B, Beitler JJ, Vikram B. Intensity-modulated radiation therapy for head and neck cancer: emphasis on the selection and delineation of the targets. Semin Radiat Oncol. 2002;12:238–49.
2. Cianchetti M, Mancuso A, Amdur RJ, Werning JW, Kirwan J, Morris CG, et al. Diagnostic evaluation of squamous cell carcinoma metastatic to cervical lymph nodes from an unknown head and neck primary site. Laryngoscope. 2009;119:2348–54.
3. Pavlidis N, Briasoulis E, Hainsworth J, Greco F. Diagnostic and therapeutic management of cancer of an unknown primary. Eur J Cancer. 2003;39:1990–2005.
4. Nasopharyngeal Cancer Treatment Concensus Guidelines. 2013. http://www. albertahealthservices.ca/info/cancerguidelines.aspx. Accessed 28 Sept 2015.
5. Mendenhall WM, Mancuso AA, Parsons JT, Stringer SP, Cassisi NJ. Diagnostic evaluation of squamous cell carcinoma metastatic to cervical lymph nodes from an unknown head and neck primary site. Head Neck. 1998;20:739–44.
6. Galloway TJ, Ridge J. Management of Squamous cancer metastatic to cervical nodes with an unknown primary site. J Clin Oncol. 2015;33:3328–37.
7. Grau C, Johansen LV, Jakobsen J, Geertsen P, Andersen E, Jensen BB. Cervical lymph node metastases from unknown primary tumours. Results from a national survey by the Danish Society for Head and Neck Oncology. Radiother Oncol. 2000;55:121–9.
8. Guntinas-Lichius O, Peter Klussmann J, Dinh S, Dinh M, Schmidt M, Semrau R, et al. Diagnostic work-up and outcome of cervical metastases from an unknown primary. Acta Otolaryngol. 2006;126:536–44.
9. Calabrese L, Jereczek-Fossa B, Jassem J, Rocca A, Bruschini R, Orecchia R, et al. Diagnosis and management of neck metastases from an unknown primary. Acta Otorhinolaryngol Ital. 2005;25:2–12.
10. Randall D, Johnstone P, Foss RD, Martin PJ. Tonsillectomy in diagnosis of the unknown primary tumor of the head and neck. Otolaryngol Head Neck Surg. 2000;122:52–5.
11. Regelink G, Brouwer J, De Bree R, Pruim J, Van Der Laan BF, Vaalburg W, et al. Detection of unknown primary tumours and distant metastases in patients with cervical metastases: value of FDG-PET versus conventional modalities. Eur J Nucl Med. 2002;29:1024–30.
12. Rudmik L, Lau HY, Matthews TW, Bosch JD, Kloiber R, Molnar CP, et al. Clinical utility of PET/CT in the evaluation of head and neck squamous cell carcinoma with an unknown primary: a prospective clinical trial. Head Neck. 2011;33:935–40.
13. Hagen B, O'Beirne M, Desai S, Stingl M, Pachnowski CA, Hayward S. Innovations in the ethical review of health-related quality improvement and research: The Alberta Research Ethics Community Consensus Initiative (ARECCI). Healthc Policy. 2007;2:e164–77.
14. Hoffman M, Ihloff A, Gorogh T, Weise J, Fazel A, Krams M, et al. p16(INK4a) overexpression predicts translational active human papillomavirus infection in tonsillar cancer. Int J Cancer. 2010;127:1595–602.
15. Fischbein NJ, Caputo GR, Kaplan MJ, Price DC, Singer MI, Dillon WP, et al. Metastatic head and neck cancer: role and usefulness of FDG PET in locating occult primary tumors. Radiology. 1998;210:177–81.
16. Lassen U, Daugaard G, Eigtved A, Damgaard K, Friberg L. 18 F-FDG whole body positron emission tomography (PET) in patients with unknown primary tumours (UPT). Eur J Cancer. 1999;35:1076–82.
17. Bohuslavizki KH, Klutmann S, Kröger S, Sonnemann U, Buchert R, Werner J, et al. FDG PET detection of unknown primary tumors. J Nucl Med. 2000;41:816–22.
18. Metastatic malignant disease of unknown primary origin: Diagnosis and management of metastatic disease of unknown primary origin 2010. https://www.nice.org.uk/guidance/cg104. Accessed 28 Sept 2015.
19. Waltonen JD, Ozer E, Hall NC, Schuller DE, Agrawal A. Metastatic carcinoma of the neck of unknown primary origin: evolution and efficacy of the modern workup. Arch Otolaryngol Head Neck Surg. 2009;135:1024–9. doi:10.1001/archoto.2009.145.
20. Durmus K, Rangarajan SV, Old MO, Agrawal A, Teknos TN, Ozer E. Transoral robotic approach to carcinoma of unknown primary. Head Neck. 2014;36:848–52.
21. Mehta V, Johnson P, Tassler A, Kim S, Ferris RL, Nance M, et al. A new paradigm for the diagnosis and management of unknown primary tumors of the head and neck: a role for transoral robotic surgery. Laryngoscope. 2013;123:146–51.
22. Hatten KM, O'Malley BW, Bur AM, Patel MR, Rassekh CH, Newman JG, et al. Transoral robotic surgery-assisted endoscopy with primary site detection and treatment in occult mucosal primaries. JAMA Otolaryngol Head Neck Surg. 2017;143:267–73.
23. Schwetschenau E, Kelley DJ. The adult neck mass. Am Fam Physician. 2002;66:831–8.
24. Fahimi F, Müller O, Hoffmann TK. Neck mass. Merk Man. 2013;61:8–10.
25. Thandar M, Jonas N. An approach to the neck mass. AJOL. 2004;22:266–72.
26. Gleeson M, Herber A, Richards A. Management of lateral neck masses in adults. BMJ. 2000;320:1521–4.
27. Pfister DG, Spencer S, Brizel DM, Burtness B, Busse PM, Caudell JJ, et al. Head and Neck Cancers, Version 1.2015. J Natl Compr Canc Netw. 2015;13: 847–55. quiz 856.
28. Shack L, Lau HY, Huang L, Doll C, Hao D. Trends in the incidence of human papillomavirus-related noncervical and cervical cancers in Alberta, Canada: a population-based study. C Open. 2014;2:E127–32.
29. Haynes J, Arnold KR, Aguirre-Oskins C, Chandra S. Evaluation of neck masses in adults. Am Fam Physician. 2015;91:698–706.
30. Lo C-P, Chen C-Y, Chin S-C, Lee K-W, Hsueh C-J, Juan C-J, et al. Detection of suspicious malignant cervical lymph nodes of unknown origin: diagnostic accuracy of ultrasound-guided fine-needle aspiration biopsy with nodal size and central necrosis correlate. Can Assoc Radiol J. 2007;58:286–91.

4

Evolution of gender representation among Canadian OTL-HNS residents: a 27-year analysis

Sarah Chorfi[1], Joseph S. Schwartz[2], Neil Verma[1*], Meredith Young[3,4], Lawrence Joseph[5] and Lily H. P. Nguyen[2,3]

Abstract

Background: The proportion of females enrolling into medical schools has been growing steadily. However, the representation of female residents among individual specialties has shown considerable variation. The purpose of this study was to compare the trends of gender representation in Otolaryngology – Head and Neck Surgery (OTL-HNS) residency programs with other specialty training programs in Canada. In order to contextualize these findings, a second phase of analysis examined the success rate of applicants of different genders to OTL-HNS residency programs.

Method: Anonymized data were obtained from the Canadian Residency Matching Service (CaRMS) and from the Canadian Post-M.D. Education Registry (CAPER) from 1988 to 2014. The differences in gender growth rates were compared to other subspecialty programs of varying size. Descriptive analysis was used to examine gender representation among OTL-HNS residents across years, and to compare these trends with other specialties. Bayesian hierarchical models were fit to analyze the growth in program rates in OTL-HNS based on gender.

Results: CaRMS and CAPER data over a 27 year period demonstrated that OTL-HNS has doubled its female representation from 20% to 40% between 1990 and 1994 and 2010-2014. The difference in annual growth rate of female representation versus male representation in OTL-HNS over this time period was 2.7%, which was similar to other large specialty programs and surgical subspecialties. There was parity in success rates of female and male candidates ranking OTL-HNS as their first choice specialty for most years.

Conclusions: Female representation in Canadian OTL-HNS residency programs is steadily increasing over the last 27 years. Large variation in female applicant acceptance rates was observed across Canadian universities, possibly attributable to differences in student body or applicant demographics. Factors influencing female medical student career selection to OTL-HNS require further study to mitigate disparities in gender representation and identify barriers to prospective female OTL-HNS applicants.

Keywords: Gender, Female, Diversity, Minority, Otolaryngology, Residents

Background

The proportion of female students pursuing postgraduate medical education has grown steadily [1]. Conversely, there has been considerable variation in the proportion of female residents across individual specialties. Studies have found that gender has an influential role in future career and residency program choices, more so than life goals, career motivation and personality traits [1–7].

There are several advantages of gender equity among the physician workforce, including benefits to patient care. Specifically, a diverse workforce includes a broader range of physicians which increases the likelihood of addressing health inequalities and providing care to underserved populations [8]. Although the factors leading to patient satisfaction are complex, male and female physicians tend to adopt different styles of practice, which may be unique and beneficial to patient populations [9]. The benefits of having a gender balanced healthcare

* Correspondence: neil.verma90@gmail.com

Presented as a poster presentation at the annual meeting of the Canadian Society of Otolaryngology - Head and Neck Surgery in Ottawa, May 2014

[1]Faculty of Medicine, McGill University Health Centre, Montreal Children's Hospital, McGill University, Room A02.3015, 1001 Boulevard Decarie, Montreal, QC H4A 3J1, Canada

Full list of author information is available at the end of the article

team include providing a mixture of complementary interpersonal skills [9]. Research has demonstrated female leaders tend to adopt a more democratic and participative style of leadership [10], a style that is increasingly promoted as the preferred style of leadership given the shift of medicine to a system-based delivery of care. Several studies have reported that female physicians are more likely to engage in a patient-centered approach and spend a greater length of time with their patients [11, 12]. While this is not a gender-specific trait, a gender balanced medical team could thus be more likely to address the needs of a broader demographic of patients. Ultimately, gender parity within the physician workforce encourages the development of a healthcare environment that will strengthen physician-patient relationships, patient satisfaction and overall patient outcomes [13–15].

Gender equity appears to be of considerable benefit beyond obvious moral and ethical interests. Gender misrepresentation may place limitations on the quality of selected resident trainees by inherently limiting the application process to a segregated pool of applicants [5]. A specialty that is attractive to both genders would therefore present more opportunities to select the most qualified candidate. In addition, female role-models for female trainees could encourage pursuit of careers in a broad range of specialties [3, 9].

When specifically considering Otolaryngology - Head and Neck Surgery (OTL-HNS), women were underrepresented compared to larger programs despite increasing female representation in OTL-HNS within American residency training programs [16, 17]. Investigating the demographic characteristics of newly admitted residents allows for a projection of future gender representation across a variety of medical and surgical specialties, helps contextualize physician human resource planning, but also helps identify some potential barriers to increasing gender representativeness within OTL-HNS programs.

To our knowledge, there has been no published study on the nature or evolution of gender representation among Canadian Otolaryngology-Head and Neck Surgery (OTL-HNS) residents. The overarching goal of this study was to provide a descriptive analysis of the recent history of gender representation in residency training in Canada compared to OTL-HNS. We chose to compare Canadian OTL-HNS residency training programs to programs of similar and larger number of registered residents with a focus on growth rates of female trainees compared to male trainees. A secondary aim involved a comparison of acceptance rates to OTL-HNS residency training programs between male and female applicants across all Canadian institutions.

Methods

Ethics approval was not required since this study was a post-hoc analysis of publically available data. Each postgraduate Canadian OTL-HNS residency program ($n = 13$) was assigned a randomly generated number between one and 13 in order to anonymize institutions for the purposes of analysis.

Study overview

We conducted a retrospective review of two databases: the Canadian Residency Matching Service (CaRMS) and the Canadian Post-M.D. Education Registry (CAPER). The Canadian Residency Matching Service (CaRMS) provided the following data from 2006 to 2014: gender representation of Canadian residency training programs, demographics of all Canadian OTL-HNS residency training programs, and demographics of medical students applying to Canadian OTL-HNS residency training programs. The CaRMS database captures all applicants participating in the annual CaRMS residency matching process. A matched candidate refers to a candidate who is accepted into a residency program to which they applied.

CaRMS data prior to 2006 was deemed unreliable due to an incomplete data set. Therefore, the Canadian Post-M.D. Education Registry (CAPER) provided Canadian resident demographics including gender representation from 1988 to 2005. This data stems from a self-reported census completed by all resident trainees and submitted by the postgraduate medical education offices of each Canadian medical school to CAPER for archiving.

We measured female representation by analyzing self-reported gender for CAPER data and using the statistics provided by CaRMS. Trends in female representation among Canadian OTL-HNS residency programs were compared to other similarly-sized surgical subspecialties, such as cardiac surgery, neurosurgery, ophthalmology, orthopedic surgery, plastic surgery and urology. Comparisons were also made to larger training programs such as family medicine, internal medicine, general surgery, anaesthesiology, pediatrics and psychiatry. Difference in growth rates between genders in OTL-HNS programs was calculated and compared to both similarly-sized surgical subspecialties as well as larger-sized residency programs. Finally, we compared success rates of female and male applicants and analyzed differences across institutions.

Statistical analysis

Descriptive statistics and graphical trends over time were compiled for each residency training program across all years. Bayesian hierarchical Poisson regression models were fit in order to analyze trends over time and compare these trends between males and females across different residency training programs. At the first level of our hierarchical model, the count for each program within each year and for each gender were assumed to follow a Poisson distribution with a rate lambda, assumed different for each data point. Poisson rates were therefore permitted to vary for each year, program and gender. At the second level of our hierarchical model the natural logarithm of these rates followed a linear regression model, with each rate lambda regressed based on program, year, and gender. In order to account for different baseline levels within each program, different intercepts were used in the linear regression model for each program. Similarly, to account for different trends over time within each specialty, each were also given their own slope. At the third level of the hierarchical model non-informative prior densities were used for all parameters, so that the data drive the final inferences. To interpret the estimated regression coefficients on the count scale rather than on the logarithms of these counts, the exponential of the estimated coefficients were calculated. All parameters were estimated using the posterior median with 95% credible intervals. Credible intervals are the Bayeisan analogue to frequentist confidence intervals, but have the more natural interpretation that the probability of the estimated parameter is within the given interval is 95%. All analyses were carried out using WinBUGS (Version 1.4.3, MRC Biostatistics Unit, Cambridge UK).

Results
Growth rates of gender representation: OTL-HNS compared to larger programs

The proportion of females registered in a residency training program in Canada has increased within all programs included in our analysis, with female representation in OTL-HNS effectively doubling from 20%

(i.e. 8 successful female applicants out of a total of 41) to 40% (51 successful female applicants out of a total of 129) between 1990 and 1994 and 2010-2014 (Fig. 1). OTL-HNS had the lowest percentage of females (20%) between 1990 and 1994 compared to larger specialties. Pediatrics had the largest percentage of females (65%) between 1990 and 1994. To account for the increase in size of residency training programs, we analyzed the difference in female and male growth rates of all programs. The difference in growth rates between females and males in OTL-HNS was 2.7% [95% credible interval 0.9, 4.7] per year and was comparable to larger programs (Table 1). In contrast, general surgery and pediatrics had a substantial mean difference in growth rates between females and males (respectively 4.2% [3.1, 5.2] and 3.8% [2.7, 5.0]) (Table 2), which was not significantly different compared to OTL-HNS. Overall, OTL-HNS has a similar difference in female and male growth rates to larger residency training programs and programs of comparable size.

Growth rates of gender representation: OTL-HNS compared to surgical specialties

The annual growth rate of female representation in OTL-HNS was statistically comparable to most other surgical subspecialties (Fig. 2). There was no statistical difference in annual growth rates of female representation between OTL-HNS compared to cardiac surgery, neurosurgery, ophthalmology, plastic surgery or orthopedic surgery (Table 2). No statistically significant difference was found between female and male growth rates between different surgical subspecialties (Table 2).

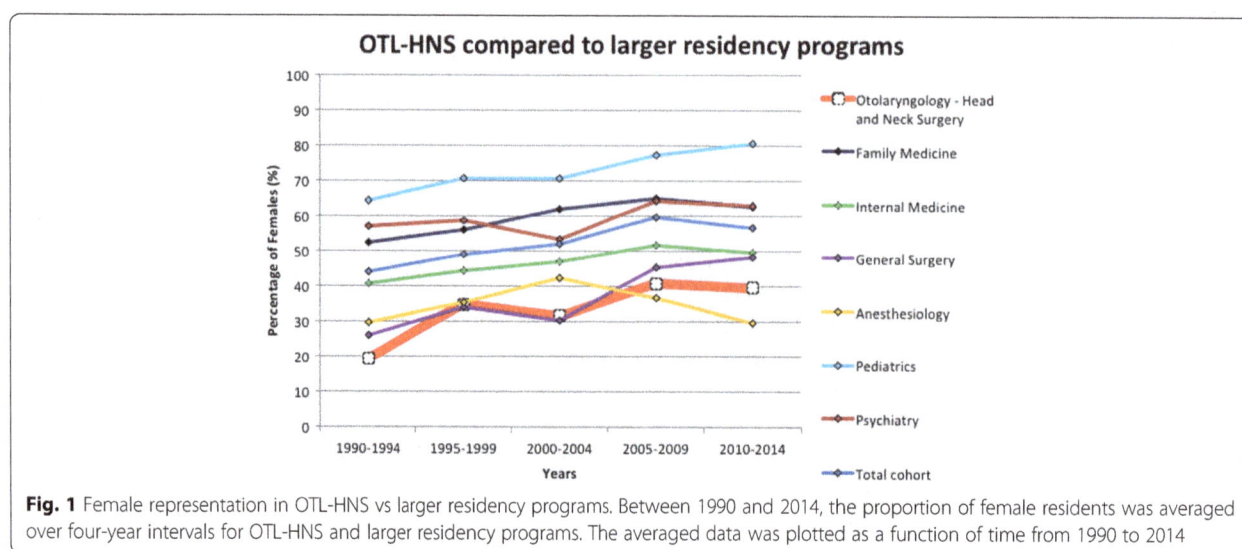

Fig. 1 Female representation in OTL-HNS vs larger residency programs. Between 1990 and 2014, the proportion of female residents was averaged over four-year intervals for OTL-HNS and larger residency programs. The averaged data was plotted as a function of time from 1990 to 2014

Table 1 Gender-specific growth rates in OTL-HNS versus larger residency programs

Specialty	Annual growth rates (percentage/year) [95% credible intervals]		
	Female	Male	Difference
OTL-HNS	8.2 [6.5, 10.1]	5.5 [4.1, 6.9]	2.7 [0.9, 4.7]
Anesthesiology	6.8 [5.8, 7.7]	4.8 [4.0, 5.5]	2.0 [0.8, 3.2]
Family Medicine	4.5 [4.2, 4.7]	2.1 [1.8, 2.4]	2.4 [2.0, 2.7]
General Surgery	3.5 [2.7, 4.3]	−0.68 [−1.3, −0.1]	4.19 [3.1, 5.2]
Internal Medicine	5.0 [4.6, 5.5]	2.5 [2.1, 2.9]	2.5 [1.9, 3.1]
Pediatrics	5.6 [4.9, 6.2]	1.8 [0.8, 2.7]	3.8 [2.7 5.0]
Psychiatry	6.2 [5.6, 6.9]	4.7 [3.9, 5.4]	1.5 [0.5, 2.5]

Data collected from both CaRMS and CAPER regarding the number of female and male applicants in OTL-HNS and selected larger residency programs was averaged between 1990 and 2014. Gender-specific differences in growth rate were calculated for each specific program

Acceptance rates of first-choice applicants to OTL-HNS

Acceptance rates among first choice applicants varied among female applicants from year to year, with a decrease compared to male applicant acceptance rates in 2013 and 2014 (Fig. 3). During this period, 12.5% and 28.6% of women ranking OTL-HNS as their first choice were accepted compared to 51.8% and 43.5% of men, respectively (Fig. 4). There was an average of 19 female first-choice applications per year compared to 26 male first-choice applications between 2006 and 2014 (Table 3). The range of acceptance rates for men was 30% to 51.8% and the range for women was 12.5% to 48%. In the 9 years studied, six of these years had a greater acceptance rate of male applicants, and 3 years had a greater acceptance rate of female applicants. Of note, in 2006, 46.6% of females ranking OTL-HNS as their first choice (7 successful candidates out of 15 total candidates) were accepted compared to 30% of males (6 successful candidates out of 20 total candidates). However, no significant differences were found between the acceptance rates of females and males throughout the years studied.

Female representation and acceptance rates of applicants to OTL-HNS programs

Between 2006 and 2014, acceptance rates of female applicants to OTL-HNS varied significantly between universities with a range of 16% to 65%. (Fig. 5). Female representation across institutions was largely above 40% with three programs having less than 30% of their residents being female. One institution had female residents accouting for only 18% of all trainees. However, six of the 13 surveyed institutions had greater than 50% of their residents being female.

Discussion

To our knowledge, our study is the first to examine the current state and evolution of gender representation among Canadian OTL-HNS training programs in comparison to other postgraduate training programs. Our results document that, currently, OTL-HNS continues to have a lower female resident representation compared to larger training programs, while having similar gender representation in comparison to similarly-sized surgical subspecialties. Interestingly, annual growth rates for female OTL-HNS residents significantly exceeds the rates seen in larger residency programs and the majority of surgical subspecialties. Finally, there exists significant variability in female representation amongst the individual Canadian OTL-HNS residency programs.

Research has explored the role of gender in medical students' choice of specialty [1–7], with the role model hypothesis suggests that the establishment of gender congruent role models may influence a medical trainee's choice of specialty. A lack of female role models in certain specialties likely accounts for fewer females in those fields [3, 9], and the impact of resident role models exceeds that of faculty role models, possibly due to greater frequency of interactions and a greater sense of identification with residents than with faculty members [18]. However, it is conceivable that a female medical student from a gender balanced OTL-HNS faculty might have

Table 2 Gender-specific growth rates in OTL-HNS versus surgical subspecialty programs

Specialty	Annual growth rates (percentage/year) [95% credible intervals]		
	Female	Male	Difference
OTL-HNS	8.2 [6.5, 10.1]	5.5 [4.1, 6.9]	2.7 [0.9, 4.7]
Cardiac surgery	5.1 [1.4, 9.2]	2.4 [−0.88, 5.7]	2.7 [0.3, 5.7]
Neurosurgery	6.0 [3.4, 8.5]	3.9 [2.2, 5.6]	2.2 [−0.5, 4.1]
Ophthalmology	6.9 [5.3, 8.5]	4.5 [3.2, 5.7]	2.5 [0.6, 4.2]
Orthopedics	9.2 [7.5, 10.9]	6.4 [5.5, 7.3]	2.8 [1.1, 4.6]
Plastic surgery	8.8 [6.4, 11.6]	5.1 [3, 7.1]	3.6 [1.5, 7]
Urology	8.0 [5.8, 10.2]	5.7 [4.3, 7.1]	2.4 [0.1, 4.4]

Data collected from both CaRMS and CAPER regarding the number of female and male applicants in OTL-HNS and selected surgical specialty programs was averaged between 1990 and 2014. Gender-specific differences in growth rate were calculated for each specific program

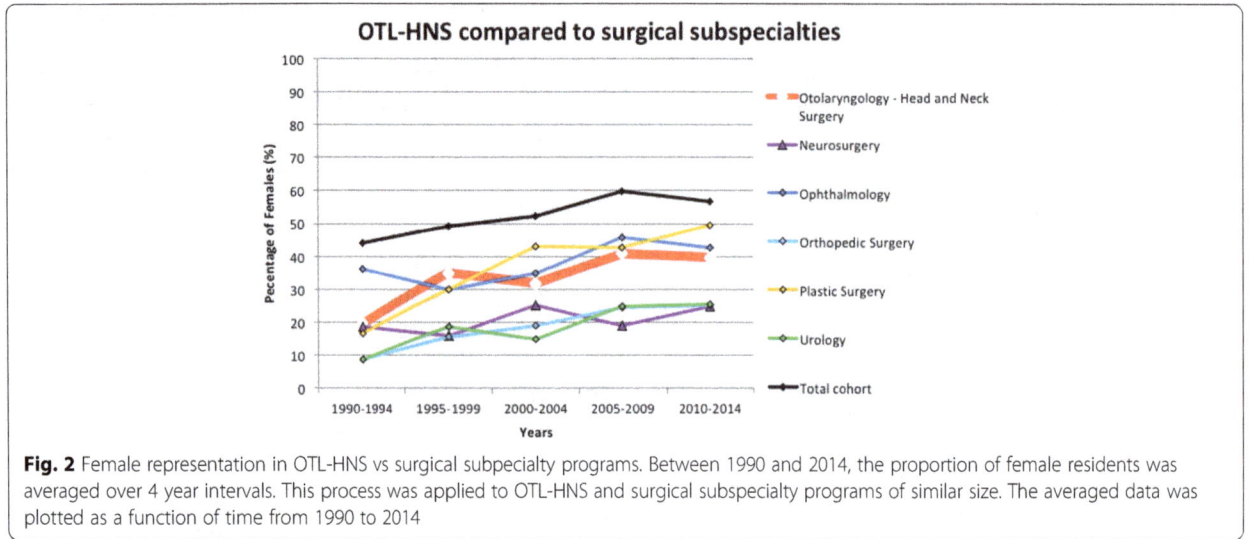

Fig. 2 Female representation in OTL-HNS vs surgical subpecialty programs. Between 1990 and 2014, the proportion of female residents was averaged over 4 year intervals. This process was applied to OTL-HNS and surgical subspecialty programs of similar size. The averaged data was plotted as a function of time from 1990 to 2014

been accepted to a program with a paucity of female resident trainees. The impact of gender congruent role models would require an analysis of the gender makeup of faculty encountered during applicants' medical school training and current residency program, but is a factor worthy of consideration. This represents an important additional avenue for future investigation to ultimately better understand trends gender representation and to develop gender parity in our healthcare workforce.

In addition, surgical specialties have been rated poorly with respect to work-life balance and this has been traditionally suggested to explain the lack of female representation in surgical specialties [19, 20]. The perception of worse lifestyle in surgery can be associated with the number of working hours, training years prior to certification as well as the acute, stressful nature of the work involved [21, 22]. However, it is unclear how much influence the perception of a poorer lifestyle has on deterring prospective applicants or if this influence is gender-specific [9]. Assumptions regarding lifestyle preferences and gender may not be universally supported, as obstetrics and gynecology attracts a greater number of female applicants despite being known for a less than favorable lifestyle [23].

The reinforcement of gender roles expressed through subtle and unconscious gender beliefs may also influence an applicant's choice of specialty - male medical students may be more likely to be advised to prioritize specialty

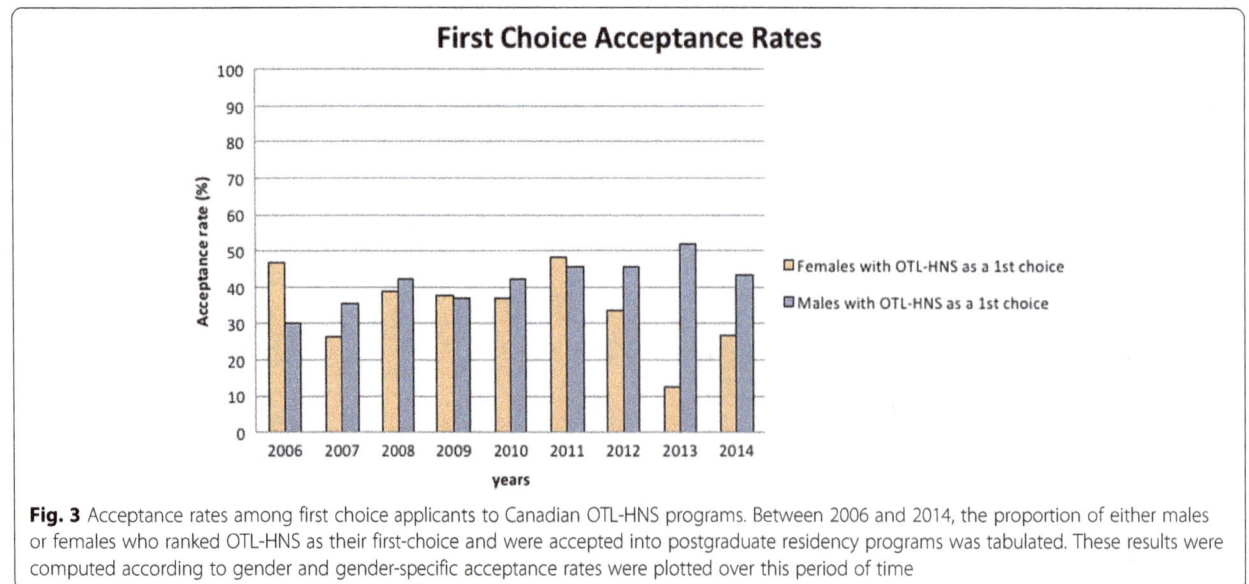

Fig. 3 Acceptance rates among first choice applicants to Canadian OTL-HNS programs. Between 2006 and 2014, the proportion of either males or females who ranked OTL-HNS as their first-choice and were accepted into postgraduate residency programs was tabulated. These results were computed according to gender and gender-specific acceptance rates were plotted over this period of time

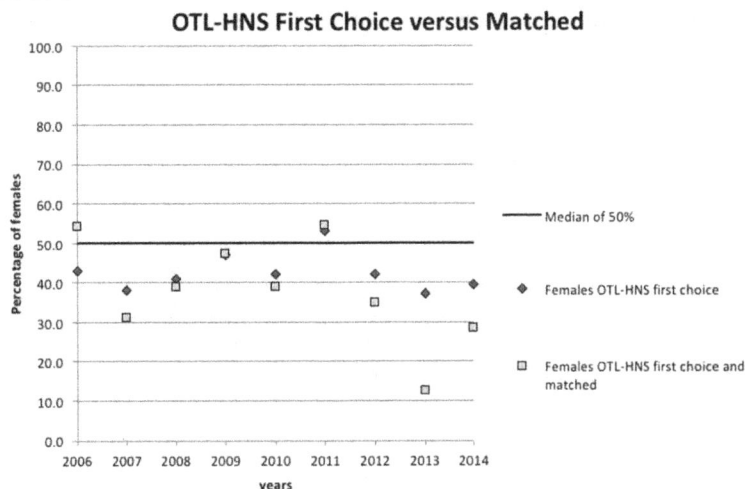

Fig. 4 Trends of female representation and acceptance rates in OTL-HNS. Between 2006 and 2014, the proportion of females among all applicants that ranked OTL-HNS as their first choice was calculated and plotted. The proportion of female applicants to OTL-HNS that successfully matched to OTL-HNS postgraduate residency programs was also plotted between 2006 and 2014. The average of all acceptance rates between 2006 and 2014 was also plotted

preference over familial consideration compared to females [24]. Selection of career choices may also be related to the evaluations of medical students, which may be gender-specific. For example, the student evaluations tend to emphasize particular qualities in trainees that were gender-specific; males have been shown to receive evaluations which reinforce their technical abilities, whereas female candidates receive evaluations which highlight their humanistic attributes [25]. The importance of technical abilities for a career in surgery may disadvantage and discourage applicants who do not

Table 3 Acceptance rates among first choice applicants to OTL-HNS programs

Year	Applicant 1st Choice		Matched 1st Choice		Success Rate Female (%)	Success Rate Males (%)
	Female	Male	Female	Male		
2006	15	20	7	6	46.7	30.0
2007	19	31	5	11	26.3	35.5
2008	18	26	7	11	38.9	42.3
2009	24	27	9	10	37.5	37.0
2010	19	26	7	11	36.8	42.3
2011	25	22	12	10	48.0	45.5
2012	24	33	8	15	33.3	45.5
2013	16	27	2	14	12.5	51.9
2014	15	23	4	10	26.7	43.5
Average	19.4	26.1	6.8	10.9	34.1	41.5

Between 2006 and 2014, the proportion of either males or females who ranked OTL-HNS as their first-choice and were accepted into postgraduate residency programs was tabulated. Gender-specific success rates were calculated for each year along with an average success rate

receive positive feedback regarding those skills from applying to surgical post-graduate training programs.

The variation in female representation in OTL-HNS residents across Canadian institutions is large and may be attributable to certain factors particular to institutions. With the majority of institutions reaching near parity in female and male representation, the presence of significant underrepresentation in certain institutions suggest that their individual qualities may be more contributory than the characteristics of OTL-HNS as a specialty. Female representation in undergraduate medical education programs and the lack of postgraduate role models across the country may help explain differences in gender representation at the postgraduate level, however this remains speculative at best. The differences in gender composition of the student body may also be in due to differences in recruitment and admissions policies, and remains an important avenue for future research. Further studies may be of benefit to postgraduate OTL-HNS program directors in so far as facilitating gender parity among recruited trainees, including the identification of barriers at the application and admissions stages of post graduate medical education.

Strengths of our study include analysis over a prolonged time frame to allow assessment of growth of female representation. Contextualization of gender representation in OTL-HNS was possible through comparison with larger programs and smaller surgical subspecialty programs, which share a number of similar characteristics with OTL-HNS. The main limitation of this study was the assessment of gender representation trends in smaller programs, as there are very few admitted candidates per year.

Female acceptance rates across Canadian universities

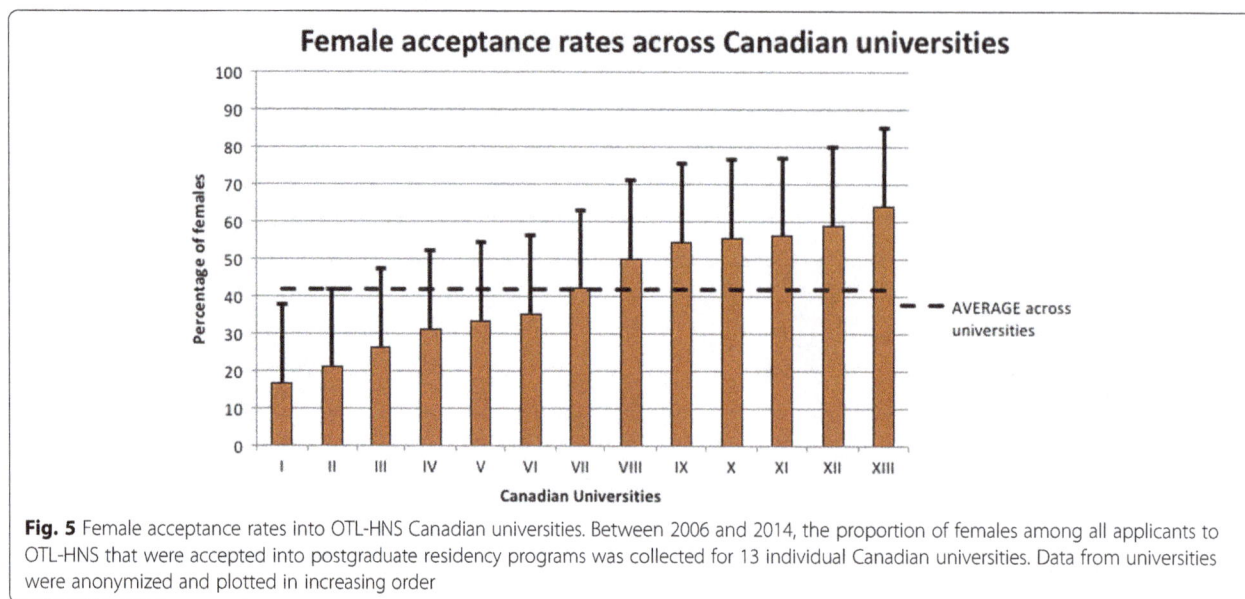

Fig. 5 Female acceptance rates into OTL-HNS Canadian universities. Between 2006 and 2014, the proportion of females among all applicants to OTL-HNS that were accepted into postgraduate residency programs was collected for 13 individual Canadian universities. Data from universities were anonymized and plotted in increasing order

OTL-HNS and other surgical subspecialty programs have a relatively small number of trainees, such that minor changes in the number of female trainees may translate to a large change in the rate of female representation across time. As a result, it is difficult to determine the significance of increased growth rates in female representation in OTL-HNS residency, particularly when comparisons are made to larger programs. Small changes in gender composition of the trainees may lead to large variation in measured female representation and growth rates of female applicants, however our results demonstrated relative consistency across time. The incorporation of two separate sources of data (CAPER and CaRMS) for our analysis with CAPER being a self-reported census represents an additional limitation of this study.

Future work may include investigating the influence of medical curriculum and role model exposure on trainees' selection of career paths during pre-clinical years. The investigations of other contributory factors such as gender role models, applicant perception of the given specialty, perception of lifestyle within the given specialty and the recruitment techniques employed by residency programs also represent interesting avenues of future study, and could provide explanations for the findings described here.

Conclusion

Female representation in OTL-HNS continues to improve with a large variability in the success rate of female applicants across Canadian institutions. Despite progress towards gender parity in OTL-HNS residency programs in Canada, certain institutions continue to report underrepresentation of female residents, possibly due to certain characteristics unique to those residency programs. A better understanding of these trends may allow us to identify supports and barriers of gender parity in surgical training programs and ultimately suggest appropriate recommendations. This will lead to the most qualified trainees being selected, gender parity within the OTL-HNS workforce, and ultimately improved patient outcomes. Ensuring the presence of gender congruent role models and addressing the negative perception of work-life balance within subspecialty surgery could reduce barriers to female medical student trainees applying to OTL-HNS residency training programs, and careful monitoring or admissions practices may facilitate the matching of the most appropriate candidates, regardless of gender.

Abbreviations
CAPER: Canadian Post-M.D. Education Registry; CaRMS: Canadian Residency Matching Service; OTL-HNS: Otolaryngology – Head and Neck Surgery

Acknowledgements
Not applicable.

Funding
Not applicable.

Authors' contributions
SC was responsible for the creation and designing of the study with JS and LN providing input into the design of the study and supervision of the project. LJ provided statistical expertise and analysis for the collected data and MY provided input into the design of the study, appropriate review of the literature and revisions to the manuscript. NV was responsible for drafting the manuscript, tabulating and organizing data. All authors read and approved the final manuscript.

Competing interests

The authors declare that they have no competing interests.

Author details

[1]Faculty of Medicine, McGill University Health Centre, Montreal Children's Hospital, McGill University, Room A02.3015, 1001 Boulevard Decarie, Montreal, QC H4A 3J1, Canada. [2]Department of Otolaryngology-Head and Neck Surgery, McGill University, Montreal, Canada. [3]Centre for Medical Education, McGill University, Montreal, Canada. [4]Department of Medicine, McGill University, Montreal, Canada. [5]Department of Epidemiology and Biostatistics, McGill University, Montreal, Canada.

References

1. Canadian Post-MD Education Registry (CAPER). Annual Census Of Post-MD Trainees 2015–2016. https://caper.ca/~assets/documents/pdf_2015_16_ CAPER_Census.pdf.
2. Baxter N, Cohen R, McLeod R. The impact of gender on the choice of surgery as a career. Am J Surg. 1996;172(4):373–6.
3. Boyd JS, Clyne B, Reinert SE, Zink BJ. Emergency medicine career choice: a profile of factors and influences from the Association of American Medical Colleges (AAMC) graduation questionnaires. Acad Emerg Med. 2009;16(6): 544–9.
4. Buddeberg-Fischer B, Klaghofer R, Abel T, Buddeberg C. Swiss residents' speciality choices–impact of gender, personality traits, career motivation and life goals. BMC Health Serv Res. 2006;6:137.
5. Fitzgerald JE, Tang SW, Ravindra P, Maxwell-Armstrong CA. Gender-related perceptions of careers in surgery among new medical graduates: results of a cross-sectional study. Am J Surg. 2013;206(1):112–9.
6. Riska E. Gender and medical careers. Maturitas. 2011;68(3):264–7.
7. Schwartz JS, Young M, Velly AM, Nguyen LH. The evolution of racial, ethnic, and gender diversity in US otolaryngology residency programs. Otolaryngol Head Neck Surg. 2013;149(1):71–6.
8. Rabinowitz HK, Diamond JJ, Veloski JJ, Gayle JA. The impact of multiple predictors on generalist physicians' care of underserved populations. Am J Public Health. 2000;90(8):1225–8.
9. Roter DL, Hall JA. Physician gender and patient-centered communication: a critical review of empirical research. Annu Rev Public Health. 2004;25:497–519.
10. Eagly AH, Johnson BT. Gender and leadership-style - a Metaanalysis. Psychol Bull. 1990;108(2):233–56.
11. Jefferson L, Bloor K, Birks Y, Hewitt C, Bland M. Effect of physicians' gender on communication and consultation length: a systematic review and meta-analysis. J Health Serv Res Policy. 2013;18(4):242–8.
12. Roter DL, Hall JA, Aoki Y. Physician gender effects in medical communication: a meta-analytic review. JAMA. 2002;288(6):756–64.
13. Bertakis KD, Franks P, Azari R. Effects of physician gender on patient satisfaction. J Am Med Womens Assoc. 2003;58(2):69–75.
14. Cooper-Patrick L, Gallo JJ, Gonzales JJ, Vu HT, Powe NR, Nelson C, et al. Race, gender, and partnership in the patient-physician relationship. JAMA. 1999;282(6):583–9.
15. Jahng KH, Martin LR, Golin CE, DiMatteo MR. Preferences for medical collaboration: patient-physician congruence and patient outcomes. Patient Educ Couns. 2005;57(3):308–14.
16. Association of American Medical Colleges. Canadian Medical Graduation Questionnaire 2015 https://www.aamc.org/data/cgq/.
17. Viola KV, Bucholz E, Yeo H, Piper C, Bell RH Jr, Sosa JA. Impact of family and gender on career goals: results of a national survey of 4586 surgery residents. Arch Surg. 2010;145(5):418–24.
18. McCord JH, McDonald R, Leverson G, Mahvi DM, Rikkers LF, Chen HC, et al. Motivation to pursue surgical subspecialty training: is there a gender difference? J Am Coll Surg. 2007;205(5):698–703.
19. Dorsey ER, Jarjoura D, Rutecki GW. The influence of controllable lifestyle and sex on the specialty choices of graduating U.S. medical students, 1996-2003. Acad Med. 2005;80(9):791–6.
20. Newton DA, Grayson MS, Thompson LF. The variable influence of lifestyle and income on medical students' career specialty choices: data from two U. S. medical schools, 1998-2004. Acad Med. 2005;80(9):809–14.
21. Baldwin DC Jr, Daugherty SR, Tsai R, Scotti MJ Jr. A national survey of residents' self-reported work hours: thinking beyond specialty. Acad Med. 2003;78(11):1154–63.
22. Shanafelt TD, Balch CM, Bechamps GJ, Russell T, Dyrbye L, Satele D, et al. Burnout and career satisfaction among American surgeons. Ann Surg. 2009; 250(3):463–71.
23. Wendel TM, Godellas CV, Prinz RA. Are there gender differences in choosing a surgical career? Surgery. 2003;134(4):591–6. discussion 6-8.
24. Johansson EE, Hamberg K. From calling to a scheduled vocation: Swedish male and female students' reflections on being a doctor. Medical Teach. 2007;29(1):e1–8.
25. Pamies RJ, Woodard LJ, Blair CR, Roetzheim RG, Herold AH. The influence on students' specialty selections of faculty evaluations and mini-board scores during third-year clerkships. Acad Med. 1992;67(2):127–9.

5

Delayed facial nerve decompression for severe refractory cases of Bell's palsy : a 25-year experience

Ilyes Berania[1], Mohamed Awad[1], Issam Saliba[1], Jean-Jacques Dufour[1] and Marc-Elie Nader[1,2]*

Abstract

Background: This study aims to assess the effectiveness of delayed facial nerve decompression for Bell's palsy (BP).

Methods: We performed a retrospective case review of all patients having undergone facial nerve decompression for severe refractory BP between 1984 and 2009 at our tertiary referral center. Demographics, timing between onset of symptoms and surgical decompression, degree of facial nerve dysfunction pre- and post-operatively, follow-up length after surgery and postoperative complications were recorded. Facial nerve dysfunction was assessed using the House-Brackmann (HB) scale. Electroneuronography, electromyography and imaging results were assessed when available.

Results: Eighteen patients had surgery between 21 and 60 days after onset of BP (group I), and 18 patients had surgery more than 60 days after onset of symptoms (group II). In group II, 11 patients had surgery between 61 and 89 days and 7 patients after 90 days. Groups I and II showed similar functional gain and rates of improvement to HB 3 or better (11/18 vs. 11/18, $p > 0.05$). In group II, patients operated 60 to 89 days after onset of BP showed a significantly higher rate of improvement to HB 3 or better (9/11 vs. 2/6, $p = 0.049$) with higher functional gain compared to those operated after 90 days ($p = 0.0293$).

Conclusions: When indicated, facial nerve decompression for BP is usually recommended within the first 2 weeks of onset of facial paralysis. Nonetheless, our results suggest that patients with severe BP could benefit from decompression surgery within 90 days after onset of symptoms in the absence of an opportunity to proceed earlier to surgery. Further investigation is still required to confirm our findings.

Keywords: Bell's palsy, Surgical decompression, Facial nerve, Functional outcomes

Background

Idiopathic facial paralysis, also defined as Bell's palsy (BP), is the most common peripheral mono-neuropathy affecting approximately 20–30 per 100,000 individuals annually [1]. This condition causes an acute dysfunction of the facial nerve, which may be partial or complete. The disorder is typically unilateral and affects mainly voluntary facial muscle contraction [2]. Motor dysfunction may lead to incomplete eyelid closure, predisposing to corneal abrasion,

exposure keratitis or corneal ulcerations [3]. Patients with Bell's palsy may also complain of xerostomia, dysgeusia and aural pain. These symptoms seem associated with a poorer nerve recovery prognosis [4]. Although most cases are self-limited, about 4% of patients remain with severe and persistent facial nerve dysfunction [5].

While there is strong evidence for initial conservative medical treatment in patients with BP [6–8], surgical decompression of the facial nerve remains a more controversial subject. Varying opinions exist in regards to the optimal surgical approach, extent of nerve decompression and timing of surgery. Both, the transmastoid and middle fossa approaches have their proponents. Some authors have argued that the transmastoid approach is an effective

* Correspondence: mnader@mdanderson.org
[1]Division of Otolaryngology - Head and Neck Surgery, Université de Montréal, Centre Hospitalier de l'Université de Montréal (CHUM) – Hôpital Notre-Dame, 1560 Sherbrooke Street, Montreal, QC H2L 4M1, Canada
[2]Department of Head and Neck Surgery, Unit 1445, The University of Texas MD Anderson Cancer Center, 1515 Holcombe Blvd, Houston, TX 77030, USA

treatment option that allows sufficient access to the facial nerve with low complication rates [9]. They have described techniques to decompress the geniculate ganglion and the distal labyrinthine segment while avoiding temporal lobe compression. Others have abandoned that procedure in favor of the middle fossa approach. They believe it offers better access to the facial nerve medial to the geniculate ganglion while having an acceptable complication risk profile [10]. The controversy around the choice of the surgical approach is closely related to the debate regarding the extent of nerve decompression. Some authors have recommended to decompress specifically the labyrinthine and meatal segments of the facial nerve [10]. These recommendations are based on studies showing that these two segments are the narrowest portions of the temporal bone at which nerve conduction blockage commonly occurs [11, 12]. Others have recommended instead subtotal decompression from the labyrinthine segment to the stylomastoid foramen based on their results showing reduced recurrences of BP and improved recovery [13]. Regarding timing of surgery, it is generally accepted that most favorable outcomes are obtained when decompression is performed within the first 14 days after onset of symptoms [14]. However, some studies have suggested potential benefits from delayed decompression anywhere from 1 month up to 4 months following the onset of BP [9, 15, 16]. Determining the role of delayed decompression is clinically relevant, especially considering the reality of the Canadian Healthcare system where patients may experience significant delays before being assessed by a neurotologist.

The benefits of surgical decompression in BP still need to be further clarified because of the lack of randomized reports addressing the subject and the potential significant surgical risks. More precisely, the role of delayed surgical decompression remains unclear. The present study reports clinical outcomes of patients with persistent and severe Bell's palsy who underwent delayed facial nerve decompression surgery at our institution.

Methods

After obtaining institutional review board approval (University of Montreal Hospital Center, IRB# 2016–6154, CE 15.154 – CA), we conducted a retrospective case review that included all patients having undergone facial nerve decompression between 1984 and 2009 for severe refractory BP at our tertiary care center. A total of 36 patients were selected based on the following inclusion criteria: 1) Early onset facial paralysis concordant with a diagnosis of Bell's palsy, 2) age ≥ 18 years, 3) patients with a persistent House-Brackmann (HB) grade V or VI in early assessments prior to surgical intervention, 4) initial management with high-dose steroids with or without antiviral agents or clinical surveillance only (i.e. no oral steroids).

Patients presenting early, within 2 weeks of onset of BP, were treated medically with oral corticosteroids. Those diagnosed within 3 days of onset also received antiviral therapy. Surgical decompression was systematically offered to patients with persistent facial paralysis HB grade 5 or 6 who showed more than 90% denervation on electroneuronography (ENoG). A certain proportion of our patients could not undergo ENoG testing, either because they presented more than 21 days after onset of symptoms or testing was unavailable. It was the practice of the senior neurotologist (JJD) to offer surgery to those patients after an in-depth discussion about the controversies and uncertainty of this treatment option in the absence of electrophysiological testing.

All 36 patients underwent transmastoid decompression surgery. A surgical technique similar to the one described by Yanagihara et al. was followed [17]. In summary, after completing a mastoidectomy, the vertical segment of the facial nerve was identified, and the facial recess was drilled out. The incudostapedial joint was carefully disarticulated, and the incus was temporarily removed. Air cells anterior to the superior bony semicircular canal were widely dissected, allowing access to the geniculate ganglion and distal labyrinthine segment. Through this transmastoid approach, the facial nerve was decompressed 180 degrees from the distal labyrinthine segment to the stylomastoid foramen, including the geniculate ganglion. The epineurium was carefully incised using a fine Beaver blade. At the end of the procedure, a tympanomeatal flap was elevated, and the incus was interposed. Two patients also underwent a middle fossa exposure in addition to a transmastoid approach. This change in surgical technique reflected the individual preference of one of the neurotologists (IS) who joined our institution in 2003.

Patients who underwent surgical decompression were classified according to the time between the onset of facial paralysis, determined during the first visit with a neurotologist, and day of the surgery; group I included patients who had surgery 21 to 60 days after onset of symptoms while group II comprised those with surgery performed >60 days. The second group was further divided as group IIa for patients having undergone surgery between 61 and 89 days and group IIb for those operated 90 days or more after onset of symptoms. Our study did not identify any patients who had early surgery within 21 days of initial diagnosis.

For each patient, the following data was obtained: demographic parameters, initial use of conservative therapy, timing between onset of symptoms and surgical decompression, degree of facial nerve dysfunction pre- and post-operatively, follow-up visits after surgery, and post-operative complications. Facial nerve dysfunction was assessed using the House-Brackmann (HB) grading scale.

Electroneuronography, EMG and imaging results were assessed when available.

Functional improvement of facial nerve was reported using three methods: 1) Proportion of patients with a final HB grade of 3 or better; 2) Simple functional gain was defined as the algebraic difference between pre and postoperative HB grades; 3) Weighted functional gain relied on a point-based scale more reflective of the clinical function of the facial nerve. It was based on postoperative HB grades (Table 1), and it allowed us to give more importance to HB 1 and 2 results compared to the simple functional gain method. Also, as opposed to the simple function gain calculation, no points were given if HB scores went from 6 to 5, as this degree of change did not represent a clinically significant improvement.

Statistical analysis

All statistical analyses were performed using SPSS version 19.0 (SPSS, Chicago, IL, USA). Data presented as ratios was analyzed using the Pearson χ^2 test or Fisher exact 2-tailed test if there were fewer than 10 patients in any cell of a 2×2 grid. Parametric demographic and clinical data were analyzed using the ANOVA and t-test. Simple and weighted functional gains were evaluated using the Mann-Whitney test as these represented non-parametric data. Correlation between the length of follow-up and facial nerve improvement was evaluated using linear regression analysis. A p value <0.05 was considered statistically significant.

Results

Our studied population included 19 males (52.7%) and 17 (47.2%) female patients. The mean age at diagnosis was 47.0 ($\pm$ 14.4) years. Three (8.6%) patients had a recurrent condition at the time of assessment. Among our group of patients, 26 (72.2%) patients presented total facial paralysis (HB VI). ENoG studies were available for 13 (36.1%) patients, all of whom had 0% residual nerve

function on testing. Follow-up visits of patients were between 30 days and 8 years post-operatively. A mild correlation was noted between length of follow-up and improvement in facial nerve function when using final HB grade (R squared = 0.31, p < 0.01) and weighted functional gain (R squared = 0.30, p < 0.01) as our measures of facial nerve improvement. No correlation was noted between length of follow-up and simple functional gain. (R squared = 0.06, p = 0.1454). Additional parameters are shown in Table 2.

Our study population included 18 (50.0%) patients who underwent surgery 21 to 60 days (group I) and 18 (50.0%) patients who had surgery >60 days (group II) after onset of symptoms. Within group II, 11 (61.1%) cases underwent surgical decompression between 60 and 89 days (group IIa) and 7 (38.9%) patients after 89 days (group IIb). Post-operative clinical improvement to HB 3 or better at the last follow-up visit was observed for 11 (61.1%) patients in group I and 11 (61.1%) patients in group II. In the second group, 9 (81.8%) patients in group IIa and 2 (28.6%) patients in group IIb, showed favorable recovery (p = 0.049). Additional parameters including final HB grading and preoperative studies are available in Table 3.

Comparison of clinical improvement scores revealed no significant difference between surgical decompression in patients who underwent surgery 21 to 60 days (group I) compared to patients operated after 60 days (group II, p = 0.9862). However, we noted that patients who underwent surgical decompression between 60 and 89 days (group IIa) showed a statistically significant higher clinical improvement score in comparison to those operated past 90 days (group IIb) for simple functional gain and weighted functional gain (p = 0.0293 and p = 0.0314, respectively) (Table 3).

We performed an additional subgroup analysis of only those subjects who had been initially managed with oral steroids. This analysis also excluded the two patients who underwent middle fossa decompression as to have a more homogenous population. No significant difference in clinical improvement scores was noted between group I (11 patients) and group II (eight patients) (Table 4).

The most commonly encountered surgical complication was tympanic membrane perforation following tympanomeatal flap elevation in 4/36 patients (11.1%). The other reported complications were post-operative hematoma (2/36, 5.6%) and surgical site infection (1/36, 2.8%). Audiogram results were not systematically available, and no conclusions could be drawn regarding the rate of hearing loss. Review of the operative reports did not reveal any instances of damage to the bony labyrinth or increased difficulty decompressing the distal labyrinthine segment of the facial nerve.

Table 1 Weighted functional gain scale

Pre and post-operative HB score	Improvement points attributed
6 to 6	0
5 to 5	0
6 to 5	0
5 to 4	1
6 to 4	1
6 to 3	2
5 to 3	2
6 to 2	3
5 to 2	3
6 to 1	4
5 to 1	4

Table 2 Demographic data and clinical characteristics of patients

Characteristic	Total (n = 36)	Decompression, 21–60 days (n = 18)	Decompression, 60–89 days (n = 11)	Decompression, ≥ 90 days (n = 7)	P value
Age (mean ± SD)	47.0 ± 14.4	46.0 ± 12.9	47.7 ± 17.1	50.6 ± 16.3	P = 0.767
Male/female ratio	19/17	9/9	7/4	3/4	P = 0.6529
Median months of follow-up (range)	12.2 (1.0–97.3)	7.7 (1.0–24.3)	17.6 (1.0–97.3)	15.0 (2.0–84.0)	P = 0.164
Affected side (Right/Left)	17/19	9/9	4/7	4/3	P = 0.6529

SD standard deviation

Discussion

To our knowledge, the present study represents one of the largest assessments of patients who underwent delayed surgical decompression for severe BP refractory to medical treatment. While no significant differences were noted between the two main comparison groups, the subgroup analysis suggests that patients with severe BP may benefit from decompression surgery up to 90 days after the onset of symptoms in the absence of an opportunity to proceed earlier to surgery.

Previous studies have reported variable results following delayed facial nerve decompression in patients with refractory BP. Similar to our findings, Bodenez et al. have reported favorable outcome with delayed facial nerve decompression in 13 patients with advanced facial paralysis who were operated between 1 to 4 months from the onset of BP [15]. At a one-year follow-up assessment, all their patients had showed clinical recovery to HB grade III or better. Yanagihara et al. reached similar conclusions [9].

They reported outcomes following transmastoid decompression done between 15 and 120 days after the onset of BP. Although they noted optimal results when surgery was performed early, their data suggested that delayed decompression up to 3 months may still be beneficial. They noted that 38.1% of patients operated between 31 to 60 days after onset achieved HB grade 1 compared to only 23.2% in the control group. Also, all patients treated after 60 days achieved a score of HB 3 or better compared to 86% in the nonsurgical group. On the other hand, other studies have not found delayed decompression to be as effective. Li et al. examined the outcome of transmastoid decompression 2 months after the onset of symptoms in refractory BP patients who were initially treated with corticosteroids [18]. Patients who underwent surgery between 2 and 3 months after onset of symptoms had an initial higher rate of facial function improvement compared to the control group at the three-month follow-up. However, that difference was not present at the 12-month follow-up

Table 3 Pre- and postoperative clinical parameters

Parameters	Total (n = 36)	Decompression, 21–60 days (n = 18) (Group I)	Decompression, 60–89 days (n = 11) (Group IIa)	Decompression, ≥ 90 days (n = 7) (Group IIb)	P value
Patients treated with preoperative steroids (no, %)	19 (52.8)	11 (61.1)	6 (54.5)	2 (28.6)	P = 0.4130
Preoperative EMG (no, %)	11 (30.6)	5 (27.8)	4 (36.4)	2 (28.6)	P = 0.8810
Preoperative ENoG (no, %)	13 (36.1)	7 (38.9)	4 (36.3)	2 (28.6)	P = 0.8900
Delay before surgery (Mean days, range)	63 (21–205)	38 (21–57)	68 (62–79)	127 (90–205)	
Initial Facial Function (HB mean, ± SD)	5.7 ± 0.6	5.7 ± 0.6	5.6 ± 0.7	5.7 ± 0.5	P = 0.5200
Final Facial Function (HB mean, ± SD)	3.3 ± 0.9	3.2 ± 0.7	2.9 ± 1.0	4.0 ± 0.8	P = 0.0772
Simple Functional Gain (mean gain, ± SD)	2.4 ± 1.0	2.4 ± 1.0	2.8 ± 0.8	1.7 ± 1.1	#P = 0.0293
Weighted Functional Gain (mean gain, ± SD)	1.7 ± 0.9	1.7 ± 0.8	2.1 ± 1.0	1.0 + 0.8	*P = 0.0314
Final HB score 3 or better (no, %)	22 (61.1)	11 (61.1)	9 (81.8)	2 (28.6)	**P = 0.049
Final HB score 2 or better (no, %)	6 (16.7)	3 (16.7)	3 (27.3)	0 (0)	P = 0.3531

No number
% percentage
SD standard deviation
HB House-Brackmann score
#Statistical significance, simple functional gain between Group IIa (decompression 60–89 days) and Group IIb (≥ 90 days) in Mann-Whitney test (p = 0.0293)
*Statistical significance, weighted functional gain between Group IIa (decompression 60–89 days) and Group IIb (≥ 90 days) in Mann-Whitney test (p = 0.0314)
** Statistical significance, final HB score 3 or better between Group IIa (decompression 60–89 days) and Group IIb (≥ 90 days) in Fisher exact test (p = 0.049)

Table 4 Pre- and postoperative clinical parameters of patients initially treated with oral steroids

Parameters	Total (n = 19)	Decompression, 21–60 days (n = 11) (Group I)	Decompression, >60 days (n = 8) (Group II)	P value
Preoperative EMG (no, %)	5 (26.3)	3 (27.3)	2 (25.0)	P = 0.9116
Preoperative ENoG (no, %)	6 (31.6)	4 (36.4)	2 (25.0)	P = 0.5988
Delay before surgery (mean days, range)	55 (24–113)	40 (24–57)	76 (62–113)	
Initial Facial Function (HB mean, ± SD)	5.9 ± 0.3	6.0 ± 0.0	5.7 ± 0.5	P = 0.3681
Final Facial Function (HB mean, ± SD)	3.2 ± 0.7	3.2 ± 0.8	3.3 ± 0.7	P = 0.9045
Simple Functional Gain (mean gain, ± SD)	2.5 ± 1.0	2.5 ± 1.1	2.4 ± 0.8	P = 0.8103
Weighted Functional Gain (mean gain, ± SD)	1.7 ± 0.8	1.7 ± 0.9	1.8 ± 0.7	P = 1.0
Final HB score 3 or better (no, %)	12 (63.2)	7 (63.6)	5 (62.5)	P = 0.9596
Final HB score 2 or better (no, %)	3 (15.8)	2 (18.2)	1 (12.5)	P = 0.7374

No number
% percentage
SD standard deviation
HB House-Brackmann score

visit. Similarly, Kim et al. evaluated the effectiveness of delayed transmastoid facial nerve decompression between 3 weeks and 2 months in 12 patients with BP [19]. Their study did not demonstrate any significant difference in facial nerve function between the surgical and control groups. Another study has recently reported recovery outcomes following delayed surgery done 2 weeks after diagnosis for patients with facial paralysis not responding to conservative management. It showed better functional gain when nerve decompression was performed within 2 weeks of onset of BP compared to delayed surgery beyond 26 days or medical treatment alone. Some beneficial effects were observed when surgery was done between 15 and 25 days [16]. Finally, Gantz et al. found greater recovery rates to HB grade I-II from facial paralysis if surgery was performed within 14 days of onset of BP [14]. Except for the study by Li et al., the other papers did not include a subgroup analysis comparing patients who underwent surgery beyond 90 days to those operated 14 to 90 days after onset of symptoms. Therefore, findings similar to ours may not have been identified in these studies because of this absence of subgroup analysis.

The current clinical practice guidelines strongly recommend the early use of oral steroids in the treatment algorithm of BP [2]. Several reports have showed greater recovery in nerve function with high dose oral steroids with or without anti-viral medication compared to placebo. In a recent double-blind randomized controlled study, Sullivan et al. reported that early treatment with prednisolone significantly improved the potential of complete recovery, up to 94.4% within 9 months compared to 81.6% for patients not taking steroids [6]. These findings have been further supported by a recent Cochrane review [20]. Our study did not include a control arm of subjects treated conservatively with medical therapy alone. Nonetheless, part of our data can be compared

to outcomes of conservative management available in the literature. For this comparison, it would be most appropriate to include the subset of our patients who had both oral steroids pre-operatively and a follow-up of at least 6 months. Eleven of our 36 subjects fill these criteria. Of these, 45.5% (5/11) achieved HB grade 2 or better and 100% HB 3 or better. Control groups of previous studies have had recovery to HB 2 or better between 41.7 and 65% and improvement to HB 3 or better between 81.1 and 94.4% [9, 14, 19]. This comparison may suggest that delayed decompression helps avoid severe persistent facial paralysis of HB grade 4 or worse. In turn, it would help reduce the most undesired sequelae of BP, namely incomplete eye closure and the resulting ocular complications.

The pathophysiologic mechanism of BP and findings at surgery by some authors may help explain the role of delayed facial nerve decompression in refractory BP. Although a clear causative mechanism remains to be determined, viral pathogens, notably herpes simplex virus (HSV) have been identified as potential triggers causing nerve inflammation and conduction dysfunction [21]. The inflammatory response occurring along the facial nerve appears to induce an intrinsic compression at its narrowest anatomical passage in the labyrinthine segment. Supporting this theory, facial nerve inflammation and edema has been reported as common intraoperative findings in BP patients [9, 15]. Interestingly, Bodenez et al. consistently noted inflammatory changes of the facial nerve in all of their 13 patients who underwent delayed surgical decompression, even in those operated 4 months following onset of facial paralysis [15]. Yanagihara et al. also noted edematous swelling of the facial nerve in most of their patients up to 3 months after onset [9]. Based on these findings and the results of our study, we could hypothesize that the inflammatory process may persist up to or even beyond 90 days following BP. Alternatively, our results may also be suggestive of a fibrotic remodeling process following inflammation that can maintain intrinsic compression on the nerve, which would then be relieved following surgical decompression [22].

A mild correlation was found between length of follow-up and improvement in facial nerve function. This finding corroborates the clinical observation that facial nerve function can still improve up to 6 months after an episode of Bell's palsy [5].

The optimal surgical approach to decompress the facial nerve is still debated. According to Cannon et al., facial nerve decompression should be achieved within 2 weeks of onset of BP using the middle fossa approach. Their study revealed improvement rates of 71% with low morbidity [10]. Other studies have reported good results and improved nerve recovery with the transmastoid approach [9, 13, 23–25]. In our study, all patients underwent transmastoid surgical decompression surgery as it was the preferred approach of the senior neurotologist (JJD).

Our study shows several limitations including its retrospective nature, a low proportion of patients having had pre-operative ENoG and EMG evaluations, and the absence of a control group treated with medical management alone. Electrophysiological assessment of facial nerve function was not available for all patients due to limited resources in primary and secondary centers in addition to delayed referral to our tertiary care center. We were not able to confirm that all our patients had >90% denervation prior to surgery. There is therefore a risk of overestimating the impact of delayed decompression. Moreover, although considered the most commonly used tool for the clinical assessment of facial nerve function, the HB grading scale has inherent limitations regarding its subjectivity, reliability, and longitudinal applicability [26]. These limitations of the HB scale were partially offset by having all the patients assessed by the same surgeon pre and post-operatively. Finally, the risk of hearing loss associated with facial nerve decompression is an important consideration to discuss with patients prior to surgical intervention. Significant traumatic sensorineural hearing loss is estimated between 2 and 5% [19]. In the present study, hearing assessment data was not consistently available, and no conclusions could be drawn regarding the rate of postoperative hearing loss.

Conclusion

The present study offers additional evidence that may support the role of delayed decompression surgery for BP. We recommend facial nerve decompression for BP within the first 2 weeks when indicated. Nonetheless, our results suggest that patients with severe BP may benefit from decompression surgery up to 90 days after the onset of symptoms in the absence of an opportunity to proceed earlier to surgery. Further investigation is still required to confirm our findings and to better define the role of delayed surgical intervention in the treatment algorithm of BP, especially for patients with persistent paralysis beyond 3 months.

Abbreviations
BP: Bell's palsy; EMG: Electromyography; ENoG: Electroneuronography; HB: House-Brackmann

Acknowledgements
Not applicable.

Funding
This study had no findings sources.

Authors' contributions
IB was involved in data analysis/interpretation, drafting and correction of the manuscript. MA was involved in data acquisition and interpretation. IS was involved in data interpretation and manuscript revision. JJD was involved in manuscript revision. MEN was involved in data analysis/interpretation and manuscript revision. All authors read and approved the final manuscript.

Competing interests
The authors declare that they have no competing interests.

References
1. Marson AG, Salinas R. Bell's palsy. West J Med. 2000;173(4):266–8.
2. Baugh RF, Basura GJ, Ishii LE, Schwartz SR, Drumheller CM, Burkholder R, et al. Clinical practice guideline: Bell's palsy. Otolaryngol Head Neck Surg. 2013; 149(3 Suppl):S1–27.
3. Bhatti MT, Schiffman JS, Pass AF, Tang RA. Neuro-ophthalmologic complications and manifestations of upper and lower motor neuron facial paresis. Curr Neurol Neurosci Rep. 2010;10(6):448–58.
4. De Seta D, Mancini P, Minni A, Prosperini L, De Seta E, Attanasio G, et al. Bell's palsy: symptoms preceding and accompanying the facial paresis. ScientificWorldJournal. 2014;2014:801971.
5. Peitersen E. Bell's palsy: the spontaneous course of 2,500 peripheral facial nerve palsies of different etiologies. Acta Otolaryngol Suppl. 2002;549:4–30.
6. Sullivan FM, Swan IR, Donnan PT, Morrison JM, Smith BH, McKinstry B, et al. Early treatment with prednisolone or acyclovir in Bell's palsy. N Engl J Med. 2007;357(16):1598–607.
7. Engstrom M, Berg T, Stjernquist-Desatnik A, Axelsson S, Pitkaranta A, Hultcrantz M, et al. Prednisolone and valaciclovir in Bell's palsy: a randomised, double-blind, placebo-controlled, multicentre trial. Lancet Neurol. 2008;7(11):993–1000.
8. Salinas RA, Alvarez G, Daly F, Ferreira J. Corticosteroids for Bell's palsy (idiopathic facial paralysis). Cochrane Database Syst Rev. 2010;3:CD001942.
9. Yanagihara N, Hato N, Murakami S, Honda N. Transmastoid decompression as a treatment of bell palsy. Otolaryngol Head Neck Surg. 2001;124(3):282–6.
10. Cannon RB, Gurgel RK, Warren FM, Shelton C. Facial nerve outcomes after middle fossa decompression for Bell's palsy. Otol Neurotol. 2015;36(3):513–8.
11. Ge XX, Spector GJ. Labyrinthine segment and geniculate ganglion of facial nerve in fetal and adult human temporal bones. Ann Otol Rhinol Laryngol Suppl. 1981;90(4 Pt 2):1–12.
12. Gantz BJ, Gmur A, Fisch U. Intraoperative evoked electromyography in Bell's palsy. Am J Otolaryngol. 1982;3(4):273–8.
13. Wu S-h, Chen X, Wang J, Liu H, X-z Q, Pan X-I. Subtotal facial nerve decompression in preventing further recurrence and promoting facial nerve recovery of severe idiopathic recurrent facial palsy. Eur Arch Otorhinolaryngol. 2015;272(11):3295–8.

14. Gantz BJ, Rubinstein JT, Gidley P, Woodworth GG. Surgical management of Bell's palsy. Laryngoscope. 1999;109(8):1177–88.

15. Bodenez C, Bernat I, Willer J, Barre P, Lamas G, Tankere F. Facial nerve decompression for idiopathic Bell's palsy: report of 13 cases and literature review. J Laryngol Otol. 2010;124(03):272–8.

16. Kim J, Moon IS, Lee WS. Effect of delayed decompression after early steroid treatment on facial function of patients with facial paralysis. Acta Otolaryngol. 2010;130(1):179–84.

17. Yanagihara N, Gyo K, Yumoto E, Tamaki M. Transmastoid decompression of the facial nerve in Bell's palsy. Arch Otolaryngol. 1979;105(9):530–4.

18. Li Y, Sheng Y, Feng G-D, Wu H-Y, Gao Z-Q. Delayed surgical management is not effective for severe Bell's palsy after two months of onset. Int J Neurosci. 2016;126(11):989–95.

19. Kim SH, Jung J, Lee JH, Byun JY, Park MS, Yeo SG. Delayed facial nerve decompression for Bell's palsy. Eur Arch Otorhinolaryngol. 2016;273(7):1755–60.

20. Madhok VB, Gagyor I, Daly F, Somasundara D, Sullivan M, Gammie F, et al. Corticosteroids for Bell's palsy (idiopathic facial paralysis). Cochrane Database Syst Rev. 2016;7:CD001942.

21. McCormick DP, Spruance SL. Herpes simplex virus as a cause of Bell's palsy. Rev Med Virol. 2000;10(5):285.

22. Lundberg G. Nerve injury and repair. 2nd ed. Edinburgh: Churchill Livingstone; 2004.

23. Yasumura S, Watanabe Y, Aso S, Asai M, Ito M, Mizukoshi K. Result of decompression surgery in late-stage severe facial paralysis. Acta Otolaryngol Suppl. 1993;504:134–6.

24. Pulec JL. Total facial nerve decompression: technique to avoid complications. Ear Nose Throat J. 1996;75(7):410–5.

25. Doshi J, Irving R. Recurrent facial nerve palsy: the role of surgery. J Laryngol Otol. 2010;124(11):1202–4.

26. Fattah AY, Gurusinghe AD, Gavilan J, Hadlock TA, Marcus JR, Marres H, et al. Facial nerve grading instruments: systematic review of the literature and suggestion for uniformity. Plast Reconstr Surg. 2015;135(2):569–79.

6

Factors associated with lingual tonsil hypertrophy in Canadian adults

Matthew S. Harris[1], Brian W. Rotenberg[1,2], Kathryn Roth[1,2] and Leigh J. Sowerby[1,2]*

Abstract

Background: Hypertrophy of the lingual tonsil tissue in the adult patient is thought to contribute to the pathophysiology of obstructive sleep apnea. The underlying etiology of lingual tonsil hypertrophy (LTH) in the adult patient is unclear and likely multifactorial. Previous studies have suggested that the lingual tonsils may undergo compensatory hyperplasia post-tonsillectomy in children, although it is unknown if this occurs or persists into adulthood. The purpose of this study was to determine what factors are associated with LTH in a population of Canadian adults.

Methods: Adult patients presenting for consultation to an academic Rhinology/General Otolaryngology practice were eligible for enrollment. Demographic data including age, body mass index (BMI), Reflux Symptom Index (RSI), history of allergy, and history of tonsillectomy was collected via questionnaire. Endoscopic photographs of the base of tongue and larynx were captured. These were graded for LTH and Reflux Finding Scale (RFS) by blinded examiners. Statistical analysis was performed by comparing the mean LTH value to the variables of interest using two-tailed T-test. $P < .05$ was considered significant.

Results: One hundred two subjects were enrolled. Age ranged from 18 to 78. 28 patients had previous tonsillectomy. This was not associated with a significant increase in lingual tonsil tissue ($r = -0.05$, $p = 0.61$). RFS >7 or RSI >13 was considered positive for laryngopharyngeal reflux. There was no difference in LTH based on RSI positivity ($p = 0.44$). RFS positivity correlated with increased lingual tonsil tissue ($p < 0.05$). BMI >30 was associated with increased lingual tonsil hypertrophy ($p < 0.05$).

Conclusions: An elevated body mass index and positive Reflux Finding Score are associated with lingual tonsil hypertrophy in adults. Reflux symptom index, history of allergy and history of childhood tonsillectomy are not associated with LTH.

Keywords: Laryngopharyngeal reflux, Reflux symptom index, Reflux finding score, Body mass index, Tonsillectomy, Lingual tonsil

Background

The lingual tonsils are composed of reactive lymphoid tissue at the base of the tongue. Hypertrophy of the lingual tonsils can present clinically as globus, dysphagia, and cause difficultly with exposure of the glottis during intubation. Lingual tonsil hypertrophy (LTH) can also contribute to obstructive sleep apnea (OSA) at the level of the oropharynx. In children, compensatory LTH has been observed after routine tonsillectomy [1]. Recently, Sung et al. examined factors that were associated with lingual tonsil hypertrophy in Korean patients with OSA. Obesity and endoscopic evidence of reflux were found to be associated with LTH [2]. More recently, Friedman et al. have further studied endoscopic examination of the lingual tonsils in order to standardize a grading scale [3].

To date, no study has examined with relationship with tonsillectomy as a child and LTH as an adult. There is also an emerging body of evidence that suggests environmental allergies may cause laryngeal symptoms, however, the symptom overlap and comorbidity between

* Correspondence: leigh.sowerby@sjhc.london.on.ca

Previously presented at the Triological Society Meeting at the Combined Otolaryngology Spring Meeting, April 2015 in Boston, MA as a poster presentation.

[1]Department of Otolaryngology – Head & Neck Surgery, Schulich School of Medicine & Dentistry, Western University, London, ON, Canada

[2]St. Joseph's Healthcare, Western University, 268 Grosvenor Street, London, ON N6A 4 V2, Canada

allergy and LTH has yet to be fully elucidated [4, 5]. The purpose of this study was to determine what factors are associated with LTH in a population of Canadian adults.

Methods

Research ethics board approval was obtained at Western University (London, Ontario, Canada) for this project (HSREB # 104994). A prospective cross-sectional study enrolling consecutive patients presenting for routine consultation at an academic Rhinology and General Otolaryngology – Head & Neck Surgery practice was performed from March 2014 to June 2014. All patients older than 18 and requiring flexible nasopharyngoscopy as part of their physical examination were considered eligible for inclusion. Exclusion criteria included age less than 18, non-English speaking, illiteracy, and a history of previous sleep apnea surgery as an adult. Patients completed a questionnaire for demographic data, and completed the Reflux Symptom Index (RSI). An RSI of greater than 13 was considered positive for reflux [6]. Demographic factors examined included age, body mass index (BMI), history of diagnosed OSA, history of environmental allergies and history of childhood tonsillectomy. Tonsillectomy was considered to have been performed in childhood if the patient had tonsillectomy performed before the age of 18.

During routine nasopharyngoscopy, photographs of the base of tongue and larynx were captured for each patient. This was done with the patient in a standardized "sniffing" position with the tongue protruded. All photographic images were captured by a single surgeon and were standardized in distance from larynx and base of tongue. The nasopharyngoscope was positioned just past the soft palate and a photograph was taken with view of the base of tongue and posterior wall of the pharynx with the larynx centered in the photograph. Three blinded examiners reviewed the clinical photographs of the larynx and base of tongue in a randomized fashion. The blinded reviewers were all Fellows of the Royal College of Physicians and Surgeons of Canada in Otolaryngology with practices in general otolaryngology and rhinology, and none had sub-specialty interest or expertise in laryngology. The photographs of the larynx were evaluated to calculate the Reflux Finding Scale (RFS) score (Table 1) [6]. These were averaged to create a mean RFS score, which was considered positive if the score was greater than 7 [6]. The photographs of the base of tongue were graded for LTH based on the scale published by Sung (Table 2) [2]. Mean LTH values were subsequently also calculated for each patient.

Statistical analysis was performed by comparing the mean LTH value to the variables of interest using two-tailed T-test. These included BMI (>30 vs. <30), endoscopic evidence of reflux (RFS > 7 vs. RFS < 7), Reflux

Table 1 Reflux Finding Score developed by *Belafsky* et al. [4]

Subglottic Edema	2 = present
	0 = absent
Ventricular Obliteration	2 = partial
	4 = complete
Erythema/Hyperemia	2 = arytenoids only
	4 = diffuse
Vocal Fold Edema	1 = mild
	2 = moderate
	3 = severe
	4 = polypoid
Diffuse Laryngeal Edema	1 = mild
	2 = moderate
	3 = severe
	4 = obstructing
Posterior Commissure Hypertrophy	1 = mild
	2 = moderate
	3 = severe
	4 = obstructing
Granuloma/Granulation	2 = present
	0 = absent
Thick Endolaryngeal Mucous	2 = present
	0 = absent

Symptom Index (RSI > 13 vs. RSI <13), and history of childhood tonsillectomy. Kolmogorov-Smirnov test confirmed normal distribution for age, BMI, RSI and mean RFS values. Fleiss' Kappa for multiple observers was calculated for the grading of LTH and RFS scoring by the blinded reviewers. Linear regression was performed to determine if age correlated to lingual tonsil size.

Results

One hundred and two patients were enrolled in the study (49 men, 53 women). Mean age was 48.0 years (19–78). Mean BMI was 28.2 (18.5–41.8). A previous diagnosis of gastroesophageal reflux disease or OSA was present in 20 (20%) and 15 (15%) participants respectively. Twenty-

Table 2 Lingual Tonsil Grading Scale used by *Sung* et al. [1]

Grade	Description
0	No lingual tonsil tissue
1	Spotted lingual tonsil tissue
	Base of tongue vasculature visible
2	Base of tongue vasculature obscured
	Vallecula visible
3	Vallecula obscured
4	Epiglottis obscured

seven patients (26%) had a previous childhood tonsillectomy. Patient demographics are shown in Table 3.

There was no correlation between age and lingual tonsil size ($r = -0.05$, $p = 0.61$). History of childhood tonsillectomy did not demonstrate a significant difference in LTH grading ($p = 0.51$). Patients with a BMI >30 had a significantly larger mean lingual tonsil grade than patients with BMI <30 (2.26 vs. 1.83, $p = 0.035$). Inter-rater agreement between blinded reviewers was graded as fair with Fleiss' Kappa for both the Reflux Finding Score ($\kappa = 0.34$) and lingual tonsil hypertrophy grade ($\kappa = 0.41$). A positive Reflux Finding Score was also associated with significant increase in mean lingual tonsil grade (2.31 vs. 1.76, $p = 0.008$). A positive Reflux Symptom Index showed no significant difference in lingual tonsil grading ($p = 0.44$). History of allergy also failed to demonstrate a significant difference in lingual tonsil grading (1.86 vs. 1.97, $p = 0.52$). Results are summarized in Table 4.

Discussion

Lingual tonsil hypertrophy can play a major role in OSA and in difficult intubations, yet little attention has been paid to the etiology. There appears to be a complex interplay with laryngopharyngeal reflux (LPR) emerging as a strong potential contributor to LTH and, subsequently, OSA. Previous authors have also demonstrated an association between LTH and OSA, BMI, age and smoking, but there has not been general agreement [1, 7]. This study adds further support to an association between a positive reflux finding score and BMI with lingual tonsil hypertrophy, but does not support a history of childhood tonsillectomy or age being associated with lingual tonsil size in adults.

Sung et al. demonstrated a correlation between BMI, reflux finding score and lingual tonsil hypertrophy in OSA patients [1]. A trend was also seen for a negative correlation with age, but was not statistically significant. This association has also been supported by Friedman's group in Chicago, where a statistically significant association was found between increasing LTH and decreasing age, RSI >10 and positive smoking status [7]. Interestingly, they did

not, however, find an association with BMI, PPI use or allergy medication use. Our study failed to identify any trend or correlation between age and LTH. Part of the discrepancy may be related to the scoring scale used by the respective authors. In this study, the LTH scoring scale described by Sung et al. was used because Friedman's scale was not yet published at the time of study [8]. Previous methods of measurement using both CT and MRI have also been described, but given the expense are not justified for routine evaluation in a universal-payer system such as in Canada [1]. Both Sung and Friedman's scales have demonstrated similarly good inter-rater agreement. The kappa for Sung's grading scale was reported to be 0.73, while Friedman's grading scale had a reported kappa of 0.78 for the video assessment and 0.87 for live assessment. An advantage of Friedman's scale is the use of video and various positions of the tongue, which appears to allow for greater inter-rater agreement and consistency and may be a source of some of our inter-rater disagreement. Sung's group did, however, demonstrate good correlation with measurements on MRI suggesting validity of their scale and the use of standardized photography for grading [1]. Lastly, although lingual tonsil hypertrophy has been observed in pediatric patients with prior adenotonsillectomy, a post-mortem study examining 497 corpses found only 16 (3.2%) had LTH. Of those, 6 (37.5%) had evidence of previous tonsillectomy versus 119 (23.9%) of the whole study sample, but formal statistical analysis was not performed [9].

It is likely there is a complex interplay between obesity, OSA, LPR and LTH. DelGaudio et al. demonstrated increasing severity of LTH with more severe nasopharyngeal reflux on PH probe testing, but also found that those with mild LTH had a BMI that was 8 points lower than those in the moderate and severe groups. They did not assess for OSA in the studied population [10]. It is known that OSA creates negative intra-thoracic pressure that can exacerbate reflux, but other evidence suggests that a vasovagal reflex arc may be triggered by refluxate [11]. Two previous studies have demonstrated that treatment of reflux can help in the treatment of OSA. Friedman demonstrated an average reduction in AHI from 38 to 29 in patients with a negative pH study after treatment with proton pump therapy [12]. Senior found that the apnea index decreased by 31% and respiratory disturbance index decreased by 25% with treatment with omeprazole and lifestyle modifications after one month of therapy in patients with confirmed reflux on pH probe testing [13].

Limitations of this study include the cross-sectional nature of the study and lack of confirmation of OSA or LPR by objective testing. A recent study by Chang et al. examining the reliability of the RFS score among general otolaryngologists found only fair agreement and would

Table 3 Patient Demographics

Demographic	Male	Female	Total
n	49	53	102
Age	46.7 (20–78)	49.1 (19–77)	48.0 (19–78)
BMI	28.6 (23.1–40.90)	27.8 (18.5–41.8)	28.2 (18.5–41.8)
Hx of Reflux	8 (16%)	12 (23%)	20 (20%)
Hx of Allergies	20 (41%)	28 (53%)	48 (47%)
Hx of OSA	11 (22%)	4 (8%)	15 (15%)
Hx of Childhood Tonsillectomy	15 (31%)	12 (23%)	27 (26%)

Table 4 Results of Two Tailed T-tests

Variable	BMI <30	BMI >30	BMI	Lingual Tonsil Grade
	$n = 73$	$n = 29$		
Mean Age	47.4	49.8	<30	1.83 ± 0.85
Tonsillectomy	19 (26%)	8 (28%)	>30	2.26 ± 0.85
RSI	13.5	15.2		$p = 0.035$
RFS	6.3	6.0		
LTH	1.83	2.26		
Variable	RFS <7	RFS >7	RFS	Lingual Tonsil Grade
	$n = 58$	$n = 44$		
Mean Age	45.1	52.1	<7	1.76 ± 0.82
Tonsillectomy	20 (34%)	7 (16%)	>7	2.31 ± 0.85
BMI	28.7	27.7		$p = 0.008$
RSI	14.2	14.4		
LTH	1.76	2.31		
Variable	RS1 < 13	RSI >13	RSI	Lingual Tonsil Grade
	$n = 56$	$n = 46$		
Mean Age	45.3	50.6	<13	1.99 ± 0.84
Tonsillectomy	15 (27%)	12 (26%)	>13	1.95 ± 0.90
BMI	28.0	28.6		$p = 0.44$
RFS	6.3	6.2		
LTH	1.99	1.95		
Variable	No Tonsillectomy	Previous Tonsillectomy	Palatine Tonsils	Lingual Tonsil Grade
	$n = 75$	$n = 27$		
Mean Age	44.7	56.5	Yes	2.08 ± 0.78
BMI	28.8	28.1	No	$1.93 \pm .91$
RSI	12.8	14.2		$p = 0.51$
RFS	6.5	6.1		
LTH	2.08	1.93		
Variable	Allergy	No Allergy	Allergy	Lingual Tonsil Grade
	$n = 29$	$n = 73$		
Mean Age	44.2	49.5	Yes	1.86 ± 0.73
BMI	28.4	28.1	No	1.97 ± 0.75
RSI	15.6	12.2		$p = 0.035$
RFS	6.3	5.8		
LTH	1.86	1.97		

suggest it is not reliable among non-expert users [14]. This has been the case with other studies as well [4]. Unfortunately, a more reliable endoscopic grading tool does not yet exist and use of it may have contributed to error in this study. The sample size of this study also potentially risks a type II error but no trend was present in the tonsillectomy and LTH data, making this unlikely. The p-value of the previously mentioned cadaveric study examining tonsillectomy and LTH was calculated using Fisher's exact test to be 0.25, with a sample size of almost 500 [9]. With no previously published studies finding an association between adult LTH and childhood tonsillectomy, establishing the required sample size a priori was not possible. We performed a sample size calculation assuming that tonsillectomy would produce an LTH difference similar to what was seen in this study with the RFS and BMI. This gave a sample size of 68 with a beta of 0.8. A further refinement of this study would have involved collecting specific data regarding the age at which childhood tonsillectomy was performed.

Conclusion

Our study is in agreement with previous studies that have demonstrated a correlation between obesity, endoscopic evidence of reflux and lingual tonsil hypertrophy. There does not appear to be a relationship between lingual tonsil hypertrophy and a history of previous childhood tonsillectomy.

Abbreviations
BMI: Body mass index; HSREB: Health sciences research ethics board; LPR: Laryngopharyngeal reflux; LTH: lingual tonsil hypertrophy; OSA: Obstructive sleep apnea; RFS: Reflux finding score; RSI: Reflux symptom index

Acknowledgements
Nil.

Funding
This project was funded through departmental and personal funds.

Competing interests
The authors declare that they have no competing interests.

Authors' contributions
MSH analyzed data, drafted the original manuscript and performed the literature search done prior to the study, as well as for discussion. BWR participated in data collection, editing the manuscript and providing assistant/performing the statistical analysis. KR participated in data collection, editing the manuscript and drafting the discussion. LJS conceived the idea for the study, completed ethics submission, performed patient recruitment and data collection, edited the manuscript and supervised the project. All authors read and approved the final manuscript.

References
1. Acar GO, Cansz H, Duman C, et al. Excessive reactive lymphoid hyperplasia in a child with persistent obstructive sleep apnea despite previous tonsillectomy and adenoidectomy. J Craniofac Surg. 2011;22(4):1413–5.
2. Sung MW, Lee WH, Wee JH, et al. Factors Associated With Hypertrophy of the Lingual Tonsils in Adults with Sleep-Disordered Breathing. JAMA Otolaryngol Head Neck Surg. 2013;139(6):596–603.
3. Friedman M, Yalamanchali S, Gorelick G, Joseph NJ, Hwang MS. A Standardized Lingual Tonsil Grading System: Inter-examiner Agreement. Otolaryngol Head Neck Surg. 2015;152(4):667–72.
4. Eren E, Arslanoglu S, Aktas A, Kopar A, Ciger E, Onal K, Katilmis H. Factors confusing the diagnosis of laryngopharyngeal reflux: the role of allergic rhinitis and inter-rater variability of laryngeal findings. Eur Arch Otorhinolaryngol. 2014;271(4):743–7. doi:10.1007/s00405-013-2682-y.
5. Roth DF, Ferguson BJ. Vocal allergy: recent advances in understanding the role of allergy in dysphonia. Curr Opin Otolaryngol Head Neck Surg. 2010; 18(3):176–81. doi:10.1097/MOO.0b013e32833952af.
6. Belafsky PC, Postma GN, Koufman JA. The Validity and Reliability of the Reflux Finding Score. Laryngoscope. 2001;111:1313–7.
7. Hwang MS, Salapatas AM, Yalamanchali S, Joseph NJ, Friedman M. Factors Associated with Hypertrophy of the Lingual Tonsils. Otolaryngol Head Neck Surg. 2015;152(5):851–5.
8. Friedman M, Wilson MN, Pulver TM, et al. Measurements of adult lingual tonsil tissue in health and disease. Otolaryngol Head Neck Surg. 2010;142(4): 520–5.
9. Breitmeier D, Wilke N, Schulz Y, et al. The lingual tonsillar hyperplasia in relation to unanticipated difficult intubation: is there any relationship between lingual tonsillar hyperplasia and tonsillectomy? Am J Forensic Med Pathol. 2005;26:131–5.
10. DelGaudio JM, Naseri I, Wise JC. Proximal pharyngeal reflux corre- lates with increasing severity of lingual tonsil hypertrophy. Otolaryngol Head Neck Surg. 2008;138:473–8.
11. Mansfield LE, Stein MR. Gastroesophageal reflux and asthma: a possible reflex mechanism. Ann Allergy. 1978;41:224–6.
12. Friedman M, Gurpinar B, Lin HC. Impact of treatment of gastroesophageal reflux on obstructive sleep apnea-hypopnea syndrome. Ann Otol Rhinol Laryngol. 2007;116:805–11.
13. Senior BA, Khan M, Schwimmer C, et al. Gastroesophageal reflux and obstructive sleep apnea. Laryngoscope. 2001;111:2144–6.
14. Chang BA, MacNeil SD, Morrison MD, Lee PK. The reliability of the Reflux Finding Score among general otolaryngologists. J Voice. 2015;29(5):572–7.

7

Reliability and construct validity of the Ottawa valve collapse scale when assessing external nasal valve collapse

Hedyeh Ziai[1] and James P. Bonaparte[2*]

Abstract

Background: Nasal valve collapse is a common cause of nasal obstruction in otolaryngology practice. Common examination methods, such as the Cottle Maneuver and modified Cottle Maneuver are available. However, these methods are dichotomous and do not provide ordinal severity information. The Ottawa Valve Collapse Scale (OVCS) is a grading system for assessing and easily grading external nasal valve collapse in patients with a septal deviation. The primary objective was to assess the test-retest reliability and construct validity of the OVCS grading scale. A secondary objective was to perform the same assessments on the Cottle Maneuver.

Methods: Patients with a septal deviation who were requesting surgical correction were prospectively enrolled in the study. All patients were assessed using both the Cottle Maneuver and the OVCS by one otolaryngologist at two visits separated by one month. The phi coefficient was calculated to assess the test-retest reliability of the instruments. Results of the Nasal Obstruction Symptom Evaluation (NOSE) Score was compared to determine construct validity.

Results: Ninety-two patients met our inclusion criteria. The phi coefficient was 0.62 for the OVCS and 0.32 for the Cottle Maneuver. The scores on the NOSE instrument were positively associated with the OVCS scores ($p = 0.01$) while there was no association with the Cottle Maneuver ($p = 047$).

Conclusion: This current preliminary analysis suggests that the novel Ottawa Valve Collapse Scale has good test-retest reliability and construct validity. This scale may help clinicians grade external nasal valve collapse in patients with a septal deviation. Future studies are required to determine if this scale assists surgeons in determining which patients need formal nasal valve surgery in addition to a standard septoplasty.

Keywords: Nasal obstruction, Cottle maneuver, Reliability, Nasal airway surgery, Septoplasty

Background

Nasal obstruction is a common presenting complaint in otolaryngology practice. Nasal valve collapse (NVC) is recognized as a significant contributor to nasal airway obstruction [1–3]. Although there is a wide range of symptom severity, nasal obstruction has been associated with impairment in patients' quality of life in nearly all domains [4]. Successful corrections can result in significant improvements in patient satisfaction [5].

Nasal valve collapse is often underdiagnosed in patients undergoing septoplasty and if unrecognized, can result in high rates of surgical failure [4–9]. Importantly, NVC often coexists with a septal deviation [10, 11] and the accurate preoperative evaluation and diagnosis of valve dysfunction is an essential requisite for optimal surgical planning to ensure best possible results for patients undergoing nasal airway surgery.

The preoperative diagnosis of nasal valve dysfunction is commonly based on physical examination findings [12]. Particularly, the anatomic areas involving the internal and external valves require examination. Common techniques which aid in the diagnosis include the Cottle Maneuver (CM) and the modified Cottle Maneuver [13–15].

* Correspondence: drjames.bonaparte@gmail.com
This work was presented at the Canadian Society of Otolaryngology- Head and Neck Surgery Annual Meeting in Saskatoon, Canada.
[2]Department of Otolaryngology–Head and Neck Surgery, University of Ottawa, 1919 Riverside Drive, Suite 309, Ottawa, ON K1H 7W9, Canada
Full list of author information is available at the end of the article

The Cottle Maneuver is the most commonly used test to diagnose clinically relevant nasal valve competency requiring surgical correction [2, 12]. Despite its widespread use, to our knowledge it has never been validated using patient centered outcomes, nor has it been confirmed to be a reliable test [16–18]. Additionally, the test only allows for a dichotomous assessment and does not provide information on valve collapse severity nor does it differentiate between external and internal valve collapse. This limitation was overcome by the modified Cottle Maneuver and can be used to differentiate between internal and external nasal valve collapse [15]. This test may predict surgical outcomes in patients undergoing a functional rhinoplasty; however similar to the CM, it provides dichotomous data for each nasal valve and does not provide an assessment of severity. Additionally, it is unknown if this test has adequate construct validity in patients with a co-morbid septal deviation.

Most [13, 14] divided the nasal sidewall into the upper zone (overlying the traditional area defined as the internal nasal valve) and lower zone (overlying the external nasal valve). The authors developed and validated a 4-point severity scale for the upper zone. However, grading was not provided for the location corresponding to the external nasal valve [14]. Recently, Lindsay et al. [19] developed a useful nasal anatomic worksheet to identify areas of concern in patients with nasal airway obstruction. Although this worksheet demonstrated good reliability, there were no details regarding the specifics of grading scores.

To overcome some of the deficiencies of the other methods of external nasal valve assessment, our team has developed a new scale, the Ottawa Valve Collapse Scale (OVCS). The OVCS allows clinicians to grade external nasal valve collapse under normal physiological conditions without altering the patients' anatomy. The OVCS is an ordinal scale and thus allows for grading of symptom severity from mild to severe. The scale was developed with considerations of the principles of flow dynamics. Specifically, treating the entire nose as a single system and not two isolated systems (right and left nasal cavities). Modeling the nose in this manner may help to differentiate disease severity in patients with a septal deviation and thus potentially guide treatment decisions.

The principal aim of this paper was to assess the test-retest reliability of the Ottawa Valve Collapse Scale and determine its construct validity. As a secondary objective, we will assess the same outcomes for the Cottle Maneuver.

Methods

Patients and treatment

This was a prospective case series of patients presenting to an Otolaryngology- Head and Neck Clinic in Ottawa with nasal obstruction between November 1st, 2014 and November 1st, 2016. This study was approved by our institutional ethics review board (20140735-01H) and all patients consented to inclusion.

Patients were included if they had nasal obstruction caused by a septal deviation (with or without evidence of nasal valve collapse). Patients were enrolled consecutively into the prospective protocol from the clinical practice of the supervising author (JB), a practice focusing in General Otolaryngology and Facial Plastic and Reconstructive Surgery. Inclusion criteria for the study were as follows: patients at least 18 years of age, a septal deviation, symptoms lasting at least 12 months and symptoms continuing after a minimum one-month trial of intranasal corticosteroids. Patients were excluded if they were under the age of 18 years, a Nasal Obstruction Symptom Evaluation (NOSE) [1] score of ≤1, if they had a prior septal or nasal surgery, a known traumatic cause of a septal deviation, nasal obstruction due to allergic rhinitis, chronic, or a neoplastic or autoimmune process.

Sample size calculation

A sample size calculation was performed to determine the number of patients required to compare differences between grades using an Kruskal-Wallis Test. Assuming a 95% power with a significant difference defined as 5%, we determined a difference in the NOSE score of 2 as significant with a standard deviation of 3. A minimum of 24 patients were required per group.

Protocol

Patients were assessed at two visits separated by a minimum of 1 month using a standard pre-operative clinical evaluation of the nasal airway. This included the administration of the nasal obstruction symptom evaluation (NOSE) questionnaire, flexible endoscopic examination, the Cottle Maneuver and the Ottawa Valve Collapse Scale. All examinations were performed without decongestant applied. The examiner was blinded to the results of the first visit on the subsequent visit.

To conduct the Cottle Maneuver, the clinician placed their left and right thumb on the cooresponding left and right cheek skin near the alar facial groove on the patients face. The clinician then applied a lateral force with each thumb, thereby lateralizing the cheek soft tissue and adjacent nasal wall. The patient was asked to breathe in through his/her nose at maximum effort. A patient was defined as having a positive CM if they reported subjective improvement in breathing compared to breathing without the CM.

To assess for external nasal valve collapse using the OVCS, patients were asked to breathe in through his/her nose at maximum effort. The maneuver was performed by viewing the nose aided by a light source from the basal view. The caudal edge of the lower lateral cartilage was used as the lateral boundary with the septum used as the medial boundary. Collapse was graded by viewing the degree of collapse and resulting alteration in airflow.

The degree of nasal valve collapse was graded according to the following classification: *Grade 0:* No external nasal valve collapse; *Grade I:* Unilateral Partial Collapse (≤99%); *Grade II:* Bilateral Partial collapse (≤99%) or Unilateral Complete Collapse (100%); or *Grade III:* Bilateral Complete Collapse (100%). Partial collapse was defined as active narrowing of the external nasal valve occurring during deep nasal inspiration without complete airflow blockage or contact with the septum. Complete collapse was defined as complete blockage of airflow and nasal side alar or mucosa overlying the lower lateral cartilage contacting the septum medially.

Statistical analysis

Statistical analysis was carried out using Minitab 17 (Minitab Inc.). The changes in NOSE score were reported as absolute values (raw scores from the NOSE instrument). The phi coefficient was calculated to assess for test-retest reliability of the instruments. To determine the construct validity, a Kruskal-Wallis Test was performed to compare the results of the NOSE questionnaire between severity grades for each physical examination. A value of $p < 0.05$ was considered statistically significant.

Results

Patients

Between November 1st, 2014 and November 1st, 2016, 92 patients consened to the study, a sample of convenience. Thirty patients (33%) were female and 62 (67%) were male. The mean (±SD) age was 40.4 (±15.3) years. The mean (±SD) baseline NOSE score was 14.1 (±4.0).

Cottle maneuver

Sixty-eight (74%) patients had a positive Cottle result on the initial exam, while 62 (67%) patients had a positive Cottle Maneuver on the second exam. Of these, 52 were Cottle positive on both visits, and 14 were Cottle negative on both visits (Table 1). The remaining patients had discordant examinations (Table 1). The phi coefficient for the CM was 0.32, signifying a weak test re-test reliability.

Ottawa valve collapse scale

The results of the OVCS during the two visits are included in Table 2. The phi coefficient for the test-retest reliability of the OVCS was 0.62, signifying a moderate strength positive reliability.

Construct validity

There was no difference in NOSE scores between patients who were positive or negative on the CM ($p = 0.47$) (Table 3). There was a significant difference between NOSE scores between OVCS grades, with higher NOSE scores occurring in higher OVCS grades ($p = 0.012$) (Table 4).

Discussion

The Ottawa Nasal Valve Scale was developed to assist clinicians in quickly grading nasal valve collapse in patients with a septal deviation. Although patients with a septal deviation may also have evidence of nasal valve collapse, determining which patients require nasal valve surgery, in addition to a septoplasty, can be difficult. The results of this study demonstrate that as the grade of nasal valve collapse increases, the patients' symptom severity increases suggesting worsening symptoms with worsening degrees of nasal valve collapse.

Although other methods to assess nasal valve collapse exist, they are often limited as they provide dichotomous data and do not allow for grading of symptom severity. Common tests, such as the CM, is patient-reported and examiner dependent and may explain the low test-retest reliability. Factors such patient biases, non-measurable factors (i.e. current status of the nasal cycle) and clinician factors (i.e. performance of the exam, pressure on the skin) may influence scores. Some of these factors may have been relieved in the OVCS, wherein the physician is assessing the valve collapse in a dynamic situation without any physical alteration of the nose.

Previous studies have attempted to grade nasal valve collapse. Most [13] originally described a three-point grading system similar to our method. This was later validated by Tsao et al. [14] Although the authors use this system to grade the lateral wall collapse, it corresponds to what is commonly described as the area overlying the internal nasal valve and not the external nasal valve. Similar to our method, the authors focused on the

Table 1 Cottle Maneuver Test-Retest Results

		Visit 1 Score		
		Positive	Negative	Total
Visit 2 Score	Positive	52	16	68
	Negative	10	14	24
	Total	62	30	92

Table 2 The Ottawa Valve Collapse Scale Test-Retest Results

	Visit 1 Score			
Visit 2 Score	0	1	2	3
0	28	7	2	0
1	5	10	5	0
2	2	6	20	3
3	0	0	2	2

Table 3 NOSE Score for the Cottle Maneuver

CM	n	Mean	SD	Median
Negative	30	13.8	3.4	15
Positive	66	14.2	4.2	14

p = 0.47

dynamic collapse of the nasal sidewall relative to its resting state. The authors noted good inter-rater and intra-rater reliability.

Similarly, Poirrier et al. [20] used a 4-point grading system that was applied to both the left and right side of the nose. Similar to the OVCS, it measured collapse under dynamic situations, but also considered static narrowing. The results of the study were similar to ours; however, the OVCS attempts to treat the nasal cavity as a complete system with one grade for overall breathing as opposed to bilateral scores. Our team believes that it is important to treat the nose as a complete system, particularly when deciding which treatments or combination of treatments are required.

The correct preoperative evaluation of valvular dysfunction is an essential requisite for optimal surgical planning to ensure best possible results for patients undergoing nasal airway surgery. In a retrospective series of patients who presented with failed septoplasty, 51% had significant NVC [9]. Missed preoperative dynamic nasal valve collapse has been suggested as the most common cause of septoplasty failure [1, 21–23]. A recent study suggested that nasal valve dysfunction should be considered in all patients with a septal deviation undergoing septoplasty [5]. However, as noted by Schalek and Hahn [24], unilateral nasal valve collapse without bilateral collapse is adequately corrected by a septoplasty alone if a septal deviation is present, while patients with evidence of bilateral collapse are likely more resistant to a single treatment. The OVCS aims to differentiate these patients and assist with determining which patients require nasal valve repair at the time of a septoplasty.

The NOSE questionnaire was selected as it is the most widely used validated questionnaire; [12] it is a responsive and disease-specific assessment tool that can quantitatively assess nasal obstructive symptoms in our study cohort [4, 5, 25–27]. The NOSE instrument been recently used in patients undergoing nasal valve correction

Table 4 NOSE Score for each grade of the OVCS

OVCS Grade	n	Mean	SD	Median
0	30	12.1	4.4	12
1	24	14	3	14
2	34	14.6	4.1	14
3	8	18.2	2.1	19

p = 0.012

surgery in evaluating for subjective improvements in nasal obstructive symptoms [7, 8, 28–31].

Ultimately, our aim was to develop a scale that may be used to grade external nasal valve dysfunction with the future goal of allowing clinicians to predict which patients may benefit from a more extensive nasal airway surgery including nasal valve correction. A simple tool may be the most practical in the clinical setting; however, there is no study that demonstrates which outcome measure (or combination of outcome measures) may accurately and precisely identify those patients who may benefit from nasal valve surgery, particularly when other comorbid diagnosis (septal deviation) are present. Those with more severe scores may benefit from more extensive nasal airway surgery, including nasal valve correction surgery, however future studies are required to assess this.

Although this study achieved both of its objectives, there were some limitations and important points to consider. The goal of this paper was to assess the validity and reliability of the OVCS in terms of patient symptom severity and not its ability to predict which patients require specific surgical procedures. However, this current study should serve as a basis for future research that may use the OVCS to diagnose and grade nasal valve collapse. In turn, this research should evaluate if the OVCS assists in determining which patients may require nasal valve correction surgery in addition to a septoplasty. This is important as it remains unclear if the use of the OVCS may help direct surgical planning and lead to improved patient outcomes. In addition to this, future research should assess whether combination of physical examination (ie OVCS, Cottle Maneuver, Modified Cottle) will result in the ability to predict what surgical procedure or combination of procedures are required. Future efforts may also focus on assessing criterion validity of the scale with evaluations of nasal valve collapse including objective measurement of objective nasal airflow.

The median follow-up time between the two visits was 2 months. There may have changes in patients' symptoms that may have underestimated the reliability of the instruments. That being said, the range of follow-up was random and thus we believe the error associated with this would also be random and not bias our findings. This study's findings are based on a single surgeon's assessments who is also involved in the development of the Ottawa Valve Collapse Scale. Although the surgeon was blinded to the results of the first visit, there may have been some element of recall bias and/or situational bias. Furthermore, there is no gold standard for determining NVC symptoms, and thus we used the nasal obstruction score as determined by the NOSE [32] instrument to determine the construct validity. In addition, this present study was performed on English-speaking Canadians in a single tertiary care center in Ottawa, and may limit its application to other populations. Finally, although the scale was based on application of flow dynamic principles, there was no confirmation using objective measures.

Perhaps most importantly, at this point only one physician has performed an assessment of test-retest and construct validity. Although the study met our stated objectives, we are currently in the process of completing a study assessing the inter-rater reliability as well as a multi-rated assessment of intra-rater reliability of the scale.

Conclusion

To the best of our knowledge, the present study is the first attempt to ascertain the test-retest reliability of the Cottle Maneuver and the OVCS, and the construct validity of the maneuver in assessing nasal obstruction symptoms. This current preliminary analysis suggests that the novel Ottawa Valve Collapse Scale may have improved test-retest reliability when compared to the Cottle Maneuver for diagnosing nasal valve collapse, and improved validity for patient-reported nasal obstruction. The OVCS may serve as a means in the future in diagnosing nasal valve collapse in patients undergoing nasal airway surgery.

Abbreviations

CM: Cottle Maneuver; NOSE: Nasal Obstruction Severity Evaluation; NVC: Nasal Valve Collapse; OVCS: Ottawa Valve Collapse Scale

Funding

None

Authors' contributions

HZ contributed to: the conception and design of the project; the analysis and interpretation of data; drafting the work and revising it; final approval of the version to be published; agreement to be accountable for all aspects of the work in ensuring that questions related to the accuracy or integrity of any part of the work are appropriately investigated and resolved. JP Bonaparte contributed to: conception and design of the work; acquisition, analysis and interpretation of data for the work; drafting the work and revising it; final approval of the version to be published; agreement to be accountable for all aspects of the work in ensuring that questions related to the accuracy or integrity of any part of the work are appropriately investigated and resolved.

Competing interests

The authors declare that they have no competing interests.

Author details

[1]Faculty of Medicine, University of Ottawa, Ottawa, ON, Canada. [2]Department of Otolaryngology–Head and Neck Surgery, University of Ottawa, 1919 Riverside Drive, Suite 309, Ottawa, ON K1H 7W9, Canada.

References

1. Fraser L, Kelly G. An evidence-based approach to the management of the adult with nasal obstruction. Clin Otolaryngol. 2009;34:151.
2. O'Halloran LR. The lateral crural J-flap repair of nasal valve collapse. Otolaryngol Head Neck Surg. 2003;128:640.
3. Kiyohara N, Badger C, Tjoa T, Wong B. A comparison of over-the-counter mechanical nasal dilators: a systematic review. JAMA Facial Plast Surg. 2016; 18:385.
4. Stewart M, Ferguson B, Fromer L. Epidemiology and burden of nasal congestion. Int J Gen Med. 2010;3(3):37–45.
5. Chambers KJ, Horstkotte KA, Shanley K, Lindsay RW. Evaluation of improvement in nasal obstruction following nasal valve correction in patients with a history of failed Septoplasty. JAMA Facial Plast Surg. 2015; 17(5):347–50.
6. Stewart MG, Smith TL, Weaver EM, et al. Outcomes after nasal septoplasty: results from the nasal obstruction Septoplasty effectiveness (NOSE) study. Otolaryngol Head Neck Surg. 2004;130:283–90.
7. Rhee JS, Poetker DM, Smith TL, Bustillo A, Burzynski M, Davis RE. Nasal valve surgery improves disease-specific quality of life. Laryngoscope. 2005;115:437–40.
8. Sofia OB, Neto NPC, Katustani FS, Mitre EI, Dolci JE. Evaluation of pre- and post-pyriform plasty nasal airflow. Braz J Otorhinolaryngol. 2017;523:1–9.
9. Becker SS, Dobratz EJ, Stowell N, Barker D, Park SS. Revision septoplasty: review of sourcse of persistent nasal obstruction. Am J Rhinol. 2008;22:440–4.
10. Bloching MB. Disorders of the nasal valve area. GMS Curr Top Otorhinolaryngol Head Neck Surg. 2007;6:Doc07.
11. Spielmann PM, White PS, Hussain SS. Surgical techniques for the treatment of nasal valve collapse: a systematic review. Laryngoscope. 2009;119(7):1281–90.
12. Goudakos JK, Fishman JM, Patel K. A systematic review of the surgical techniques for the treatment of internal nasal valve collapse: where do we stand? Clin Otolaryngol. 2017;42(1):60–70.
13. Most SP. Trends in functional rhinoplasty. Arch Facial Plast Surg. 2008; 10:410–3.
14. Tsao GJ, Fijalkowski N, Most SP. Validation of a grading system for lateral nasal wall insufficiency. Allergy Rhinol (Providence). 2013;4:e66–8.
15. Fung E, Hong P, Moore C, Taylor SM. The effectiveness of modified cottle maneuver in predicting outcomes in functional rhinoplasty. Plast Surg Int. 2014;2014:618313.
16. Gruber RP, Lin AY, Richards T. Nasal strips for evaluating and classifying Valvular nasal obstruction. Anesh Plast Surg. 2011;35:211–5.
17. Ahmet I, Necmi A, Aslan FS, Hatice C, Munir D, Hadul O. Reconstruction of the internal nasal valve: modified splay graft technique with endonasal approach. Laryngoscope. 2008;118:1143–739.
18. Mehdi D, Aram A, Hamid K. Reconstruction of the internal nasal valve with a splay conchal graft. Plast Reconstr Surg. 2005;116:712–20.
19. Lindsay RW, George R, Herberg ME, Jackson P, Brietzke S. Reliability of a standardized nasal anatomic worksheet and correlation with subjective nasal airway obstruction. JAMA Facial Plast Surg. 2016;18(6):449–54.
20. Poirrier AL, Ahluwalia S, Kwame I, Chau H, Bentley M, Andrews P. External nasal valve collapse: validation of novel outcome measurement tool. Rhinology. 2014;52(2):127–32.
21. Wittkopf M, Wittkopf J, Ries WR. The diagnosis and treatment of nasal valve collapse. Curr Opin Otolaryngol Head Neck Surg. 2008;16(1):10–3.
22. Ricci E, Palonta F, Preti G, et al. Role of nasal valve in the surgically corrected nasal respiratory obstruction: evaluation through rhinomanometry. Am J Rhinol. 2001;15(5):307–10.
23. Nouraei SA, Virk JS, Kanona H, Zatonski M, Koury EF, Chatrath P. Non-invasive assessment and symptomatic improvement of the obstructed nose (NASION): a physiology-based patient-centred approach to treatment selection and outcomes assessment in nasal obstruction. Clin Otolaryngol. 2016;41(4):327–40.
24. Schalek P, Hahn A. Anterior septal deviation and contralateral alar collapse. B-ENT. 2011;7:185–8.

25. Lachanas VA, Tsiouvaka S, Tsea M, Hajiioannou JK, Skoulakis CE. Validation of the nasal obstruction symptom evaluation (NOSE) scale for greek patients. Otolaryngol Head Neck Surg. 2014;151(5):819–23.

26. Marro M, Mondina M, Stoll D, de Gabory L. French validation of the NOSE and RhinoQOL questionnaires in the management of nasal obstruction. Otolaryngol Head Neck Surg. 2011;144(6):988–93.

27. Mozzanica F, Urvani E, Atac M, Scotta G, Luciano K, Bulgheroni C, De Cristofaro V, Gera R, Schindler A, Ottaviani F. Reliability and validity of the Italian nose obstruction symptom evaluation (I-NOSE) scale. Eur Arch Otolaryngol Suppl. 2013;270(12):3087–94.

28. Yeung A, Hassouneh B, Kim DW. Outcome of nasal valve obstruction after functional and aesthetic-functional Rhinoplasty. JAMA Facial Plast Surg. 2016;18(2):128–34.

29. Most SP. Analysis of outcomes after failed rhinoplasty using a disease specific quality of life instrument. Arch Facial Plast Surg. 2006;8(5):306–9.

30. Lindsay RW. Disease specific quality of life outcomes in functional rhinoplasty. Laryngoscope. 2012;122(2):254–9.

31. Balikci HH, Furdal MM. Satisfaction outcomes in open functional septorhinoplasty: prospective analysis. J Craniofac Surg. 2014;25(2):377–9.

32. Stewart MG, Witsell DL, Smith TL, Weaver EM, Yueh B, Hannley MT. Development and validation of the nasal obstruction symptom evaluation (NOSE) scale. Otolaryngol Head Neck Surg. 2004;130:157–63.

8

Clinical implications of the BRAF mutation in papillary thyroid carcinoma and chronic lymphocytic thyroiditis

Woon Won Kim[1], Tae Kwun Ha[2]* [iD] and Sung Kwon Bae[3]

Abstract

Background: The purpose of this study was to examine the possible prognostics and clinicopathologic characteristics underlying the BRAFV600E mutation and papillary thyroid carcinoma (PTC) coexisting or in absence of chronic lymphocytic thyroiditis (CLT).

Methods: This study was conducted on 172 patients who had undergone total thyroidectomy or unilateral total thyroidectomy for PTC; the patients were then examined for the BRAFV600E mutation using specimens obtained after their surgery from January 2013 to August 2015.

Results: BRAF mutations were found in 130 of 172 patients (75.6%). CLT was present in 27.9% of patients (48/172). The incidence of the BRAFV600E mutation was significantly increased in the group with no CLT ($P = 0.001$). The findings of the multivariate analysis pertaining to the coexistence of CLT and PTC showed no significant correlation other than the BRAFV600E mutation. No significant difference was noted in the clinicopathologic factors between the two groups based on the coexistence of CLT in univariate and multivariate analyses.

Conclusions: The BRAFV600E mutation is less frequent in PTC coexisting with CLT presumably because CLT and the BRAFV600E mutation operate independently in the formation and progression of thyroid cancer.

Keywords: BRAF mutation, Chronic lymphocytic thyroiditis, Papillary thyroid carcinoma

Background

Papillary thyroid carcinoma (PTC) is the most common type of thyroid cancer and accounts for approximately 80- 85% of malignant neoplasms of the thyroid gland. It has a 10-year survival rate 93% in the United States, which is relatively favorable compared to that of malignant tumors [1]. The major factors underlying the prognosis of PTC include patient age, gender, tumor size, histological findings, extrathyroidal extension, clinical lymph node metastasis and remote metastasis [2]. BRAF gene mutations have also been reported to be factors that can most accurately predict lymph node metastasis, extrathyroidal extension, advanced disease stages III and IV, and disease recurrence [3]. Among the various isoforms of Raf kinase, the B-type RAF V600E (BRAFV600E) mutation is the most commonly observed genetic abnormality in PTC that induces excessive proliferation and differentiation of tumor cells at the initial tumor stage. It is involved in, not only tumorigenesis but also in the conversion to aggressive, non-differentiated cancer [4].

Chronic lymphocytic thyroiditis (CLT) is a common autoimmune thyroid disorder in which the thyroid gland is attacked by various antibodies and cell-mediated immune processes [5]. Dailey et al. reported the coexistence of CLT in thyroid cancer for the first time in 1955 [6]. The ratio of coexistence has varied between 10.7% and 27.6% in 2008, respectively [7]. The role that CLT plays as a prognostic factor in thyroid cancer is controversial, but it is known that PTC is approximately three times in the presence of CLT [8]. Recent studies have reported an association between Hashimoto's thyroiditis, the BRAFV600E mutation, and clinicopathologic features in patients with PTC [9]. PTC with coexisting CLT

---

* Correspondence: hasus@hanmail.net
[2]Department of General Surgery, Busan Paik Hospital, Inje University College of Medicine, 75, Bokji-ro, Busanjin-gu, 614-735 Busan, Republic of Korea
Full list of author information is available at the end of the article

was less associated with extrathyroidal extension and lymph node metastasis; CLT antagonizes PTC progression when accompanying a positive BRAFV600E mutation [10]. However, this issue is still controversial as more studies are needed on the correlation between CLT and the BRAFV600E mutation as a prognostic factor for PTC. This study reviews the frequency of the BRAFV600E mutation in thyroid tissues extracted after surgery on the thyroid gland and examines the relationship between the BRAFV600E mutation and CLT as well as the correlation with prognostic factors to review clinicopathologic characteristics.

Methods

This study was conducted on 172 patients who had undergone total thyroidectomy or unilateral total thyroidectomy for PTC; the patients were then examined for the BRAFV600E mutation using specimens obtained after surgery in the Busan Paik Hospital from January 2013 to August 2015. Our institutional review board approved this retrospective study and waived the need for informed consent based on the retrospective design. CLT is an autoimmune disease characterized by widespread lymphocyte infiltration, fibrosis and parenchyma atrophy of thyroid tissue. Pathologically proven CLT was defined as the presence of diffuse lymphocytic and plasma cell infiltrate, oxyphilic cells and the formation of lymphoid follicles or reactive germinal centers in the area of normal thyroid tissue [11]. To confirm the clinicopathologic differences in PTC in the presence or absence of CLT and the BRAFV600E mutation, the patient's age and sex, size of tumor, multiplicity or bilaterality of the tumor, presence of extrathyroidal extension, cervical or lateral cervical lymph node metastasis, and TNM staging (AJCC 7th) were analyzed. If there were multiple tumors, the size of the largest tumor was measured. Regardless of the number of tumors, cases in which there was more than one malignant tumor present in both lobes were defined as bilateral.

DNA extraction & detection of the BRAFV600E mutation

Genomic DNA was extracted from the tumor using the QIAmap DNA formalin fixed paraffin-embedded extraction kit (Qiagen, Hilden, Germany) according to the manufacturer's instructions. The extracted DNA was measured by UV absorption (Nanodrop; Thermo Scientific, Wilmington, DE). For every specimen, a total of 41mg of genomic DNA was typically extracted. The T1799A mutation in BRAF exon 15 leads to a substitution of V for E at residue 600 in PTCs. The T1799A transversion was detected using the Anyplex BRAF V600E real-time detection system (Seegen Inc., Seoul, Korea). Real-time PCR was performed using a CFX96 real-time PCR system (Bio-Rad, Hercules, CA). The

cycle threshold (Ct) of real-time PCR was defined as the number of amplification cycles at which the level of fluorescent signal exceeded the threshold for the presence of the BRAF mutation. This cut-off value was determined based on the average Ct value found in 100 repeats of low-positive concentrations of the $BRAF^{V600E}$ plasmid DNA for which a positive rate of 100% was achieved. The Ct value of the target and the internal control was 533 and 30, respectively, and each run consisted of both positive and negative controls.

Statistical analysis

SPSS Version 21(SPSS Inc., Chicago, IL, USA) was used for statistical analyses of the data. The univariate variable between each group was analyzed using the chi-square test or T-test, and the corrected univariate variables were analyzed using logistic regression analysis. The statistical significance level was set at $P<0.05$.

Results

The mean age of the 172 PTC patients (20 males and 152 females) was 49.1±11.35 years (range 18–79), and the mean tumor size was 0.91 ± 0.72 cm (range 0.2–4.5 cm). Papillary thyroid microcarcinomas measuring <1 cm in size were observed in 124 cases (72.1%). The BRAFV600E mutation was confirmed in 130 PTC patients (75.6%). Metastasis in the central lymph node (N1a) was observed in 74 patients (43.0%), whereas metastasis in the lateral cervical lymph node (N1b) was confirmed in 18 patients (10.5%). Forty-eight of the 172 PTC patients (27.9%) had CLT, and the remaining 124 patients (72.1%) did not have CLT. Forty-three patients (25.0%) had multiple tumors on one lobe, whereas 33 patients (19.2%) had bilateral PTC. Of the 62 patients (36.0%) with extrathyroidal extension. Two patients showed airway, esophageal, or recurrent laryngeal nerve invasion. Overall, 106 patients (60 aged <45 years and 46 cases aged>45 years) had TNM stage 1, whereas 51 cases (29.7%) had TNM stage 3, and 14 (8.1%) had TNM stage 4a (Table 1).

Clinicopathologic factors depending on the presence of CLT in PTC

The patients with CLT were younger than those without CLT ($P = 0.06$), and the number of women was high but did not show a statistically significant difference ($P = 0.171$). No statistically significant difference was noted in the size of PTC, its multiplicity or bilaterality, extrathyroidal extension, or the frequencies of cervical and lateral cervical lymph node metastasis.

The incidence of the BRAFV600E mutation was observed significantly more in the group with no CLT (82.3%) ($P = 0.001$, Table 2).

Table 1 Demographic characteristics of 172 patients with papillary thyroid carcinoma

Characteristics	Value (%)
Total number	172(100.0)
Gender	
Female	152 (88.4)
Male	20 (11.6)
Age (year) at diagnosis (Mean ±S.D)	49.1±11.35
< 45	60 (34.9)
≥ 45	112(65.1)
Tumor size (mm)(Mean±S.D)	0.91 ± 0.47
1 cm	124(72.1)
≥ 1 cm	48(27.9)
Multifocality	
Unifocal	129 (75.0)
Multifocal	43 (25.0)
Bilaterality	
Unilateral	139 (80.8)
Bilateral	33 (19.2)
Extra thyroidal extension	
Absent	110 (64.0)
Present	62 (36.0)
Central lymph node metastasis	
Absent	98 (57.0)
Present	74 (43.0)
Lateral lymph node metastasis	
Absent	154 (89.5)
Present	18 (10.5)
Stage	
I	106(61.6%)
II	1 (0.6%)
III	51 (29.7)
IVa	14 (8.1)
Chronic lymphocytic thyroiditis	
Absent	124 (72.1)
Present	48 (27.9)
BRAF mutation	
Absent	42 (24.4)
Present	130 (75.6)

S.D Standard deviation

Multivariate analysis pertaining to the correlation between CLT and BRAFV600E mutation

Univariate analysis of the relationship between PTC and clinicopathologic factors in the presence and absence of CLT was conducted. According to the analysis, the presence of the BRAF mutation showed a noticeable interdependence. In the presence of the BRAF mutation, CLT was found at a lower frequency. This finding suggests that the presence of CLT has no association with BRAF- mutated PTC (*P*=0.001) (Table 2).

The gender and age variants, which appeared to potently influence the relationship between CLT and PTC, and the BRAF mutation were included in the logistic regression analysis. Only the BRAFV600E mutation had a statistically significant correlation with the coexistence of CLT and PTC in the multivariate analysis (*P*=0.002) (Table 3).

Comparison of PTC cases with the BRAFV600E mutation based on the presence of CLT

Of 130 PTC patients with the BRAFV600E mutation, 28 (21.5%) had CLT. No significant difference was noted in the clinicopathologic factors between the two groups categorized based on the coexistence of CLT in univariate and multivariate analyses.

Discussion

PTC is the most common thyroid cancer and gradually leads to remote metastasis, accounting for 88% of thyroid cancer cases. PTC has an overall favorable prognosis with an average 10-year survival rate of 93%, although up to 10% of patients eventually die as a result of the disease [12]. However, the frequency of coexisting CLT in patients with PTC has been reported to range from 0.5%-38% [13]. CLT is one of the autoimmune diseases that shrinks the thyroid parenchyma through infiltration or fibrosis and is the most common inflammatory thyroid disease with a frequency of 22 in 100,000 patients. CLT is 15–20 times more likely to occur in women and is more frequently seen in patients between the age of 30 and 50 years; however, it is observed in all age groups. CLT may exhibit no symptoms or a slight deterioration in thyroid function as a major cause of goiter but is not accompanied by pain. Our study shows a 27.9% coexistence between PTC and CLT, which is similar to previous studies. The correlation between the two diseases is still controversial. Some suggest that there is a positive correlation with CLT, as the activated inflammatory response present in CLT creates a favorable setting for malignant transformation. The inflammatory response may cause DNA damage through the formation of reactive oxygen species, resulting in mutations that eventually lead to the development of PTC. However, it is unclear whether CLT may lead to PTC in patients; or that CLT may be a secondary finding with PTC; or CLT and PTC may be part of a host tumor response system [14].

This study examined whether BRAFV600E is associated with CLT and PTC. BRAFV600E is only observed in anaplastic carcinoma originated from PTC or papillary carcinoma and not in other thyroid cancers, including follicular carcinoma. BRAF is a B-type Raf kinase

Table 2 Clinicopathologic factors related to chronic lymphocytic thyroiditis in 172 patients with PTC

	CLT(-)		CLT(+)		X^2/t-test	P-value
	Count	%	Count	%		
Gender						
Female	107	(13.7)	45	(6.3)	1.874	0.171
Male	17	(86.3)	3	(93.8)		
Age (Mean ±S.D)	50.06±11.51		46.44±10.62		1.893	0.060
< 45	39	(31.5)	21	(43.8)	2.304	0.129
≥ 45	85	(68.5)	27	(56.3)		
Tumor Size(mm)(Mean ±S.D)	0.92 ±0.73		0.88±0.69		0.383	0.702
< 1.0 cm	90	(72.6)	34	(70.8)	0.908	0.635
≥ 1.0 cm	34	(27.4)	14	(29.2)		
Multifocality						
Absent	94	(75.8)	35	(72.9)	0.154	0.695
Present	30	(24.2)	13	(27.1)		
Bilaterality						
Absent	101	(81.5)	38	(79.2)	0.117	0.733
Present	23	(18.5)	10	(20.8)		
Extrathyroidal extension						
Absent	76	(61.3)	34	(70.8)	1.367	0.242
Present	48	(38.7)	14	(29.2)		
Central LM metastasis						
Absent	66	(53.2)	32	(66.7)	2.550	0.110
Present	58	(46.8)	16	(33.3)		
Lateral LM metastasis						
Absent	110	(88.7)	44	(91.7)	0.323	0.570
Present	14	(11.3)	4	(8.3)		
TNM stage						
I & II	71	(57.3)	36	(75.0)	5.770	0.056
III	40	(32.3)	11	(22.9)		
IVa	13	(10.5)	1	(2.1)		
BRAF mutation						
Negative	22	(17.7)	20	(41.7)	10.732	0.001
Positive	102	(82.3)	28	(58.3)		

LN Lymph node, *TNM* Tumor/node/metastasis

Table 3 Multivariate analysis of clinicopathologicfactors associated with the BRAF mutation in papillary thyroid carcinoma with or without CLT

	B	S.E	Sig.	Exp (B)	95% CI	
					Lower	Upper
Gender	-0.819	0.667	0.220	0.441	0.119	1.630
Age	0.501	0.363	0.167	1.651	0.810	3.363
BRAF	1.184	0.380	0.002	3.267	1.550	6.887
Constant	-1.398	0.266	0.000	0.247		

B Significance probability, *S.E* Standard error, *Sig* Significance probability *Exp(B)* Odds ratio, *CI* Confidence interval

located on chromosome 7 and is the most potent activator of the mitogen-activated protein kinase/extracellular-signal-regulated kinase (MEK-ERK) pathway. The most common hotspot mutation in the BRAF gene is a thiamine transversion to adenine at nucleotide position 1799 (T1799A) in exon 15. This transversion causes a conversion of valine to glutamate of amino acid 600 in the BRAF protein, creating a constitutively active BRAF kinase, which has been proven to be an oncogene in human cancer [12] and is found in 40%–80% of all cases of papillary thyroid cancer [15].

Many studies have reported correlations between the aggressive clinical factors underlying the BRAFV600E mutation and papillary carcinoma. According to Liu X et al., a multi-institutional research study suggested that extra-thyroidal extension, multifocality, lymph node metastasis, and advanced TNM were associated with the BRAFV600E mutation in PTC [16]. The BRAFV600E mutation has been reported to increase not only the aggressive nature of the tumor but also the recurrence and mortality rates of the disease [17]. These findings suggest the need for more proactive surgery or radioactive iodine therapies and more careful follow-up observations. However, its value as a prognostic precursor is still debated because some studies have shown contradictory findings on the correlation between the BRAFV600E mutation and the aggressiveness and poor prognosis of PTC [18].

This study showed a significantly low frequency of the BRAFV600E mutation in PTC coexisting with CLT. The frequency of the BRAFV600E mutation in PTC with and without CLT was 58.3% and 82.3%, respectively ($P = 0.001$). This correlation was independently confirmed through a multivariate analysis that was adjusted for sex and age(OR: 0.353, 95%CI: 0.148–0.842). This finding is consistent with previous research findings on the significantly low frequency of the BRAFV600E mutation in PTC coexisting with CLT [19]. This result implies that PTC with CLT has a developmental mechanism that is different from the molecular genetic background of the BRAFV600E mutation. However, some PTC groups with CLT showed higher frequencies of the BRAFV600E mutation, while other studies reported that a group with a positive BRAFV600E mutation was an independently good prognostic factor [9].

PTC coexisting with CLT is generally known to be common among women; it has a good prognosis at early stages and a low recurrence rate. Existing literature does not show whether the presence of thyroiditis alters the biologic effect of PTC. In this study, the presence of thyroiditis seemed to lessen the invasive potential of PTC. There was less extrathyroidal extension and less multifocality and bilaterality in PTC with CLT. The presence of thyroiditis with PTC was associated with less lymph node metastasis on presentation. The characteristics of the clinicopathologic factors in the presence or absence of CLT did not exhibit statistically significant differences. Therefore, we can infer that CLT and the BRAFV600E mutation do not mutually affect PTC generation and progress.

This study is limited in the following ways: 1) positively prognostic and non-aggressive papillary microcarcinomas <1 cm in size are very frequent; 2) the short timeline of research and data collection in this study prevents possible long-term relevant findings for prognoses. Long-term follow-up studies are also required, with a larger sample of patients and from multiple institutions.

Conclusion

Given that the BRAFV600E mutation is less frequent in PTC with CLT, CLT and the BRAFV600E mutation presumably have independent mechanisms on how they affect the formation and progression of thyroid cancer.

Abbreviations

CLT: Chronic lymphocytic thyroiditis,; PTC: Papillary thyroid carcinomas; BRAF: b-type raf kinase; TNM: Tumor/node/metastasis; DNA: Deoxyribonucleic acid; UV: Ultraviolet; PCR: Polymerase chain reaction; Ct: Cycle treshold; S.D: Standard deviation; LN: Lymph node; TNM: Tumor/node/metastasis; B: Coefficient of regression,; S.E: Standard error; Sig: Significance probability; Exp(B): Odds ratio; CI: Confidence interval

Acknowledgements

None

Funding

None

Authors' contributions

WW Kim contributed to data collection. TK Ha contributed to study design, manuscript writing. SK Bae versed in medical and statistical terminology and interpreted results. All authors read and approved the final manuscript.

Competing interests

The authors declare that they have no competing interests.

Author details

[1]Department of General Surgery, Haeundae Paik Hospital, Inje University College of Medicine, Busan, Republic of Korea. [2]Department of General Surgery, Busan Paik Hospital, Inje University College of Medicine, 75, Bokji-ro, Busanjin-gu, 614-735 Busan, Republic of Korea. [3]Department of Medical Management, Kosin University, Busan, Republic of Korea.

References

1. Paschke R, Lincke T, Müller SP, Kreissl MC, Dralle H, Fassnacht M. The Treatment of Well-Differentiated Thyroid Carcinoma. Dtsch Arztebl Int. 2015; 112(26):452–8.
2. Ito Y, Miyauchi A, Kobayashi K, Kihara M, Miya A. Static and dynamic prognostic factors of papillary thyroid carcinoma. Endocrine journal. 2014; 61(12):1145–51.
3. Xing M, Haugen BR, Schlumberger M. Progress in molecular-based management of differentiated thyroid cancer. Lancet. 2013;381(9871): 1058–69.
4. Knauf JA, Sartor MA, Medvedovic M, Lundsmith E, Ryder M, Salzano M, et al. Progression of BRAF-induced thyroid cancer is associated with epithelial-mesenchymal transition requiring concomitant MAP kinase and TGFbeta signaling. Oncogene. 2011;30:3153–62.
5. Zhang Y, Ma X-p, Deng F-s, Liu Z-r, Wei H-q, Wang X-h, Chen H. The effect of chronic lymphocytic thyroiditis on patients with thyroid cancer. World J Surg Oncol. 2014;12:277.
6. Dailey ME, Lindsay S, Skahen R. Relation of thyroid neoplasm to Hashimoto disease of the thyroid gland. AMA Arch Surg. 1955;70:291–7.
7. Chang-Mo O, Park S, Lee JY, Won Y-J, Shin A, Kong H-J, et al. Increased Prevalence of Chronic Lymphocytic Thyroiditis in Korean Patients with Papillary Thyroid Cancer. PLoS One. 2014;9(6):e99054.

8. Kim KW, Park YJ, Kim EH, Park SY, Park DJ, Ahn SH, et al. Elevated risk of papillary thyroid cancer in Korean patients with Hashimoto's thyroiditis. Head & Neck. 2011;33:691–5.

9. Kim SJ, Myong JP, Jee HG, Chai YJ, Choi JY, Min HS, et al. Combined effect of Hashimoto's thyroiditis and $BRAF^{V600E}$ mutation status on aggressiveness in papillary thyroid cancer. Head Neck. 2016;38(1):95–101.

10. Marotta V, Guerra A, Zatelli MC, Uberti ED, Di Stasi V, Faggiano A, et al. BRAF mutation positive papillary thyroid carcinoma is less advanced when Hashimoto's thyroiditis lymphocytic infiltration is present. ClinEndocrinol. 2013;79:733–8.

11. Kim EY, Kim WG, Kim WB, Kim TY, Kim JM, Ryu JS, et al. Coexistence of chronic lymphocytic thyroiditis is associated with lower recurrence rates in patients with papillary thyroid carcinoma. Clin Endocrinol (Oxf). 2009;4:581–6.

12. Tufano RP, Teixeira GV, Bishop J, Carson KA, Xing M. BRAF mutation in papillary thyroid cancer and its value in tailoring initial treatment: a systematic review and meta-analysis. Medicine (Baltimore). 2012;91(5):274–86.

13. Jeong JS, Kim HK, Lee CR, Park SK, Park JH, Kang SW, Jeong JJ, et al. Coexistence of Chronic Lymphocytic Thyroiditis with Papillary Thyroid Carcinoma: Clinical Manifestation and Prognostic Outcome. J Korean Med Sci. 2012;27(8):883–8.

14. Jankovic B, Le KT, Hershman JM. Hashimoto's thyroiditis and papillary thyroid carcinoma: is there a correlation? J Clin Endocrinol Metab. 2013; 98(2):474–82.

15. Kim TH, Park YJ, Lim JA, Ahn HY, Lee EK, Lee YJ, et al. The association of the BRAF (V600E) mutation with prognostic factors and poor clinical outcome in papillary thyroid cancer: a meta-analysis. Cancer. 2012;118:1764–73.

16. Liu X, Yan K, Lin X, Zhao L, An W, Wang C. The association between BRAF (V600E) mutation and pathological features in PTC. Eur Arch Otorhinolaryngol. 2014;271(11):3041–52.

17. Xing M, Alzahrani AS, Carson KA, Viola D, Elisei R, Bendlova B, et al. Association between BRAF V600E mutation and mortality in patients with papillary thyroid cancer. JAMA. 2013;3091493–501.

18. Yim JH, Kim WG, Jeon MJ, Han JM, Kim TY, Yoon JH, et al. Association between expression of X-linked inhibitor of apoptosis protein and the clinical outcome in a BRAF V600E-prevalent papillary thyroid cancer population. Thyroid. 2014;24:689–94.

19. Lim JY, Hong SW, Lee YS, Kim BW, Park CS, Chang HS, et al. Clinicopathologic implications of the BRAF(V600E)mutation of the papillary thyroid cancer: a subgroup analysis of 3130 cases in a single center. Thyroid. 2013;23:1423–30.

9

Differences in gene expression profile between vocal cord Leukoplakia and normal larynx mucosa by gene chip

Jianhua Peng[1], He Li[1], Jun Chen[1], Xianming Wu[1], Tao Jiang[2] and Xiaoyun Chen[1*]

Abstract

Background: Long non-coding RNAs (lncRNAs) play an important role in tumorigenesis. Vocal cord leukoplakia is a precancerous lesion in otolaryngological practice. Till now, the expression patterns and functions of lncRNAs in vocal cord leukoplakia have not been well understood. In this study, we used microarrays to investigate the aberrantly expressed lncRNAs and mRNAs in vocal cord leukoplakia and adjacent non-neoplastic tissues.

Methods: Gene Ontology and pathway analyses were performed to determine the significant function and pathways of the differentially expressed mRNAs. qRT-PCR was performed to further validate the expression of selected lncRNAs and mRNAs in vocal cord leukoplakia.

Results: Our study identified 170 differentially expressed lncRNAs and 99 differentially expressed mRNAs, including 142 up-regulated lncRNAs and 28 down-regulated lncRNAs, and 54 up-regulated mRNAs and 45 down-regulated mRNAs. Among these, XLOC_000605 and DLX6-AS1 were the most aberrantly expressed lncRNAs. Furthermore, we identified an antisense lncRNA (LOC100506801), an enhancer-like lncRNA (AK057351) and three long intergenetic noncoding RNAs including XLOC_008001, XLOC_011989 and XLOC_007341.

Conclusions: Our results revealed that many lncRNAs were differentially expressed between vocal cord leukoplakia tissues and normal tissue, suggesting that they may play a key role in vocal cord leukoplakia tumorigenesis.

Keywords: Vocal cord leukoplakia, Long non-coding RNAs, Gene chip, Microarray

Background

Leukoplakia is a term to describe a mucosal white patch or plaque that cannot be easily scraped off. Vocal cord leukoplakia is a common precancerous lesion in otolaryngological practice. The annual incidence in the United States is estimated to be 10.2/100000 in males and 2.1/100000 in females. A comprehensive meta-analysis of laryngeal leukoplakia by Isenberg et al. revealed that 8.2% cases underwent malignant transformation during a follow-up period that ranged from 1 to 233 months between various studies. Overall 3.7% nondysplastic, 10.1% mild to moderate dysplastic and 18.1% severely dysplastic cases underwent malignant change [1]. Studies have identified smoking and alcohol as major causes and there is

also sufficient evidence implicating gastroesophageal reflux and human papilloma virus in the pathogenesis of the disease [2].

Vocal cord leukoplakia is clinically significant due to the potential for malignant transformation. A variety of proliferation markers, cyclin kinases, oncoproteins, tumor suppressors, mutations microsatellite loss of heterozygosity (LOH), nuclear image parameters and DNA ploidy have been investigated in laryngeal dysplasias, which has provided insight into the molecular mechanism of carcinogenesis [3–5]. Bartlett et al. also identified several genes including IGF-1, EPDR1, MMP-2, S100A4 which were differentially expressed between vocal cord leukoplakia and normal vocal cord tissues [6]. Despite many investigations, the exact mechanism of vocal cord leukoplakia tumorigenesis remains unclear.

Recently, a new class of noncoding RNAs, designated long noncoding RNAs (lncRNAs), was found to be

* Correspondence: chenxiaoyun2816@163.com
[1]Department of Otolaryngology, the First Affiliated Hospital of Wenzhou Medical University, Wenzhou, Zhejiang 325000, China
Full list of author information is available at the end of the article

frequently dysregulated in various diseases. LncRNAs are transcript RNA molecules longer than 200 nucleotides that do not encode a protein and reside in the nucleus or cytoplasm [7]. Aberrant expression of lncRNAs can lead to abnormalities in gene expression and tumorigenesis. The altered expressions of lncRNAs are a feature of many types of cancers and have been shown to promote the development, invasion, and metastasis of tumors by a variety of mechanisms [8]. Studies have shown that lncRNAs play an important role in larynx squamous cell carcinoma (LSCC) progression. Shen et al. reported that AC026166.2–001 was the most down-regulated lncRNA and RP11-169D4.1–001 was the most up-regulated lncRNA in LSCC tissue compared to normal laryngeal tissue [9]. Some other lncRNAs also have been reported to be correlated with LSCC tumorigenesis and progression [10–14]. However, the role of lncRNAs in vocal cord leukoplakia tumorigenesis remains unclear.

In this study, we used gene microarray analysis to measure the expression patterns of lncRNAs and mRNAs in vocal cord leukoplakia samples and compared them with the corresponding patterns in adjacent nontumorous tissue (NT) samples. Several of the differentially expressed lncRNAs were evaluated by SYBR RT-PCR in 100 pairs of tissue samples. Our results suggest that the dysregulation of lncRNAs might play an important role in vocal cord leukoplakia tumorigenesis.

Methods

Patients samples

Vocal cord leukoplakia samples and control normal vocal cord mucosal samples were collected from 103 patients of the Department of Otolaryngology, First Affiliated Hospital of Wenzhou Medical University, China, from June 2015 to June 2016. Three samples were used for microarray analysis of lncRNAs and 100 were used for quantitative PCR (Q-PCR) validation. The clinical characteristics of patients with leukoplakia vs normal tissue (control) used in gene microarray were shown in Table 1. The diagnosis of vocal cord leukoplakia was based on clinical history and white light laryngoscopy findings and further confirmed by histopathologic diagnosis of parakeratosis and mild to severe dysplasia. The vocal cord leukoplakia and matched normal vocal cord mucosal samples were snap-frozen in liquid nitrogen immediately after resection. This study was approved by the Institutional Ethics

Review Board of the First Affiliated Hospital of Wenzhou Medical University, and all patients provided written informed consent for this study.

RNA extraction

Vocal cord leukoplakia samples and normal vocal cord mucosal samples were obtained by biopsy under white light laryngoscopy. Total RNA was extracted using Trizol reagent (Invitrogen, Carlsbad, CA, USA), according to the manufacturer's protocol. The integrity of the RNA was assessed by electrophoresis on a denaturing agarose gel. A NanoDrop ND-1000 spectrophotometer was used for the accurate measurement of RNA concentration (OD260), protein contamination (OD 260/OD 280 ratio), and organic compound contamination (OD 260/OD 230 ratio).

Microarray and computational analysis

For microarray analysis, an Agilent Array platform (Agilent Technologies, Santa Clara, CA, USA) was employed. The microarray analysis was performed as described by our colleagues [15]. Briefly, sample preparation and microarray hybridization were performed based on the manufacturer's standard protocols with minor modifications. Briefly, mRNA was purified from total RNA after removal of rRNA by using an mRNA-ONLY Eukaryotic mRNA Isolation Kit (Epicentre Biotechnologies, USA). Then, each sample was amplified and transcribed into fluorescent cRNA along the entire length of the transcripts without 3′ bias by using a random priming method. The labeled cRNAs were hybridized onto a Human lncRNA Array v3.0 (8 × 60 K; Arraystar), which was designed for 30,586 lncRNAs and 26,109 coding transcripts. The lncRNAs were carefully constructed using the most highly respected public transcriptome databases (RefSeq, UCSC Known Genes, GENCODE, etc.) as well as landmark publications. Each transcript was accurately identified by a specific exon or splice junction probe. Positive probes for housekeeping genes and negative probes were also printed onto the array for hybridization quality control. After washing the slides, the arrays were scanned using an Agilent G2505C scanner, and the acquired array images were analyzed with Agilent Feature Extraction software (version 11.0.1.1). Quantile normalization and subsequent data processing was performed using the GeneSpring GX

Table 1 Clinical characteristics of patients with leukoplakia vs normal tissue used in gene microarray ($n = 103$)

	Age	Gender		Smoking	Alcohol Drinking	GERD
		Male	Female			
Normal	42.3 ± 5.7	97 (94.2%)	6 (5.8%)	45 (43.7%)	34 (33.0%)	6 (5.8%)
Leukoplakia	45.8 ± 6.9	99 (96.1%)	4 (4.9%)	87 (84.5%)	72 (69.9%)	37 (35.9%)

GERD: Gastroesophageal Reflux Disease

v12.0 software package (Agilent Technologies). The microarray work was performed by KangChen Bio-tech, Shanghai, People's Republic of China.

Functional group analysis

We used Gene Ontology analysis (GO: http://www.geneontology.org) and pathway analysis to determine the function and pathways of the differentially expressed mRNAs in vocal cord leukoplakia tissues compared to adjacent control vocal cord tissues. The P-value denotes the significance of GO Term enrichment in the differentially expressed mRNA list ($P < 0.05$ was considered statistically significant). The pathway analyses for the differentially expressed mRNAs were performed based on the latest Kyoto Encyclopedia of Genes and Genomes (KEGG: http://www.genome.ad.jp/kegg/). This analysis allowed us to determine the biological pathways for which a significant enrichment of differentially expressed mRNAs existed ($P < 0.05$ was considered statistically significant).

Quantitative PCR

Total RNA was extracted from frozen vocal cord leukoplakia tissues by using TRIzol reagent (Invitrogen) and then reverse-transcribed using an RT Reagent Kit (Thermo Scientific), according to the manufacturer's instructions. LncRNAs expression in vocal cord leukoplakia tissues was measured by quantitative PCR by using SYBR Premix Ex Taq and an ABI 7000 instrument. Some candidate lncRNAs were validated by SYBRP PCR, these genes' primers in the study for Q-PCR. Total RNA (2 mg) was transcribed to cDNA. PCR was performed in a total reaction volume of 20 µl, including 10 µl of SYBR Premix (2×), 2 µl of cDNA template, 1 µl of PCR forward primer (10 mM), 1 µl of PCR reverse primer (10 mM), and 6 µl of

double-distilled water. The quantitative real-time PCR reaction included an initial denaturation step of 10 min at 95 °C; 40 cycles of 5 s at 95 °C, 30 s at 60 °C; and a final extension step of 5 min at 72 °C. All experiments were performed in triplicate, and all samples were normalized to GAPDH. The median in each triplicate was used to calculate relative lncRNAs concentrations ($\triangle Ct = Ct$ median lncRNA - Ct median GAPDH), and the fold changes in expression were calculated [16].

Statistical methods

All results are represented as mean ± standard deviation. Statistical analysis was performed for the comparison of two groups in the microarray, and analysis of variance for multiple comparisons was performed the Student's t-test using SPSS software (Version 17.0 SPSS Inc.). A value of $p < 0.05$ was considered statistically significant.

The fold change and the Student's t-test were used to analyze the statistical significance of the microarray results. The false discovery rate (FDR) was calculated to correct the P-value. The threshold value used to designate differentially expressed lncRNAs and mRNAs was a fold change ≥2.0 or ≤0.5 ($P < 0.05$).

Results

Overview of lncRNA profiles

To study the potential biological functions of lncRNAs in vocal cord leukoplakia, we examined the lncRNA and mRNA expression profiles in human leukoplakia by microarray analysis (Figs. 1 and 2). In this study, authoritative data sources containing more than 30,586 lncRNAs were used to study the potential biological functions of lncRNA and mRNA expression profiles in vocal cord leukoplakia through microarray analysis. Our

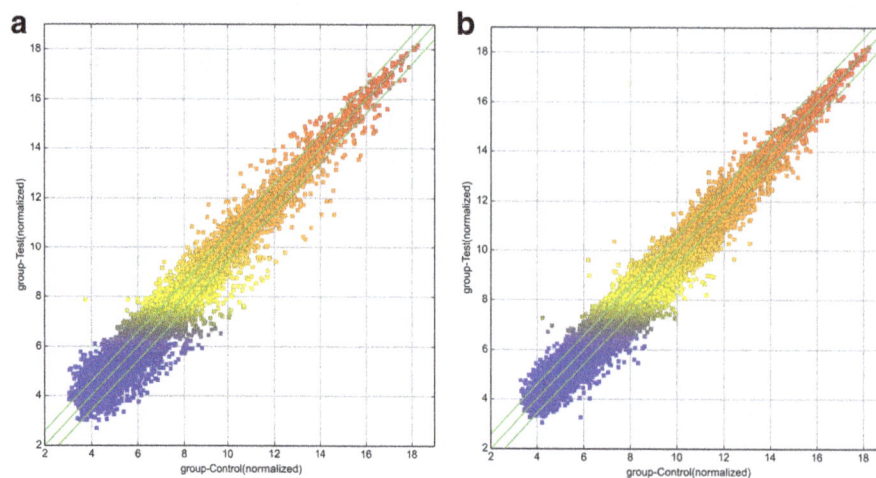

Fig. 1 a–b Scatter plots showing the variation in lncRNA (**a**) and mRNA (**b**) expression between the vocal cord leukoplakia and normal vocal cord tissue arrays. The values of the X and Y axes in the scatter plot are averaged normalized values in each group (log2-scaled). The lncRNAs above the top green line and below the bottom green line are those with a > 3-fold change in expression between the two tissues

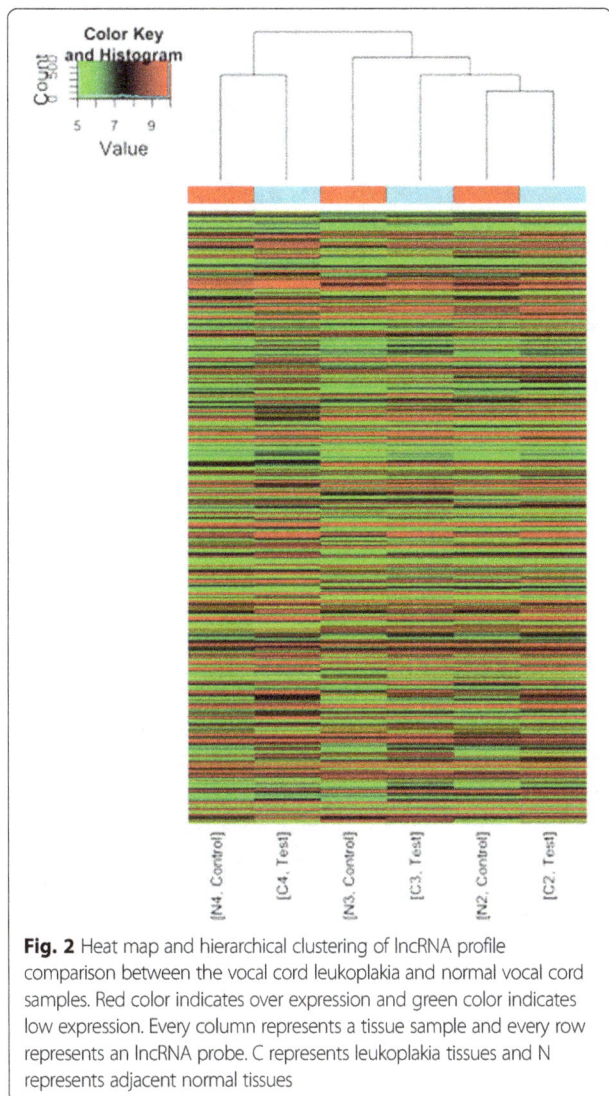

Fig. 2 Heat map and hierarchical clustering of lncRNA profile comparison between the vocal cord leukoplakia and normal vocal cord samples. Red color indicates over expression and green color indicates low expression. Every column represents a tissue sample and every row represents an lncRNA probe. C represents leukoplakia tissues and N represents adjacent normal tissues

Table 2 Top 10 differentially expressed lncRNAs in vocal cord leukoplakia tissue compared with adjacent non-tumorous tissue

up-regulated		down-regulated	
lncRNAs	Fold Change	lncRNAs	Fold Change
XLOC_000605	17.24	DLX6-AS1	4.14
RP11-187O7.3	6.17	KRT17P2	4.13
XLOC_011401	5.31	RP13-608F4.1	3.08
SACS-AS1	4.98	L25629	2.90
XLOC_011403	4.92	CTD-2382E5.1	2.63
FAM86FP	4.11	RP11-351E7.1	2.58
LOC100131138	3.96	HERC2P2	2.49
AC005152.2	3.86	SAA3P	2.48
AC004920.3	3.82	XLOC_006684	2.43
XLOC_008001	3.78	VNN2	2.36

regulatory RNAs but instead belong to multiple categories with some common features. Recent evidence indicates that antisense transcripts are frequently functional and use diverse transcriptional and post-transcriptional gene regulatory mechanisms to carry out a wide variety of biological roles [17]. In this study, LOC100506801 was the only differentially expressed antisense lncRNA (fold change ≥2.0, $P < 0.05$) between vocal cord leukoplakia and normal vocal cord samples. It was significantly up-regulated as was its nearby gene, ECE19 (fold change = 1.70, $P = 0.001$).

Differentially expressed enhancer-like lncRNAs and nearby coding genes

Ørom UA et al. found an enhancer-like function for a set of lncRNAs in human cell lines. Depletion of these lncRNAs led to decreased expression of their neighboring protein-coding genes [18]. In this study, we identified the lncRNAs with enhancer-like lncRNA functions using GENCODE annotation. Our results reveal that AK057351 was the only differentially expressed enhancer-like lncRNA (fold change ≥2.0, $P < 0.05$) between these two groups. It was up-regulated and its nearby gene was EFHA1. EFHA1 was itself up-regulated like the enhancer-like lncRNA (fold change =2.43, $P = 0.03$).

Differentially expressed lincRNAs and associated coding gene

Long intergenetic noncoding RNAs (lincRNAs) are transcribed from thousands of loci in mammalian genomes and might play widespread roles in gene regulation and other cellular processes [19]. In this study, we identified 3 differentially expressed lincRNAs and associated coding mRNAs (fold change ≥2.0, $P < 0.05$): XLOC_008001, XLOC_011989 and XLOC_007341. All of them were up-regulated as were their associated mRNAs, MSN (fold change =1.63, $P = 0.01$), RRAD

results showed that there were 170 differentially expressed lncRNAs (fold change ≥2.0 or ≤0.5; $P < 0.05$) between vocal cord leukoplakia and normal vocal cord samples. Among these, 142 lncRNAs were found to be up-regulated in the vocal cord leukoplakia group compared to the normal vocal cord mucosal group, while 28 lncRNAs were down-regulated between these two groups (Table 2 shows the top 10 differentially expressed lncRNAs). Among these, XLOC_000605 was the most significantly up-regulated lncRNA and DLX6-AS1 was the most significantly down-regulated one.

LncRNAs classification and subgroup analysis
Differentially expressed antisense lncRNAs and nearby coding genes

Mammalian genomes encode numerous natural antisense transcripts. Functional validation studies indicate that antisense transcripts are not a uniform group of

(fold change =2.69, $P = 0.04$) and TPM2 (fold change =1.68, $P = 0.007$), respectively.

Overview of mRNA profiles

Ninety-nine mRNAs were found to be differentially expressed between vocal cord leukoplakia and normal vocal cord mucosa tissue (fold change ≥ 2.0, $P < 0.05$). Among these, 54 were up-regulated and 45 were down-regulated (Table 3 shows the top 10 differentially expressed mRNAs).

GO analysis

GO analysis is a functional analysis that associates differentially expressed mRNAs. The GO categories were derived from the Gene Ontology website (www.geneontology.org) and comprised of 3 structured networks: biological processes, cellular components and molecular function. According to the GO annotation tool, the genes corresponding to the down-regulated mRNAs included 455 genes involved in biological processes, 73 genes involved in cellular components and 60 genes involved in molecular functions. The genes corresponding to the up-regulated mRNAs included 109 genes involved in biological processes, 12 genes involved in cellular components, and 21 genes involved in molecular functions.

Pathway analysis

We performed the pathway analysis based on the latest Kyoto Encyclopedia of Genes and Genomes (KEGG) database. This analysis was used to determine the biological pathways associated with the most differentially expressed mRNAs in vocal cord leukoplakia. Our results identified 5 up-regulated pathways (including Primary immunodeficiency, Glioma, Melanoma, Bile secretion, Cell cycle signaling pathways) (Fig. 3) and 14 down-regulated pathways (including ECM-receptor interaction,

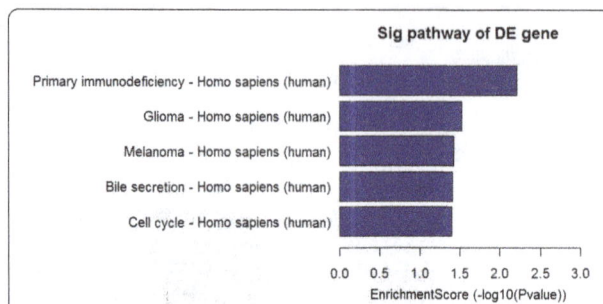

Fig. 3 Pathway analysis of upregulated mRNAs in vocal cord leukoplakia. Five upregulated pathways were identified, including Primary immunodeficiency, Glioma, Melanoma, Bile secretion, Cell cycle signaling pathways

focal adhesion, Regulation of actin cytoskeleton, Proteoglycans in cancer, TGF-beta signaling pathway, Cell adhesion molecules and PI3K-Akt signaling pathways) (Fig. 4).

Real-time quantitative PCR validation

Based on features of the differentially expressed lncRNAs such as fold difference, gene locus, and nearby encoding genes, a number of interesting candidate lncRNAs were selected for further analysis (including XLOC_000605, RP11-187O7.3, XLOC_011403, XLOC-011401, SACS-AS1, FAM86FP, DLX6-AS1, KRT17P2). We verified the expression of these lncRNAs by real-time quantitative RT-PCR by using GAPDH as a reference gene and by calculating the $2^{-\triangle\triangle CT}$ values. The results showed that the microarray results for the selected lncRNAs were consistent with the results of RT-PCR (Fig. 5).

Discussion

In recent years, researchers have focused their attention on the analysis of protein-coding transcripts to characterize patterns and potential functional roles. The development of next-generation sequencing technology has led to the discovery of a new class of non-coding RNA transcripts, lncRNAs. Numerous investigations suggest that lncRNAs perform key regulatory functions in chromatin remodeling and gene expression in many biological processes, including X-chromosome inactivation, gene imprinting, and stem cell maintenance [20, 21]. Furthermore, lncRNAs are important factors in the control of gene expression in cancer [22], and lncRNAs such as HOTAIR have been shown to play a significant role in the development and progression of tumors [8]. It has also been demonstrated that lncRNAs are differentially expressed in normal cells and tumor cells. As lncRNAs constitute an important class of gene expression regulatory factors, their aberrant expression would inevitably lead to abnormal gene expression levels, which may result in tumorigenesis. Promoters bind to many transcription factors by mechanisms such as chromosomal

Table 3 Top 10 differentially expressed mRNAs in vocal cord leukoplakia tissue compared with adjacent non-tumorous tissue

up-regulated		down-regulated	
mRNAs	Fold Change	mRNAs	Fold Change
RPL10L	3.79	GPX8	3.99
SOWAHA	3.51	WDR19	3.87
HMGCS2	3.38	SEC31A	3.45
ZSCAN1	3.17	CTSF	3.42
OR4P4	2.97	ARID4A	3.14
PDP1	2.93	KIF20A	2.99
C1orf53	2.82	DUSP6	2.89
OSGIN2	2.81	CALD1	2.86
ZNF853	2.79	PNISR	2.82
OR6C3	2.78	FIP1L1	2.81

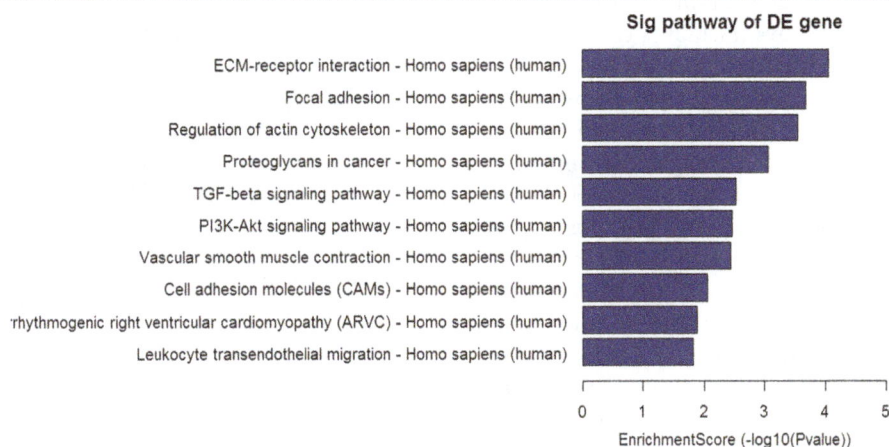

Fig. 4 Pathway analysis of downregulated mRNAs in vocal cord leukoplakia. Fifteen downregulated pathways were identified, including ECM-receptor interaction, focal adhesion, Regulation of actin cytoskeleton, Proteoglycans in cancer, TGF-beta signaling pathway, Cell adhesion molecules and PI3K-Akt signaling pathways

rearrangements and transfer elements [23]. However, the profile and the biological function of lncRNAs in vocal cord leukoplakia remain unknown.

Until now, there have been no reports describing the expression profiles of lncRNAs in vocal cord leukoplakia and there have been no studies on the association of lncRNA expression with the clinical characteristics and outcomes of in vocal cord leukoplakia. In this study, we analyzed the lncRNAs expression profiles in the tissues of vocal cord leukoplakia to uncover the potential role of lncRNAs in the pathogenesis of its tumorigenesis. High-throughput microarray techniques revealed a set of

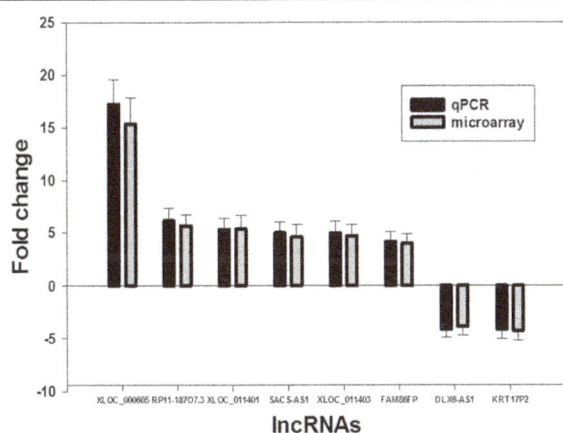

Fig. 5 Comparison between gene chip data and qPCR result. XLOC_000605, RP11-187O7.3, XLOC_011403, XLOC-011401, SACS-AS1, FAM86FP, DLX6-AS1, KRT17P2 determined to be differentially expressed in vocal cord leukoplakia samples compared with NT samples in three patients by microarray were validated by qPCR. The heights of the columns in the chart represent the log-transformed median fold changes (T/N) in expression across the three patients for each of the four lncRNAs validated. The validation results of the 8 lncRNAs indicated that the microarray data correlated well with the qPCR results

differentially expressed lncRNAs, including 142 that were up-regulated and 28 that were down-regulated in vocal cord leukoplakia tissue compared to normal vocal cord mucosa. Furthermore, we identified several subgroups of lncRNA, including antisense lncRNA, enhancer-like lncRNA, and lincRNA. Enhancers are classically defined as *cis*-acting DNA sequences that can increase the transcription of genes. They generally function independently of orientation and at various distances from their target promoter (or promoters) [24]. Ørom et al. also found some lncRNAs with enhancer-like functions in human cells [18]. In this study, we identified a significantly up-regulated enhancer-like lncRNA AK057351 and its associated gene EFHA1. Antisense lncRNAs are another subgroup of lncRNAs which can induce chromatin and DNA epigenetic changes, thus affecting the expression of sense mRNA. In this study, we identified an up-regulated antisense lncRNA LOC100506801 and its associated gene, ECE19. LincRNA are long non-coding sequences located between the protein-coding genes. More than 3500 lincRNAs have been reported in mammalian genome so far, which are involved in physiological processes through regulation of gene expression. Aberrant expression of lincRNAs has been found in both solid tumors and leukemia. The role of lincRNAs, however, remains unclear. In this study, we identified 3 significantly up-regulated lincRNAs and associated coding mRNAs. They were XLOC_008001, XLOC_011989 and XLOC_007341 and the associated mRNAs were MSN, RRAD and TPM2, respectively.

To investigate the lncRNAs' target gene function, GO analysis and KEGG pathway annotation were applied to the lncRNAs' target gene pool. GO analysis revealed that the number of genes corresponding to down-regulated mRNAs was larger than that corresponding to up-regulated mRNAs. KEGG annotation showed that there were 5 up-regulated pathways (including ethanol metabolism, viral carcinogenesis, RNA transduction, and cell cycle pathways) and 14 down-regulated pathways (including propionate metabolism and fatty acid metabolism pathways). These pathways might play important roles in vocal cord leukoplakia tumorigenesis. Further studies should be performed to investigate this hypothesis. 8 of the lncRNAs identified in the microarray analysis were confirmed by RT-PCR to be aberrantly expressed in vocal cord leukoplakia tissues. Among these lncRNAs, XLOC_000605 was the most significantly up-regulated, and DLX6-AS1 was the most significantly down-regulated. Little has been known about the function of these two lncRNAs until now. These findings may provide a potential strategy to distinguish between vocal cord leukoplakia tissue and normal vocal cord tissue. Our results suggest that these two lncRNAs might contribute to vocal cord leukoplakia tumorigenesis. Further studies of the biological function of XLOC_000605 and DLX6-AS1 will be required to confirm this potential association.

Conclusions

In conclusion, our study revealed a set of lncRNAs with differential expression in vocal cord leukoplakia compared with normal larynx mucous tissue, and also identified several subgroups of lncRNAs such as antisense lncRNAs, enhancer-like lncRNAs and lincRNAs. Moreover, we found that XLOC_000605 and DLX6-AS1 were significantly dysregulated and these two lncRNAs might contribute to vocal cord leukoplakia tumorigenesis. One limitation to this study is the small sample size, which may have been insufficient to detect every truly differentially expressed gene. In addition, we did not investigate the function of the differentially expressed genes which were identified. Further investigations directed at the lncRNAs and mRNAs identified above will be required to uncover their biological functions and their association with vocal cord leukoplakia tumorigenesis.

Abbreviations

GO: Gene Ontology; KEGG: Kyoto Encyclopedia of Genes and Genomes; lincRNA: long intergenetic noncoding RNA; lncRNA: long non-coding RNA; NT: nontumorous tissue

Acknowledgements

Not applicable.

Funding

This study was supported by a grant number 2013C33241 from Public Technology Application Research Foundation from Department of Science and Technology of Zhejiang Province and Y20110090 from Wenzhou Municipal Science and Technology Bureau Foundation.

Authors' contributions

PJ, LH, CJ, WX, JT and CX participated in the conceptualization and design of the study, analysis and interpretation of data, drafting and/or revising the manuscript, and have approved the manuscript as submitted.

Authors' information

All authors are affiliated with the First Affiliated Hospital of Wenzhou Medical University.

Competing interests

The authors declare that they have no competing interests.

Author details

[1]Department of Otolaryngology, the First Affiliated Hospital of Wenzhou Medical University, Wenzhou, Zhejiang 325000, China. [2]Institute of Translation Medicine, the First Affiliated Hospital of Wenzhou Medical University, Wenzhou, Zhejiang 325000, China.

References

1. Isenberg JS, Crozier DL, Dailey SH. Institutional and comprehensive review of laryngeal leukoplakia. Ann Otol Rhinol Laryngol. 2008;117(1):74–9.
2. Singh I, Gupta D, Yadav S. Leukoplakia of larynx: a review update. J Laryngol Voice. 2014;4:39–44.
3. Jeannon JP, Soames JV, Aston V, Stafford FW, Wilson JA. Molecular markers in dysplasia of the larynx: expression of cyclin-dependent kinase inhibitors p21, p27 and p53 tumour suppressor gene in predicting cancer risk. Clin Otolaryngol Allied Sci. 2004;29:698–704.
4. Ioachim E, Peschos D, Goussia A, Mittari E, Charalabopoulos K, Michael M, et al. Expression patterns of cyclins D1, E in laryngeal epithelial lesions: correlation with other cell cycle regulators (p53, pRb, Ki-67 and PCNA) and clinicopathological features. J Exp Clin Cancer Res. 2004;23:277–83.
5. Forastiere A, Koch W, Trotti A, Sidransky D. Head and neck cancer. N Engl J Med. 2001;345(26):1890–900.
6. Bartlett RS, Heckman WW, Isenberg J, Thibeault SL, Dailey SH. Genetic characterization of vocal fold lesions: leukoplakia and carcinoma. Laryngoscope. 2012;122(2):336–42.
7. Ponting CP, Oliver PL, Reik W. Evolution and functions of long noncoding RNAs. Cell. 2009;136(4):629–41.
8. Gupta RA, Shah N, Wang KC, Kim J, Horlings HM, Wong DJ, et al. Long non-coding RNA HOTAIR reprograms chromatin state to promote cancer metastasis. Nature. 2010;464(7291):1071–6.
9. Shen Z, Li Q, Deng H, Lu D, Song H, Guo J. Long non-coding RNA profiling in laryngeal squamous cell carcinoma and its clinical significance: potential biomarkers for LSCC. PLoS One. 2014;9(9):e108237.
10. Feng L, Wang R, Lian M, Ma H, He N, Liu H, et al. Integrated analysis of long noncoding RNA and mRNA expression profile in advanced laryngeal Squamous cell carcinoma. PLoS One. 2016;11(12):e0169232.
11. Guan GF, Zhang DJ, Wen LJ, Xin D, Liu Y, Yu DJ, et al. Overexpression of lncRNA H19/miR-675 promotes tumorigenesis in head and neck squamous cell carcinoma. Int J Med Sci. 2016;13(12):914–22.
12. Wu T, Qu L, He G, Tian L, Li L, Zhou H, et al. Regulation of laryngeal squamous cell cancer progression by the lncRNA H19/miR-148a-3p/DNMT1 axis. Oncotarget. 2016;7(10):11553–66.
13. Zhang C, Gao W, Wen S, Wu Y, Fu R, Zhao D, et al. Potential key molecular correlations in laryngeal squamous cell carcinoma revealed by integrated analysis of mRNA, miRNA and lncRNA microarray profiles. Neoplasma. 2016; 63(6):888–900.

Differences in gene expression profile between vocal cord Leukoplakia and normal larynx mucosa by gene...

61

14. Wang P, Wu T, Zhou H, Jin Q, He G, Yu H, et al. Long noncoding RNA NEAT1 promotes laryngeal squamous cell cancer through regulating miR-107/CDK6 pathway. J Exp Clin Cancer Res. 2016;35:22.

15. Xu G, Chen J, Pan Q, Huang K, Pan J, Zhang W, et al. Long noncoding RNA expression profiles of lung adenocarcinoma ascertained by microarray analysis. PLoS One. 2014;9(8):e104044.

16. Ren S, Peng Z, Mao JH, Yu Y, Yin C, Gao X, et al. RNA-seq analysis of prostate cancer in the Chinese population identifies recurrent gene fusions, cancer-associated long noncoding RNAs and aberrant alternative splicings. Cell Res. 2012;22(5):806–21.

17. Faghihi MA, Wahlestedt C. Regulatory roles of natural antisense transcripts. Nat Rev Mol Cell Biol. 2009;10(9):637–43.

18. Ørom UA, Derrien T, Beringer M, Gumireddy K, Gardini A, Bussotti G, et al. Long noncoding RNAs with enhancer-like function in human cells. Cell. 2010;143(1):46–58.

19. Ulitsky I, Bartel DP. lincRNAs: genomics, evolution, and mechanisms. Cell. 2013;154(1):26–46.

20. Mercer TR, Dinger ME, Mattick JS. Long non-coding RNAs: insights into functions. Nat Rev Genet. 2009;10(3):155–9.

21. Wang KC, Chang HY. Molecular mechanisms of long noncoding RNAs. Mol Cell. 2011;43(6):904–14.

22. Khachane AN, Harrison PM. Mining mammalian transcript data for functional long non-coding RNAs. PLoS One. 2010;5(4):e10316.

23. Loh YH, Wu Q, Chew JL, Vega VB, Zhang W, Chen X, et al. The Oct4 and Nanog transcription network regulates pluripotency in mouse embryonic stem cells. Nat Genet. 2006;38(4):431–40.

24. Pennacchio LA, Bickmore W, Dean A, Nobrega MA, Bejerano G. Enhancers: five essential questions. Nat Rev Genet. 2013;14(4):288–95.

10

Patterns of regional recurrence in papillary thyroid cancer patients with lateral neck metastases undergoing neck dissection

Jason J. Xu[1], Eugene Yu[2], Caitlin McMullen[1], Jesse Pasternak[3], Jim Brierley[4], Richard Tsang[4], Han Zhang[1], Antoine Eskander[1], Lorne Rotstein[3], Anna M. Sawka[5], Ralph Gilbert[1], Jonathan Irish[1], Patrick Gullane[1], Dale Brown[1], John R. de Almeida[1] and David P. Goldstein[1*]

Abstract

Background: Practice variability exists for the extent of neck dissection undertaken for papillary thyroid carcinoma (PTC) metastatic to the lateral neck nodes, with disagreement over routine level V dissection.

Methods: We performed a retrospective medical record review of PTC patients with lateral neck nodal metastases treated at University Health Network from 2000 to 2012. Predictive factors for regional neck recurrence, including extent of initial neck dissection, were analyzed using Cox regression.

Results: Out of 204 neck dissections in 178 patients, 110 (54%) underwent selective and 94 (46%) had comprehensive dissection including level Vb. Mean follow-up was 6.3 years (SD). Significant predictors of regional failure were the total number of suspicious nodes on preoperative imaging ($p = 0.029$), largest positive node on initial neck dissection ($p < 0.01$), and whether patients received adjuvant radiotherapy ($p = 0.028$). The 5-year ipsilateral regional recurrence rate was 8 and 9% with selective and comprehensive dissection, respectively ($p = 0.89$).

Conclusion: The extent of neck dissection did not predict the probability of regional recurrence in PTC patients presenting with lateral neck metastases.

Keywords: Papillary thyroid carcinoma, Neck dissection, Regional recurrence

Background

There is no clear consensus regarding the extent of lateral neck dissection required in the treatment of papillary thyroid carcinoma (PTC). For patients presenting with clinical, radiographic or cytologic evidence of lateral lymph node metastases, the standard of care includes lateral neck lymph node dissection [1, 2]. However, variability in clinical practice persists regarding the levels of dissection required. Some surgeons perform a comprehensive neck dissection – including a formal level Vb dissection – with the intention of potentially lowering the rate of regional

recurrence [3–5]. Others, believing that elective level Vb dissection is unwarranted and results in greater morbidity [6], argue that a formal level Vb dissection should only be performed given sufficient clinical and radiographic suspicion of disease in that level [7, 8].

A meta-analysis examining patterns of nodal metastases in patients with PTC and lateral neck metastases reported level V metastatic disease in 25.3% of cases, with Va and Vb nodal positivity in 7.9 and 21.5% of patients, respectively [3]. Based on this high rate of Vb involvement, the authors recommended a comprehensive lateral neck dissection including levels IIa, IIb, III, IV and Vb in all patients with PTC and lateral neck disease. However, the data from this meta-analysis for level Vb recurrence was pooled from only 3 uncontrolled case series with a small sample size (pooled $n = 137$). The general approach to the management of the

* Correspondence: david.goldstein@uhn.ca
The Canadian Society of Otolaryngology-Head and Neck Surgery Annual Meeting Poliquin Competition; 2016 June; Charlottetown, PE.
[1]Department of Otolaryngology—Head and Neck Surgery, University Health Network, University of Toronto, Toronto, Ontario, Canada
Full list of author information is available at the end of the article

neck for PTC at the University Health Network (Princess Margaret Cancer Center and Toronto General Hospital) has been to base the levels of neck dissection on the extent of disease as determined with preoperative ultrasound and/or cross-sectional CT imaging. Given the high reported rate of nodal metastases on pathologic examination in level Vb we sought to determine the rate and patterns of regional failure in patients undergoing neck dissection for thyroid cancer at our institution.

Methods

Study design

We conducted a retrospective review of all consecutive PTC patients with lateral neck metastases treated at the University Health Network (UHN) from January 1, 2000 to August 1, 2012. We obtained approval from the UHN Research Ethics Board. Subjects were identified by screening all patients with both a diagnosis of thyroid cancer and any billing code for lateral neck dissection. Collection of data from the charts went up to March 31, 2016. Adult patients (>18 years of age) who underwent unilateral or bilateral lateral neck dissection for regional metastases from PTC were eligible for inclusion. Neck dissections could have been performed either concurrently or no more than 5 years after the initial thyroidectomy. We excluded patients if they had any pathology other than PTC (including insular cell carcinoma or Hurthle cell carcinoma), a history of previous neck dissection, no metastases identified in the neck dissection specimen on histopathology, received ≥2 radioactive iodine (RAI) treatments prior to neck dissection, incomplete operative notes where the extent or type of neck dissection could not be determined, or if they were lost to follow up within the first 12 months after surgery.

The general approach to neck dissection for PTC at the University Health Network has been to perform a resection of the levels of the neck with radiographic or clinical suspicion of metastases; however, the extent of dissection was determined ultimately at the discretion of the treating surgeon. General indications for performing a comprehensive dissection of level Vb in the absence of radiographic evidence of metastases included bulky nodal metastases and/or large nodal disease, significant level IV metastases or surgeon preference.

We extracted data on patient demographics, the extent of neck dissection performed, pathology results including nodal ratio of dissection specimens, adjuvant treatment given and development of regional recurrence. A staff radiologist reviewed all pre- and post operative computerized tomography (CT) images and collected data on the location, size and total number of nodes suspicious for PTC metastases. Nodes were deemed suspicious if any of the following features were present: cystic and enhancing with small foci of calcifications,

enhancing internal solid components and necrotic and enhancing. The size requirement of suspicious lymph nodes were 1.5 cm for level 1B and jugulo-diagastric nodes and 1 cm for all other lymph nodes, taken in context with the aforementioned suspicious features.

Two study authors independently reviewed operative notes to determine the extent of neck dissection performed by level. Disagreements were reconciled through consensus or with the surgeon who performed the case. Patients were separated into two cohorts depending on the extent of the neck dissection they received. The selective dissection group was defined as those that received a neck dissection comprised of levels IIa (+/−IIb), III, IV and often the anterior aspect of level Vb. The comprehensive neck dissection group received formal IIa (+/−IIb) to Vb dissection, which included dissecting the posterior accessory nerve to the anterior border of trapezius and resecting all the nodal tissue below.

Outcomes and statistics

Our primary outcome was regional recurrence of PTC in the ipsilateral lateral neck. For patients with bilateral neck disease, we analyzed each side separately. Patients were recorded as having a regional recurrence if they had histologically proven PTC in a lymph node on fine needle aspiration (FNA) or salvage neck dissection, or had CT and ultrasound findings consistent with nodal recurrence (based on the above mentioned criteria) with or without elevated or rising thyroglobulin levels. We only classified patients as regional recurrence if they recurred in the lateral neck, and thus we did not count patients with isolated thyroid bed or central compartment recurrences for the purposes of this study. The location of neck recurrence was determined based on imaging.

Comparison of clinical features between selective and comprehensive neck dissection was performed using the Chi-squared test or Fisher's exact test for categorical variables and Student's T-test or Wilcoxon rank sum test for continuous variables. Time to neck recurrence was analyzed using the Kaplan-Meier method. Univariate and multivariate analysis was conducted using Cox proportional hazards regression model. Statistical significance was defined as $p < 0.05$. Statistical analysis was performed using SAS version 9.4 and R 3.1.2.

Results

Baseline comparison between selective and comprehensive neck dissection groups

After review, 178 patients who underwent 204 neck dissections met the inclusion criteria. Of note, we excluded 11 potentially eligible patients due to incomplete operative notes,16 due to being lost to follow-up, 19 because they had two or more prior RAI treatments, and 14 who presented >5 years with neck disease after their initial thyroidectomy. Of the 204 neck dissections that met inclusion criteria, 110 (54%) were selective and 94 (46%) were comprehensive dissections. There were 26 patients who underwent bilateral neck dissections. Concurrent total thyroidectomy was performed in 169 cases (83%), concurrent completion thyroidectomy was performed in 6 cases (3%), and 29 cases had prior thyroidectomy (14%). The mean age was 44.8 years (SD = 14.9) with 45% (n = 91) of patients being older than 45 years of age. The majority of patients (60%, n = 123) were female. There were no significant differences between the selective neck dissection patient group and the comprehensive neck dissection group in terms of patient demographics.

On pre-operative staging, 4% (n = 4) of patients undergoing selective neck dissection and 19% (n = 18) patients undergoing a comprehensive neck dissection had radiographic evidence of level V disease ($p < 0.001$). Patients undergoing a comprehensive neck dissection had a greater mean number of radiographic suspicious nodes (3.6 vs 2.6, p = 0.034) and greater diameter in the largest node (2.4 cm vs. 1.6 cm, $p < 0.01$) compared with those who underwent selective neck dissection. On pathologic assessment of neck dissection specimens (Table 1), the comprehensive dissection group had a greater mean number of positive nodes (6.7 vs. 5.2, p =0.03) and greater number of total nodes removed (34.8 vs. 27.8, $p < 0.01$) compared with the selective neck dissection group, but no significant difference in whether there were nodes with extracapsular extension, nodal ratio or mean diameter of the largest node.

In terms of adjuvant treatment, almost all patients received adjuvant radioactive iodine. There were no differences between the neck dissection groups in terms of RAI dose, number of treatments and whether external beam radiotherapy was received (Table 2).

Outcomes

The mean length of follow up was 75.6 months (SD = 33.7). Mean follow up for the selective and comprehensive groups were 67 and 86 months, respectively. There were a total of 20 regional recurrences in the

overall cohort, with 12 in the selective neck dissection group and 8 in the comprehensive neck dissection group. In terms of regional recurrences, 14 were based on pathologic assessment (13 salvage neck dissection pathology and 1 FNA biopsy) and 6 were based on imaging alone without pathologic assessment. Of the latter group, 5 had increasing thyroglobulin levels in addition to suspicious imaging features, while 1 had positive anti-thyroglobulin antibodies.

The 5-year ipsilateral regional control rate for the entire cohort was 92% (95% CI: 88–96%). The results of the univariate analysis are listed in Table 3. The significant predictors of regional failure were the total number of suspicious nodes on preoperative imaging (p = 0.029), largest positive node on initial neck dissection ($p < 0.01$), and whether patients received external

Table 1 Neck dissection specimen pathology

	Full Sample (n = 204)	Comprehensive (n = 94)	Selective (n = 110)	P-value
Extracapsular Extension (ECE)	49 (24%)	22 (23%)	27 (25%)	0.87
Positive Nodes[a]	5.9 (4.8)	6.7 (5.5)	5.2 (4.1)	**0.03**
Total Nodes[a]	31 (17.3)	34.8 (18)	27.8 (16)	**0.004**
Nodal Ratio	21.6%	21.1%	21.9%	0.74
Nodal Size (cm)[a]	2.5 (1.2)	2.7 (1.3)	2.4 (1.1)	0.12

[a]Mean (SD)
Significant p values are captured in bold

Table 2 Adjuvant treatment

	Full Sample (n = 204)	Comprehensive (n = 94)	Selective (n = 110)	P-value
Received RAI	203 (100)	94 (100)	109 (99)	0.99
RAI Dose[a]	135 (42)	132 (38.2)	138 (45.1)	0.39
Multiple RAI Doses	8 (4)	2 (2)	6 (5)	0.29
Received EBRT	13 (6)	7 (7)	6 (5)	0.58

[a]Mean (SD)

Table 3 Univariate analysis–Cox proportional hazards regression for regional recurrence

Variable	HR (95%CI)	Global p-value
Selective Neck Dissection (Ref: Comprehensive)	0.94 (0.39,2.27)	0.89
Age ≥ 45 (Ref: <45)	0.93 (0.39,2.26)	0.88
Concurrent Thyroidectomy (Ref:No)	0.66 (0.21,2.06)	0.48
Extracapsular Extension	1.89 (0.75,4.74)	0.17
Level V Disease (Ref:No)	1.91 (0.64,5.72)	0.25
Total Nodes (CT)	1.26 (1.02,1.55)	**0.029**
Largest Node (CT)	1.24 (0.81,1.89)	0.32
Total Nodes (Path)	1.04 (0.97,1.11)	0.29
Largest Node (Path)	1.56 (1.19,2.05)	**0.0015**
Nodal Ratio (Path)	5.11 (0.38,68.66)	0.22
RAI (Ref: No)	3296373.77 (0,Inf)	1
RAI Dose	1 (0.99,1.01)	0.66
Multiple RAI (Ref: No)	0 (0,Inf)	1
EBRT (Ref: No)	3.45 (1.14,10.37)	**0.028**
Male (Ref: Female)	0.93 (0.38,2.27)	0.87
Age	1 (0.97,1.03)	0.91
Follow-Up (months)	1 (0.98,1.01)	0.61

Significant p values are captured in bold

beam radiotherapy (EBRT, $p = 0.028$). The type of neck dissection was not predictive of regional recurrence (Fig. 1). The 5-year regional control rate was 91% (86–97) for the selective dissection group and 92% (87–98) for the comprehensive dissection group ($p = 0.89$). Multivariate Cox regression model adjusted for significant factors identified on univariate analysis found that the hazard ratio of selective neck dissection for neck recurrence was 2.55 (95% CI: 0.63–10.38, $p = 0.19$). Multivariate analysis was performed excluding patients who received EBRT and found that selective neck dissection was still not significantly associated with regional recurrence ($p = 0.26$, Table 4).

A subgroup analysis was performed for those patients who did not have positive level V disease on pre-operative imaging. There were 106 and 76 cases in the selective and comprehensive groups, respectively. Similarly, the type of neck dissection was not predictive of regional recurrence (Fig. 2), with a 5-year regional control rate of 94% (95% CI: 90–99) and 92% (95% CI: 86–98) for the selective and comprehensive groups, respectively ($p = 0.63$).

The location of regional recurrence by type of neck dissection is listed in Table 5. In the selective group, 6 of 12 cases of recurrence (50%) were considered "out-of-neck dissection field" failures, with 5 cases involving level V and 1 case involving in level IIb. For the comprehensive group, 3 of 8 cases of recurrence (37.5%) contained "out-of-field" failures, all in level IIb. The comprehensive and selective groups had no significant difference in the rate of level Vb recurrence (2% vs 3%, $p = 1.00$) or recurrence at any other level.

All five patients in the selective dissection group with recurrence in level V did not have any suspicious level V adenopathy on their pre-operative CT. These patients had on average 7 positive lymph nodes on their initial neck dissection specimen, with an average nodal ratio of

Table 4 Multivariate analysis–Cox PH regression model adjusted for total nodes on pre-operative CT and largest node on pathology

Variable	HR (95%CI)	Global p-value
Selective Neck Dissection (Ref: Comprehensive)	2.35 (0.53,10.41)	0.26
Total Nodes (CT)	1.29 (1.01,1.65)	**0.039**
Largest Node (Path)	2.06 (1.17,3.6)	**0.012**

Significant p values are captured in bold

0.21. The largest positive node for these patients is on average 2.5 cm. The salvage neck dissection pathology showed fewer positive nodes for the comprehensive group (1.7 vs 4, $p = 0.038$) and more total nodes removed for the selective group (13.2 vs 6.2, $p = 0.039$), but no difference in nodal ratio or size of the largest positive node (Table 6).

Discussion

The 2012 American Thyroid Association (ATA) consensus statement on lateral neck dissection for PTC states that "lateral neck dissection performed for macroscopic DTC metastases should be the selective neck dissection of levels IIa, III, IV and Vb." [1] However, while the more updated 2015 ATA guideline strongly recommends that "therapeutic lateral neck compartmental lymph node dissection should be performed for patients with biopsy-proven metastatic lateral cervical lymphadenopathy," the extent of surgery or which nodal compartments to dissect are no longer specified [2]. The approach to nodal management at the University Health Network, Princess Margaret Cancer Center generally has been to base the extent of neck dissection on the location and volume of disease seen on pre-operative imaging, and to avoid the comprehensive level Vb neck dissection where feasible in

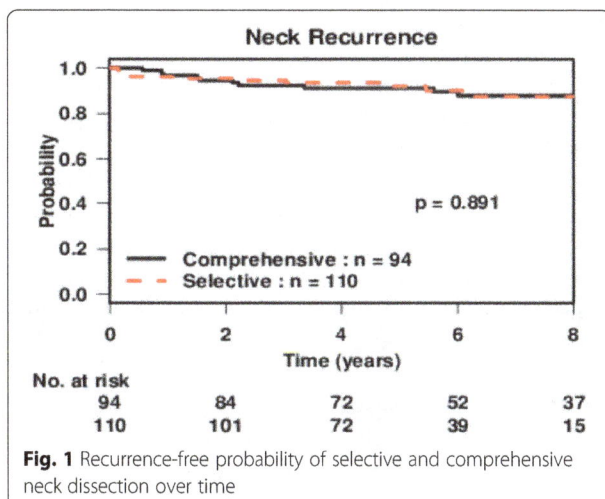

Fig. 1 Recurrence-free probability of selective and comprehensive neck dissection over time

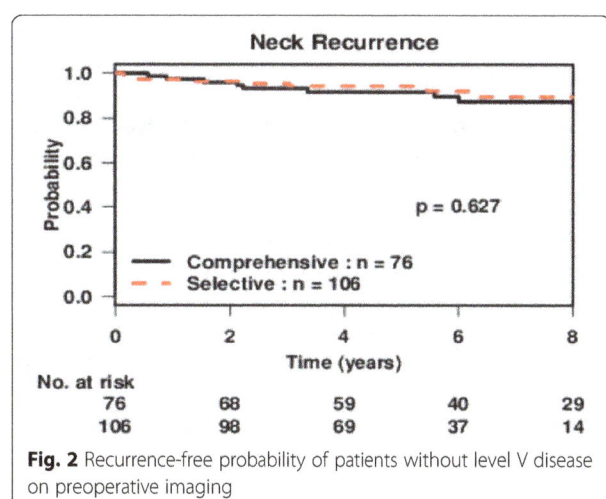

Fig. 2 Recurrence-free probability of patients without level V disease on preoperative imaging

Table 5 Location of regional recurrence by neck dissecton type

	Full Sample (n = 204)	Comprehensive (n = 94)	Selective (n = 110)	p
Level IIa Disease	9 (4%)	2 (2%)	7 (6%)	0.18
Level IIb Disease	6 (3%)	5 (5%)	1 (1%)	0.097
Level III Disease	5 (2%)	3 (3%)	2 (2%)	0.66
Level IV Disease	8 (4%)	3 (3%)	5 (5%)	0.73
Level Va Disease	2 (1%)	1 (1%)	1 (1%)	1.00
Level Vb Disease	5 (2%)	2 (2%)	3 (3%)	1.00
Total Nodes[a]	2.5 (2.8)	2.8 (3.6)	2.2 (1.6)	0.73
Largest Node[a]	1.5 (0.7)	1.4 (0.5)	1.7 (1)	0.47

[a]Mean (SD)

order to reduce potential morbidity. This conflicts with several reports in the literature, which argue that a comprehensive level Vb dissection is always necessary given a high rate of level Vb metastases ranging from 15 to 40%, with Eskander et. al. in their meta-analysis of 18 pooled studies reporting level Vb disease in 21.5% of patients [2]. Other authors since the meta-analysis have also argued for routine level V comprehensive dissection based on similar findings. One such example is Javid et. al. who reported a series of 241 lateral neck dissections for PTC and found level V involvement in 16.9% of cases [9]. Their series had a recurrence rate of 10.9%, all in patients who had comprehensive dissection of levels II–V, with 3 cases of recurrence involving level V. Again, these authors argue that level V dissection is always necessary as there is disease involvement in about one-fifth of cases.

There are several limitations to consider though when interpreting the results of the aforementioned studies. Primarily, these studies do not specify whether the positive nodes found in level V are macroscopic or microscopic disease, the latter of which may have less impact on clinically significant outcomes [10, 11]. Secondly, the method of marking neck levels in the specimen is not always reported, and for the studies that do specify this, there are a

Table 6 Revision neck dissection specimen pathology

	Full Sample (n = 204)	Comprehensive (n = 94)	Selective (n = 110)	p
Positive Nodes[a]	2.7 (2.6)	1.7 (1.6)	4 (3.1)	**0.038**
Total Nodes[a]	9.2 (7.8)	6.2 (6.5)	13.2 (7.9)	**0.039**
Nodal Ratio	31.8%	41.9%	24.6%	0.35
Largest Node (cm)[a]	1.7 (0.9)	1.6 (0.5)	1.9 (1.1)	0.44

[a]Mean (SD)

Significant p values are captured in bold

range of different methods used which confound the results. As such, we sought to determine if a selective approach to neck management in thyroid cancer with cervical metastases is associated with high recurrence rates, particularly in those undergoing less than comprehensive neck dissection of level Vb. Of the 204 neck dissections in our series, the overall regional control rate was high at 92%. With the selective dissection group, the 5-year regional control rate was equally high at 91%, with only 5 cases of regional recurrence in level V. The incidence of regional neck recurrence was the same regardless of whether comprehensive level V dissection was performed (8% vs 9% at 5 years, p = 0.89). The only statistically significant predictors for lateral neck recurrence on univariate analysis were total number of suspicious nodes on preoperative imaging, largest positive node on initial neck dissection, and whether patients received EBRT. On multivariate analysis, there remained no statistically significant difference in recurrence between the groups after accounting for the clinicopathologic variables associated with recurrence between the cohorts.

Patients were not randomized in our study to the type of neck dissection performed, which may represent a significant confounding factor. Although neck disease in level Vb on radiographic imaging is a clear indication for comprehensive level Vb dissection, the decision to perform this type of neck dissection at our center is not solely based on this finding alone. Other factors that guide the extent of neck dissection include the volume of disease (i.e. number of nodes and size of nodes), as well as location of the positive nodes outside of level Vb. This explains why 81% of the comprehensive cases in our series did not have level V disease on pre-operative imaging, and why the comprehensive group had larger pathological nodes on preoperative imaging (2.4 cm vs. 1.6 cm, p < 0.01), more total nodes on imaging (3.6 vs. 2.6, p = 0.03), and more positive nodes on the pathology specimen (6.7 vs. 5.2, p < 0.05). There were 4 patients who received selective neck dissection only but also had level V involvement on pre-operative imaging, which did not fit with our treatment philosophy. Two of these patients developed recurrence in the lateral neck. Since we reviewed the imaging retrospectively, it is possible that the level V involvement was originally missed at the time of surgery. The surgeons at the time may also have elected to perform an incomplete rather than comprehensive level V dissection with the plan to resect the nodal metastases from an anterior approach. Due to the retrospective nature of our study, we were also unable to determine TNM stage and histologic variants of PTC on all the patients, as some patients were referred for management of their neck with prior thyroidectomy performed at an outside center.

In our series, level V failure in the selective dissection patients only occurred in 5 out of 110 dissections (4.5%). This rate is lower than would be expected based on the literature, and there are several potential explanations for this difference. Firstly, some patients in our selective cohort may have benefited from a partial level V dissection, as the surgeons in this series frequently remove nodes in the anterior portion of level V during a selective neck dissection. Much of level Vb can be approached through an anterior approach as part of a "selective neck dissection". Secondly, almost all patients in our study received adjuvant RAI as recommended in the ATA guidelines for all patients with clinical neck metastases (intermediate risk), which may reduce the rate of lateral neck recurrence in cases of microscopic nodal disease. In our series, we did not record whether the nodal metastases were microscopic or macroscopic. Micrometastatic disease may not significantly impact regional recurrence rates, independent of RAI use [10, 11].

Comprehensive level Vb neck dissection may place the spinal accessory nerve at greater risk of injury, as surgeons must dissect it from the nodal tissue of the posterior neck up to its entry into the anterior border of trapezius. Temporary or permanent injury to the nerve can occur from traction, devascularization or microtrauma and will result in shoulder-related disability characterized by shoulder droop, winged scapula, inability to shrug and dull non-localizing pain exacerbated by shoulder movement [12, 13]. We were not able to collect any data regarding shoulder morbidity in our study. However, we know from the existing literature that significant shoulder disability after comprehensive neck dissection including levels IIb and V will occur in up to 40% of patients, although much of this may be temporary [6]. Selective neck dissection, on the other hand, is associated with minimal shoulder morbidity, with patients exhibiting less shoulder impairment and fewer activity limitations when compared to comprehensive or radical neck dissections [6]. Additionally, extensive supraclavicular nodal dissection may result in increased rates of chylous fistula or seroma, and may put the brachial plexus and phrenic nerves at greater risk. If formal level Vb dissection does not improve regional recurrence rates, the surgeon would potentially avoid these additional morbidities by performing a selective, rather than comprehensive, lateral neck dissection.

Conclusion

For PTC patients presenting with lateral neck metastases, a comprehensive level V dissection did not appear to reduce the rate of lateral neck recurrence over time. A selective neck dissection strategy to remove only the levels with suspicious nodes on preoperative CT appeared to be equally effective. Selection bias within this study limits our ability to draw definitive conclusions regarding differences in regional recurrence between selective and comprehensive neck dissection.

Abbreviations
CT: Computerized tomography; EBRT: External beam radiotherapy; ECE: Extracapsular extension; PTC: Papillary thyroid cancer; RAI: Radioactive iodine

Acknowledgements
Wei Xu and Susie Su for lending their expertise on statistical analysis.

Funding
None.

Authors' contributions
JX contributed to study design, data collection, interpretation of results and drafting of the manuscript. EY provided the radiological interpretation. DG created the study design, performed data collection and interpretation of results. CM, JP, JB, RT, HZ, AE, LR, AS, RG, JI, PG, DB, JdA contributed to interpretation of results and manuscript writing. All authors read and approved the final manuscript.

Competing interests
None.

Author details
[1]Department of Otolaryngology—Head and Neck Surgery, University Health Network, University of Toronto, Toronto, Ontario, Canada. [2]Department of Medical Imaging, University Health Network, University of Toronto, Toronto, Ontario, Canada. [3]Department of Surgery, Division of General Surgery, University Health Network, University of Toronto, Toronto, Ontario, Canada. [4]Department of Radiation Oncology, University Health Network, University of Toronto, Toronto, Ontario, Canada. [5]Department of Medicine, Division of Endocrinology, University Health Network University of Toronto, Toronto, Ontario, Canada.

References
1. Stack BC, Ferris RL, Goldenberg D, et al. American thyroid association consensus review and statement regarding the anatomy, terminology, and rationale for lateral neck dissection in differentiated thyroid cancer. Thyroid. 2012;22(5):501–8. doi:10.1089/thy.2011.0312.
2. Haugen BR, Alexander EK, Bible KC, et al. 2015 American thyroid association management guidelines for adult patients with thyroid nodules and differentiated thyroid cancer. Thyroid. 2015;26(1):1. doi:10.1089/thy.2015.0020.
3. Eskander A, Merdad M, Freeman JL, Witterick IJ. Pattern of spread to the lateral neck in metastatic well-differentiated thyroid cancer: a systematic review and meta-analysis. Thyroid. 2013;23(5):583–92. doi:10.1089/thy.2012.0493.
4. Zhang X-J, Liu D, Xu D-B, Mu Y-Q, Chen W-K. Should level V be included in lateral neck dissection in treating papillary thyroid carcinoma? World J Surg Oncol. 2013;11:304. doi:10.1186/1477-7819-11-304.

5. Farrag T, Lin F, Brownlee N, Kim M, Sheth S, Tufano RP. Is routine dissection of level II-B and V-A necessary in patients with papillary thyroid cancer undergoing lateral neck dissection for FNA-confirmed metastases in other levels. World J Surg. 2009;33(8):1680–3. doi:10.1007/s00268-009-0071-x.

6. Goldstein DP, Ringash J, Bissada E, et al. Scoping review of the literature on shoulder impairments and disability after neck dissection. Head Neck. 2014; 36(2):299–308. doi:10.1002/hed.23243.

7. Caron NR, Tan YY, Ogilvie JB, et al. Selective modified radical neck dissection for papillary thyroid cancer-is level I, II and V dissection always necessary? World J Surg. 2006;30(5):833–40. doi:10.1007/s00268-005-0358-5.

8. Yu W-B, Tao S-Y, Zhang N-S. Is level V dissection necessary for low-risk patients with papillary thyroid cancer metastasis in lateral neck levels II, III, and IV. Asian Pac J Cancer Prev. 2012;13(9):4619–22.

9. Javid M, Graham E, Malinowski J, et al. Dissection of levels II through v is required for optimal outcomes in patients with lateral neck lymph node metastasis from papillary thyroid carcinoma. J Am Coll Surg. 2016;222(6): 1066–73. doi:10.1016/j.jamcollsurg.2016.02.006.

10. Bardet S, Ciappuccini R, Quak E, et al. Prognostic value of microscopic lymph node involvement in patients with papillary thyroid cancer. J Clin Endocrinol Metab. 2015;100(1):132–40. doi:10.1210/jc.2014-1199.

11. Randolph GW, Duh Q-Y, Heller KS, et al. The prognostic significance of nodal metastases from papillary thyroid carcinoma can be stratified based on the size and number of metastatic lymph nodes, as well as the presence of extranodal extension. Thyroid. 2012;22(11):1144–52. doi:10.1089/thy.2012.0043.

12. Nahum AM, Mullally W, Marmor L. A syndrome resulting from radical neck dissection. Arch Otolaryngol. 1961;74:424–8.

13. Guo C, Zhang Y, Zhang L, Zou L. Surgical anatomy and preservation of the accessory nerve in radical functional neck dissection. Zhonghua Kou Qiang Yi Xue Za Zhi. 2003;38(1):12–5.

11

Surgical site infections following oral cavity cancer resection and reconstruction is a risk factor for plate exposure

Christopher M. Yao, Hedyeh Ziai, Gordon Tsang, Andrea Copeland, Dale Brown, Jonathan C. Irish, Ralph W. Gilbert, David P. Goldstein, Patrick J. Gullane and John R. de Almeida[*]

Abstract

Background: Plate-related complications following head and neck cancer ablation and reconstruction remains a challenging problem often requiring further management and reconstructive surgeries. We aim to identify an association between surgical site infections (SSI) and plate exposure.

Methods: A retrospective study between 1997 and 2014 was performed to study the association between postoperative SSI and plate exposures. Eligible patients included those with a history of oral squamous cell carcinoma who underwent surgical resection, neck dissection, and free tissue reconstruction. Demographic and treatment related information was collected. SSI were classified based on CDC definition and previously published literature. Univariable analysis on demographic factors, smoking history, diabetes, radiation, surgical and hardware related factors; while multivariable analysis on SSI, plate height, segmental mandibulectomy defects and radiation were conducted such as using cox proportional hazard models.

Results: Three hundred sixty-five patients were identified and included in our study. The mean age of the study group was 59.2 (+/−13.8), with a predominance of male patients (61.9%). 10.7% of our patient cohort had diabetes, and another 63.8% had post-operative radiation therapy. Patients with SSI were more likely to have plate exposure (25 vs. 6.4%, $p < 0.001$). Post-operative SSI, mandibulectomy defects, and plate profile/thickness were associated with plate exposure on univariable analysis (OR = 5.72, $p < 0.001$; OR = 2.56, $p = 0.014$; OR = 1.44, $p = 0.003$ respectively) and multivariable analysis (OR = 5.13, $p < 0.001$; OR = 1.36, $p = 0.017$; OR = 2.58, $p = 0.02$ respectively).

Conclusion: Surgical site infections are associated with higher rates of plate exposure. Plate exposure may require multiple procedures to manage and occasionally free flap reconstruction.

Keywords: Surgical Site Infections, Plate-related Complications, Head and neck cancer, Plate exposure, Plate height, Mandibular reconstruction

Background

Instrumentation with titanium plates is often required following ablative surgery for oral cancer. These plates are typically used for patients who require instrumentation for the surgical approach (e.g. mandibulotomy) or for reconstruction of mandibular defects. Plate-related complications may occur in up to 0–45% of cases, and may include plate exposure (4–46%), loose screws (0.8–5.8%), or plate fractures (0–3.3%) [1–16]. These complications may result in significant health care burden such as prolonged antibiotic therapy, revision surgery and impact patients' quality of life.

Surgical site infections (SSIs) following head and neck cancer surgery may occur in as many as 10–45% of cases despite antibiotic prophylaxis [17–24]. SSIs have been defined by the Center for Disease Control and Prevention (CDC) as infection within the first 30 postoperative days with at least one of several factors, including purulent drainage, positive culture, and either a deliberate incision and drainage or presence of supporting signs and

* Correspondence: john.dealmeida@uhn.ca
Department of Otolaryngology-Head and Neck Surgery/Surgical Oncology, Princess Margaret Cancer Centre, University Health Network, 610 University Avenue, 3-955, Toronto, ON M5G 2 M9, Canada

symptoms [25]. The development of SSIs can further lead to serious complications including wound breakdown, mucocutaneous fistulae, sepsis, and death. Delayed wound healing may also result in a poor cosmetic outcome, delayed oral intake and a delay in adjuvant therapies.

Several factors have been previously shown to be associated with the development of plate-related complications including plate related factors (plate material, plate profile, type and size of screws) [2, 4, 5], patient factors (smoking, diabetes, previous radiation, previous hyperbaric oxygen) [8, 9], and surgical defect [7, 10, 15]. We hypothesize that SSIs may result in colonization of the alloplastic plate and result in subsequent plate exposure. The present study aims to understand the relationship between post-operative surgical site infections and plate-related complications.

Methods

Approval from the institutional review ethics board of the University Health Network was obtained. All patients 18 years or older who underwent an oral cavity resection and neck dissection for squamous cell carcinoma, requiring either a mandibulotomy or mandibulectomy with free flap reconstruction and osseous plating performed at the University Health Network in Toronto, Canada between 1997 and 2014 were identified. Eligible patients were identified using a pre-existing oral cavity database based off of the Cancer Registry from Princess Margaret Cancer Centre. Electronic medical records were reviewed to confirm candidacy. Patients who were treated with transoral approaches (i.e. no hardware used), or those requiring surgical management of osteoradionecrosis, and those with incomplete documentation of follow-up postoperative care were excluded.

All included patients received antimicrobial prophylaxis with cephalosporins (or clindamycin, if patient was documented with a penicillin allergy), and flagyl starting 30–60 min prior to incision and continuing for at least 24 h after surgery, although practices varied by practitioner. Surgical sites were sterilized prior to initial incision with either povidone-iodine or chlorhexidine.

Clinical information was ascertained from the electronic medical record, and paper charts for the early study period. Patient demographic information and comorbidities, treatment details, pathologic features, and oncologic outcomes were recorded. Postoperative wound infections were defined according to the Centers for Disease Control and Prevention (CDC) National Nosocomial Infections Surveillance (NNIS) system for superficial and deep incisional SSI, by criteria for post-operative wound infection following head and neck cancer surgery as described by Grandis et. al; and further included the development of an orocutaneous fistula in the presence of other infectious signs and symptoms (Table 1) [17, 25]. Distant infections

Table 1 Criteria for Surgical Site Infection

CDC Guidelines	Grandis et al. 1992 [17]
Superficial SSI: Infection within 30 days of the operation Involving Skin and Subcutaneous tissue of the incision	Presence of fever, elevated leukocyte count, appearance of wound, institution of antimicrobial therapy
At least one of: a. Purulent drainage from the incision b. Organisms identified by aseptically obtained sample c. Incision is deliberately opened by a physician AND patient has at least one of the following: pain, localized swelling, erythema or heat d. Diagnosis of SSI by physician	
The following are not included: a. Stitch abscess alone b. The diagnosis and treatment of cellulitis (erythema, warmth, swelling) alone does not meet criteria	
Deep SSI: Infection within 30–90 days of the operation Involves the deeper soft tissues of the incision	
At least one of: a. Purulent drainage b. Deep incision with spontaneous dehiscence, or is deliberately opened by surgeon and organism is cultured and patient has at least one of the following signs and symptoms: fever, localized pain, and tenderness. c. Abscess, or radiological evidence of an infection.	

such as pneumonia, or urinary tract infections were not captured in our study. Post-operative clinical notes were reviewed, and data pertaining to fevers, white count, differential, cultures, use of antibiotics, procedures including surgical debridement or incision and drainage at the bedside or in the operating room, presence of hematoma or hemorrhage were extracted. Furthermore, plate related characteristics including plate thickness, use of rescue screws, and use of locking screws were recorded. Surgical defects were categorized according to the bony and soft tissue defect. Bony defects were categorized as segmental or non-segmental mandibulectomy defects. Soft tissue defects were considered adverse if the defect involved the external skin, lip, buccal mucosa, mandibular alveolus, or retromolar trigone; sites where soft tissue resection places patients at a higher risk for plate related complications such as plate exposure. Other early post-operative wound related complications such as wound dehiscence, or flap compromise were also collected. Plate related complications (plate exposure, plate fracture) over the course of clinical follow-up were identified from clinical and operative notes. Loose screws were not captured in this study.

Patient demographic, treatment, and pathologic data were summarized using descriptive statistics. Univariable analysis determining the association between wound infection and plate-related complication was performed using cox proportional hazard ratios. Multivariable analyses using cox regression analysis was performed to account for the impact of other variables including plate height, segmental mandibulectomy defects, post-operative infection, and post-operative radiation.

Results

A total of 365 patients meeting our study criteria were identified. The mean age of the study group was 59.2 (+/-13.8), with more males (61.9%) than females (38.1%) (Table 2). A hundred and two patients (27.9%) were actively smoking at the time of diagnosis, 111 (30.4%) had a history of smoking, and some never having smoked (36.7%). Only 10.7% of our patient cohort had diabetes, and another 63.8% had post-operative radiation therapy. Patients were reconstructed with either osseous-cutaneous free flaps (58.0%), or soft-tissue free flaps (39.2%), with one patient reconstructed using a pectoralis major (0.3%). Eighty-four patients (23.0%) developed surgical site infections within 30 days of their operation. The most common SSI formed were neck abscesses (11.5%), and orocutaneous fistulae (10%). Patient were followed for an average of 25.2 months.

There were 39 (10.7%) patients who developed plate exposure post-operatively. There were no plate fractures in our population. Patients who developed post-operative SSI were more likely to develop subsequent plate exposure (25 vs. 6.4%, p <0.001). Univariable analysis performed on potential risk factors using Cox hazard ratio revealed post-operative infection (HR = 5.72, 95% CI = 3.04 – 10.80, p < 0.001), segmental mandibulectomy (HR = 2.56, 95% CI = 1.21 – 5.39, p = 0.014), and plate height (HR = 1.43, 95% CI = 1.13 – 1.82, p = 0.003) to be significantly associated with increased rates of plate exposures (Table 3). Patient characteristics such as age, sex, diabetes, post-operative radiation and smoking were not significantly associated. Other plate-related factors including use of rescue screw and locking screw; as well as adverse soft tissue defects were also not significantly associated.

In multivariable analyses (Table 4), plate height, segmental mandibulectomy defects, SSI and post-operative radiation were included. SSI (HR = 5.13, 95% CI = 2.70 – 9.77, p <0.001), segmental mandibulectomy defects (HR = 2.58, 95% CI = 1.16 – 5.76, p = 0.020), and plate height (HR = 1.36, 95% CI = 1.06 –1.75, p = 0.017) were significantly associated with plate exposures in a Cox regression analysis. Post-operative radiation was not statistically associated with rates of plate exposure.

The overall Kaplan-Meier curves for SSI and rates of plate exposure are displayed in Fig. 1. The 5-year probability of plate exposure free survival is 61.05 vs. 91.75%, (p <0.001) for patients with and without SSIs, respectively, as compared using the log-ranked test.

Majority of patients who developed plate exposure were initially reconstructed with bony osseous free flaps (74.4%) (Table 5). The overall mean time to plate exposure was 15.1 months. 59.0% of plate exposures occurred intra-orally, with 38.5% occurring externally, and 2.5% not documented. Plate exposures occurred intra-orally at a median time of 5.7 months compared with external plate exposures, which occurred at a median of 29.8 months. Twelve patients (30.7%) had concurrent bony concerns, with seven (17.9%) demonstrating non-union and five (12.8%) with concurrent bone exposure. No patients developed plate fractures in our study.

Management of these plate exposures included conservative approaches (11 patients, 28.3%), revision operations with plate removal and debridement of sequestra (9 patients, 23.1%), revision operations with plate removal and local flap (6 patients 15.3%), or revision operations with plate removal and free flap (13 patients, 33.3%) (Table 5). Of the patients managed with a free flap, 6 patients received a fibular free flap (46.2%), 4 patients received an anterolateral thigh free flap (30.8%), 2 received a radial forearm free flap (15.4%), and one received an unknown free flap (7.6%). Seven of these patients (17.9%) were re-plated after removal of the exposed plate. During the follow-up of these patients, another 7 patients (17.9%) required multiple procedures.

Discussion

In the present study we showed a strong association between SSIs and plate-related complications. As no patient in our population had plate fractures, we focused on plate exposures. Plate profile as well as segmental mandibular defects reconstructed with osseous free flaps are also associated with plate exposures. The rates of post-operative SSI and plate exposures in the present study are corroborated by previous studies (26.8% compared with 22–46% [19, 24, 26, 27] and 12.3% compared with 4–46% [1–16]). To date, however, our study is the first that demonstrates an association between SSI and plate exposures.

There are several factors that have previously been established that are associated with plate complications. In the present study, we chose a homogenous population of patients with oral cavity squamous cell carcinoma. This patient population is associated with risk factors such as smoking that in and of themselves may predispose patients to impaired healing and subsequent plate complications [28]. Other non-surgical factors such as diabetes has been shown to significantly predict plate complications [9]. In our population, commonly held non-surgical risk factors for plate-related complications including smoking, diabetes, pre-operative or post-operative

Table 2 Demographics and patient characteristics of 365 patients

	Overall (365)	Infection (84)	No Infection (281)	P-Value
Age	59.2 (18.5 – 93.0)	59.5 (+/− 13.7)	59.1 (+/− 13.0)	0.853
Missing	0			
Sex				
M	226 (61.9%)	50 (59.5%)	176 (62.6%)	0.611
F	139 (38.1%)	34 (40.5%)	105 (37.4%)	
Missing	0			
Smoking				
non-smoker	134 (36.7%)	25 (29.8%)	109 (38.8%)	0.272
Ex-smoker	111 (30.4%)	32 (38.1%)	79 (28.1%)	
Active smoker	102 (27.9%)	22 (26.2%)	80 (28.5%)	
Missing	18 (4.9%)	5 (8.3%)	13 (4.6%)	
T2DM				
yes	39 (10.7%)	10 (11.9%)	29 (10.3%)	0.794
no	325 (89.0%)	74 (88.1%)	251 (89.3%)	
missing	1 (0.3%)	0	1 (0.4%)	
Plate Factors:				
Plate Size				
10 mm	10 (2.6%)	5 (5.5%)	5 (1.7%)	0.031
15 mm	279 (72.7%)	67 (73.6%)	212 (72.4%)	
20 mm	6 (1.6%)	2 (2.2%)	4 (1.4%)	
24 mm	16 (4.2%)	7(7.7%)	9 (3.1%)	
28 mm	14 (3.6%)	1(1.1%)	13 (4.4%)	
missing	59 (15.4%)	9 (9.9%)	50 (17.1%)	
Post-op Rads				
yes	233 (63.8%)	49 (58.3%)	184 (65.5%)	0.005
no	129 (35.3%)	32 (38.1%)	97 (34.5%)	
Missing	3 (0.8%)	3 (3.6%)		
Screws				
Locking	62 (17.0%)	9 (10.7%)	53 (18.9%)	0.106
Non-locking	247 (67.7%)	66 (78.6%)	181 (64.4%)	
Missing	56 (15.3%)	9 (10.7%)	47 (16.7%)	
Rescues	76 (20.8%)	18 (21.4%)	58 (20.6%)	0.618
Non-rescue	234 (64.1%)	57 (67.9%)	177 (63.0%)	
Missing	55 (15.1%)	9 (10.7%)	46 (16.4%)	
Surgical Defect:				
Soft Tissue:				
adverse[a]	179 (49.0%)	45 (53.6%)	135 (48.0%)	0.162
non-adverse	180 (49.3%)	36 (42.9%)	143 (50.9%)	
missing	6 (1.7%)	3 (3.5%)	3 (1.1%)	
Segmental Mandibulectomy Defect:				
Yes	212 (58.1%)	44 (52.4%)	168 (59.8%)	0.482
No	149 (40.8%)	39 (46.4%)	110 (39.1%)	
missing	4 (1.1%)	1 (1.2%)	3 (1.1%)	

Table 2 Demographics and patient characteristics of 365 patients *(Continued)*

Flaps				
Osseous +/− cutaneous	212 (58.0%)	40 (47.6%)	172 (61.2%)	0.426
Soft Tissue	143 (39.2%)	41 (48.8%)	102 (36.3%)	
Local Regional	1 (0.3%)	1 (1.2%)	0 (0.0%)	
Missing	9 (2.5%)	2 (2.4%)	7 (2.5%)	
Follow-up time (Median)	25.2 months	11.1 +/− 27.6 months	30.84 +/− 31.3 months	0.005
Plate Exposure				
yes	39 (10.7%)	21 (25.0%)	18 (6.4%)	<0.001
no	324 (88.8%)	63(75.0%)	261 (92.9%)	
missing	2 (0.5%)		2 (0.7%)	

aAdverse soft-tissue defects refer to surgical defects involving the retromolar trigone, buccal mucosa, mandibular alveolus, lip, and external skin

radiation, and chemotherapy, were not significantly associated with plate-exposures. Despite not being found to be independently significant for plate exposure, the significance of these risk factors cannot be overlooked given the well-established biological processes whereby these factors can impair wound healing [29–31].

Herein we describe a strong association between SSIs and plate exposures. Infections of the head and neck following ablative surgery may lead to bacterial colonization of plates, resulting in biofilm formation, wound contamination and subsequent plate exposure requiring hardware removal to eliminate the nidus of infection [32]. Durand et al. recently reviewed their experience of SSIs following head and neck free reconstructive surgeries reporting 25% of their swabs growing normal oral flora, 44% gram-negative bacilli, 20% methicillin-resistant *Staphylococcus aureus* and 16% methicillin-sensitive *Staphylococcus aureus* [33]. The authors found that in 67% of cultures, at least one pathogen was found to be resistant to prophylactic antibiotics. These infections that are often difficult to treat corroborate our finding that surgical site infections may lead to plate exposure as they are often recalcitrant to antimicrobial therapy.

Other studies focusing on the pathophysiology of plate exposures have previously suggested both plate material and plate profile to be potential predictors [1, 2, 4]. Although multiple studies have found no significant difference between stainless steel and titanium plates in complication rates, when lower profile plates were used, plate exposure rates were found to decrease from 20 to 4% [34, 35]. These studies corroborate our finding that higher profile plates were associated with increased plate exposure in both univariable and multivariable analysis.

Surgical defect size is another potential confounding factor that may be related to plate related complications. We showed that patients with segmental mandibulectomy defects are more likely to develop plate exposures. Although there are several existing classifications schemes for the reconstruction of mandibular defects that further categorize mandibulectomy defects, we chose to dichotomize this variable as the primary outcome was the association of infections with plate exposures [36–39].

Adequate reconstruction after ablative surgery with sufficient soft tissue restoration is critical in avoiding plate exposures. For patients with mandibulectomy defects, reconstruction with vascularized bone is imperative for anterior segmental defects to avoid an "Andy Gump" deformity while for patients with lateral defects some groups propose a soft tissue reconstruction with or without a plate as an alternative to vascularized bony reconstruction depending on overall disease prognosis, age, dentition, and comorbid status [15, 16, 40, 41]. Furthermore, with larger soft tissue defects, osseocutaneous flaps may not have adequate associated soft tissue components, and two free tissue transfers may be required to optimize the reconstruction, adding to both surgical time and complexity [41]. Whichever reconstruction method is chosen, if insufficient bone and soft tissue were used to reconstruct the defect, wound contracture and steady pressure of the plate against the skin may lead to eventual plate exposure [14]. In one study, over-reconstructing medial soft tissue aspects and obliterating dead space resulted in a reduction of plate exposures from 38 to 8% even in patients reconstructed with lateral defects with a plate and soft tissue [41]. The site of mandibulectomy defect was at one point considered an important factor in eventual plate exposure, with mandibulectomy defects involving the central mandible found to have higher rates of plate exposure [7]. With improved microvascular reconstructive techniques, however, the site of the mandibulectomy defect was not found to be a significant predictor of plate exposure [5, 8, 9]. Overall, studies have found lower rates of plate exposure in patients with mandibulotomies (0–15%) [42–45]. In the present study, we showed decreased plate exposure with mandibulotomies compared to those with mandibulectomy defects. This is likely due to the length of the plate in addition to the associated soft tissue defects.

Table 3 Univariate Analysis using Cox-Regression Analysis

Variable	Proportion of post-op exposure		Hazard ratio	95% CI	P-Value
	Exposure	No exposure			
Age					
<60 years	15 (4.1%)	145 (39.7%)	1.43	0.75 – 2.74	0.274
>60 years	24 (6.6%)	181 (49.6%)			
Sex					
male	27 (7.4%)	199 (54.5%)	0.674	0.341 – 1.331	0.255
female	12 (3.3%)	127 (34.8%)			
T2DM					
yes	4 (1.1%)	35 (9.6%)	1.051	0.373 – 2.957	0.925
no	35 (9.6%)	290 (79.5%)			
missing		1 (0.2%)			
Smoking					
active smoker	11 (3.0%)	91 (24.9%)	0.986	0.668 – 1.456	0.943
ex-smoker	12 (3.2%)	99 (27.1%)			
non-smoker	15 (4.1%)	119 (32.6%)			
missing	1 (0.2%)	17 (4.9%)			
Adj radiotherapy					
yes	28 (7.7%)	205 (56.2%)	1.461	0.727 – 2.940	0.287
no	11 (3.0%)	121 (33.1%)			
Use of rescue screw					
yes	14 (35.9%)	62 (19.0%)	1.132	0.849 – 1.510	0.398
no	24 (61.5%)	210 (64.4%)			
missing	1 (2.6%)	54 (16.6%)			
Use of locking screw					
yes	10 (25.6%)	52 (16.0%)	1.06	0.731 – 1.528	0.767
no	28 (71.8%)	219 (67.2%)			
missing	1 (2.6%)	55 (16.9%)			
Segmental Mandibulectomy					
yes	30 (76.9%)	182 (55.8%)	2.556	1.212 – 5.391	0.014
no	9 (23.1%)	140 (43.0%)			
missing		4 (1.2%)			
Adverse Soft Tissue					
yes	20 (51.3%)	159 (48.8%)	1.312	0.671 – 2.565	0.427
no	15 (38.5%)	165 (50.6%)			
missing	4 (10.2%)	2 (0.6%)			
Plate Height					
10 mm	3 (7.7%)	7 (2.1%)	1.436	1.131 – 1.824	0.003
15 mm	25 (64.1%)	236 (72.4%)			
20 mm	1 (2.6%)	5 (1.5%)			
24 mm	3 (7.7%)	12 (3.7%)			
28 mm	6 (15.3%)	8 (2.5%)			
missing	1 (2.6%)	58 (17.8%)			
Post-op Infection					
yes	21 (5.8%)	63 (17.2%)	5.72	3.04 – 10.80	<0.001
no	18 (4.9%)	263(72.1%)			

Table 4 Multivariate Analysis using Cox Regression Survival Analysis

Variables	Hazard radio	95% CI	P-Value
Post-op Infection	5.13	2.70 - 9.77	0.000
Segmental Mandibulectomy	2.58	1.16 – 5.76	0.020
Plate Height	1.36	1.06 – 1.75	0.017
Post-op Rads	1.02	0.47 – 2.13	0.996

Plate exposures continue to be the most common plate-related complication in mandibular reconstructive surgery [1–16]. Although in some instances managed conservatively, many plate exposures affect patient quality-of-life and plate removal with secondary reconstruction is occasionally necessary [3]. In our study, several patients required plate removal with secondary reconstruction. In addition, some patients develop recurrent plate exposures, suggesting that there may be systemic factors leading to poor wound healing.

Plate exposures can be classified as intra-oral or extra-oral. Nicholsen et al. noted a pattern where extra-oral plate exposure occurred at a mean of ten months post-operatively, while intra-oral plate exposure occurred at a mean of six weeks – three months [7]. This pattern was also seen in our population, with intraoral exposures occurring earlier than external exposures. Given the difference in timing, it is conceivable that the pathophysiology may differ between these two entities. Although there is little evidence to support this, we hypothesize that intraoral exposures are secondary to wound breakdown and salivary contamination whereas external exposure is likely related to longstanding pressure necrosis of the surrounding soft tissues although wound infection is still a contributing factor as we have seen in the present study.

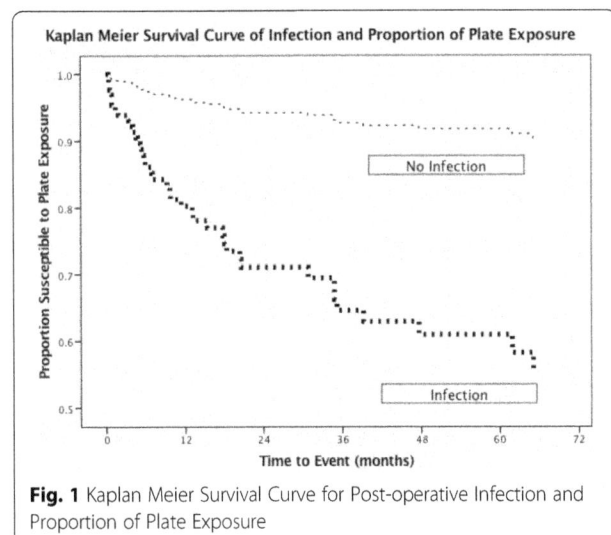

Fig. 1 Kaplan Meier Survival Curve for Post-operative Infection and Proportion of Plate Exposure

Table 5 Management of 39 patients with plate exposure

Original Flap Utilized	
Fibular Flap	25 (64.1%)
Radial Forearm Free Flap	7 (17.9%)
Anterolateral Thigh Flap	3 (7.7%)
Scapular Free Flap	4 (10.3%)
Post-operative Issues:	
flap failures (24 h take-back)	3 (7.7%)
infection	19 (48.7%)
hematoma	1 (2.6%)
Post-op Radiation:	
yes	26 (66.7%)
no	13 (33.3%)
Time to Plate Exposure:	
mean	15.1 months (0.4 – 120.8)
median	9.24 months
Exposure Location:	
intraoral	23 (59.0%)
external	15 (38.5%)
unknown	1 (2.5%)
Mean Time to Plate Exposure by Location:	
Internal	13.6 +/– 10.4 months　　p = 0.012*
External	42.3 +/– 18.0 months
Concurrent Bony Concerns:	
non-union	7 (17.9%)
bone exposure	5 (12.8%)
Management:	
Conservative	11 (28.3%) (1 palliative, 1 complete closure, ongoing monitoring)
OR Plate Removal/Debridement	9 (23.1%)
OR Plate removal + Local Flap	6 (15.3%)
OR Plate Removal + Free Flap	13 (33.3%)
Outcomes:	
Multiple Revision	7 (17.9%)
Chronic Drainage	1 (2.6%)
Recurrence	2 (5.1%)
Deceased	3 (7.7%)

*calculated using student t-test

Our study had several limitations. It is limited by a retrospective design albeit the findings of the association between SSI and plate exposure are strongly significant. Furthermore, some definitions used were subjective such as the definition of an adverse soft tissue defect. Furthermore, given the retrospective design, we were unable to study the volume of tissue extirpated and the volume of tissue reconstructive, both of which have implications on the development of plate exposures. Lastly the scope of our study did not capture several important outcome measures such as the impact of plate exposure on mastication, swallowing, speech, and quality of life. Future studies may address some of these issues.

Conclusions

Mandibular reconstruction remains a challenging task for the head and neck reconstructive surgeon. Numerous factors including the defect size, location of the defect, and presence of wound healing compromising conditions must be judiciously reviewed and considered to prevent plate-related complications. SSIs may portend a greater risk towards the development of plate exposure, as does plate height and adverse bony defects. Plate exposure may require multiple procedures to manage and occasionally free flap reconstruction.

Abbreviations

CDC: Centers for disease control and prevention; NNIS: National nosocomial infections surveillance; SSI: Surgical site infection

Acknowledgements
Not applicable

Funding
No sources of funding were sought for this study.

Authors' contributions

CY carried out the study design, data acquisition, coordination, data analysis and manuscript preparation. HZ, GT, and AC were involved with the data acquisition. JD conceived the study design, and was involved with the data analysis. All authors read and approved the final manuscript.

Competing interests

The authors declare that there are no competing interests.

References

1. Futran ND, Urken ML, Buchbinder D, Moscoso JF, Biller HF. Rigid fixation of vascularized grafts in mandibular reconstruction. Arch Otolaryngol Head Neck Surg. 1995;121(1):70–6.
2. Klotch DW, Gal TJ, Gal RL. Assessment of plate use for mandibular reconstruction: has changing technology made a difference? Otolaryngol Head Neck Surg. 1999;121(4):388–92.
3. Wei FC, Celik N, Yang WG, Chen IH, et al. Complications after reconstruction by plate and soft-tissue free flap in composite mandibular defects and secondary salvage reconstruction with osteocutaneous flap. Plast Reconstr Surg. 2003;112(1):37–42.
4. Farwell DG, Kezirian EJ, Heydt JL, Yueh B, Futran ND. Efficacy of small reconstruction plates in vascularized bone graft mandibular reconstruction. Head Neck. 2006;28(7):573–79.
5. Knott PD, Suh JD, Nabili V, Sercarz JA, Head C, Abemayor E, Blackwell KE. Evaluation of hardware-related complications in vascularized bone grafts
6. with locking mandibular reconstruction plate fixation. Arch Otolaryngol Head Neck Surg. 2007;133(12):1302–6.
6. Zavattero E, Fasolis M, Garzino-Demo P, Berrone S, Ramieri GA. Evaluation of plate-related complications and efficacy of fibula free flap mandibular reconstruction. J Craniofac Surg. 2014;25:397–9.
7. Nicholson RE, Schuller DE, Forrest A, et al. Factors involved in long- and short-term mandibular plate exposure. Arch Otolaryngol Head Neck Surg. 1997;123:217–22.
8. Maurer P, Eckert AW, Kriwalsky MS, Schubert J. Scope and limitations of methods of mandibular reconstruction: a long-term follow-up. Br J Oral Maxillofac Surg. 2010;48(2):100–4.
9. van der Rijt EE, Noorlag R, Koole R, Abbink JH, Rosenberg AJ. Predictive factors for premature loss of Martin 2.7 mandibular reconstruction plates. Br J Oral Maxillofac Surg. 2015;53(2):121–5.
10. Deleyiannis FWB, Rogers C, Lee E, Russavage J, et al. Reconstruction of the lateral mandibulectomy defect: management based on prognosis and location and volume of soft tissue resection. Laryngoscope. 2006;116:2071–80.
11. Boyd JB. Use of reconstruction plates in conjunction with soft-tissue free flaps for oromandibular reconstruction. Clinic in Plast Surg. 1994;21:69–77.
12. Urken ML, Buchbinder D, Costantino PD, et al. Oromandibular reconstruction using microvascular composite flaps: report of 210 cases. Arch Otolaryngol Head Neck Surg. 1998;124:46–55.
13. Head C, Alam D, Sercarz JA, et al. Microvascular flap reconstruction of the mandible: a comparison of bone grafts and bridging plates for restoration of mandibular continuity. Otolaryngol Head Neck Surg. 2003;129:48–54.
14. Onoda S, Kimata Y, Yamada K, Sugiyama N, Onoda T, Eguchi M, Mizukawa N. Prevention points for plate exposure in the mandibular reconstruction. J Craniomaxillofac Surg. 2012;40:e310–14.
15. Arden RL, Rachel JD, Marks SC, et al. Volume-length impact of lateral jaw resections on complication rates. Arch Otolaryngol Head Neck Surg. 1999;125:68–72.
16. Mariani PB, Kowalski LP, Magrin J. Reconstruction of large defects postmandibulectomy for oral cancer using plates and myocutaneous flaps: a long-term follow-up. Int J Oral Maxillofac Surg. 2006;35:427–32.
17. Grandis JR, Snyderman CH, Johnson JT, Yu VL, D'Amico F. Postoperative wound infection – a poor prognostic sign for patients with head and neck cancer. Cancer. 1992;70:2166–70.
18. Girod DA, McCulloch TM, Tsue TT, Weymuller JREA. Risk factors for complications in clean-contaminated head and neck surgical procedures. Head Neck. 1995;17(1):7–13.
19. de Melo GM, Ribeiro KC, Kowalski LP, Deheinzelin D. Risk factors for postoperative complications in oral cancer and their prognostic implications. Arch Otolaryngol Head Neck Surg. 2001;127(7):828–33.
20. Penel N, Fournier C, Lefebvre D, Lefebve JL. Multivariate analysis of risk factors for wound infection in head and neck squamous cell carcinoma surgery with opening of mucosa. Study of 260 surgical procedures. Oral Oncol. 2005;41(3):294–303.
21. Simo R, French G. The use of prophylactic antibiotics in head and neck oncologic surgery. Curr Opin Otolaryngol Head Neck Surg. 2006;14:55–61.
22. Lotfi CJ, Cavalcanti Rde C, Silva AM C e, Latorre Mdo R, et al. Risk factors for surgical-site infections in head and neck cancer surgery. Otolaryngol Head Neck Surg. 2008;138(1):74–80.
23. Ogihara H, Akeuchi K, Majima Y. Risk factors of postoperative infection in head and neck surgery. Auris Nasus Larynx. 2009;36(4):457–60.
24. Lee DH, Kim SY, Nam SY, Choi SH, Choi JW, Roh JL. Risk factors of surgical site infection in patients undergoing major oncological surgery for head and neck cancer. Oral Oncol. 2011;47:528–31.
25. Horan TC, Gaynes RP, Martone WJ, Jarvis WR, Emori TG. CDC definitions of nosocomial surgical site infections, 1992: a modification of CDC definitions of surgical wound infections. Am J Infect Control. 1992;20(5):271–4.
26. Mitchell RM, Mendez E, Schmitt NC, Bhrany AD, Futran ND. Antibiotic prophylaxis in patients undergoing head and neck free flap reconstruction. JAMA Otolaryngol Head Neck Surg. 2015;14(12):1096–103.
27. Yang CH, Chew KY, Solomkin JS, et al. Surgical site infections among high-risk patients in clean-contaminated head and neck reconstructive surgery. Ann Plast Surg. 2013;71:S55–60.
28. Shuman AG, Entezami P, Chernin AS, Wallace NE, Taylor JMG, Hogikyan ND. Demographics and efficacy of head and neck cancer screening. Otolaryngol Head Neck Surg. 2010;143(3):353–60.

29. Brem H, Tomic-Canic M. Cellular and molecular basis of wound healing in diabetes. J Clin Investig. 2007;117:1219–22.

30. Sorensen LT. Wound healing and infection in surgery: the pathophysiological impact of smoking, smoking cessation, and nicotine replacement therapy: a systematic review. Ann Surg. 2012;255:1069–79.

31. Haubner F, Ohmann E, Pohl F, Strutz J, Gassner HG. Wound healing after radiation therapy: review of the literature. Radiat Oncol. 2012;7:162–71.

32. Brady RA, Leid JG, Calhoun JH, William Costerton J, Shirtliff ME. Osteomyelitis and the role of biofilms in chronic infection. Pathog Dis. 2008;52:13–22.

33. Durand ML, Yarlagadda BB, Rich DL, Lin DT, Emerick KS, Rocco JW, Deschler DG. The time course and microbiology of surgical site infections after head neck free flap surgery. Laryngoscope. 2015;125:1084–9.

34. Blackwell KE, Buchbinder D, Urken ML. Lateral mandibular reconstruction using soft-tissue free flaps and plates. Arch Otolaryngol Head Neck Surg. 1996;122:672–8.

35. Blackwell KE, Lacombe V. The bridging lateral mandibular reconstruction plate revisited. Arch Otolaryngol Head Neck Surg. 1999;125:988–93.

36. Jewer DD, Boyd JB, Manktelow RT, Zuker RM, Rosen IB, Gullane PJ, et al. Orofacial and mandibular reconstruction with the iliac crest free flap: a review of 60 cases and a new method of classification. Plast Reconstr Surg. 1989;84:391–405.

37. Urken ML, Weinberg H, Vickery C, Buchbinder D, Lawson W, Biller HF. Oromandibular reconstruction using microvascular composite free flaps: report of 71 cases and a new classification scheme for bony, soft-tissue, and neurologic defects. Arch Otolaryngol Head Neck Surg. 1991;117:733–44.

38. Iizuka T, Häfl iger J, Seto I, Rahal A, Mericske-Stern R, Smolka K. Oral rehabilitation after mandibular reconstruction using an osteocutaneous fibula free flap with endosseous implants. Factors affecting the functional outcome in patients with oral cancer. Clin Oral Implants Res. 2005;16:69–79.

39. Brown JS, Barry C, Ho M, Shaw R. A new classification for mandibular defects after oncological resection. Lancet Oncol. 2016;17:e23–30.

40. Chim H, Salgado CJ, Mardini S, Chen HC. Reconstruction of mandibular defects. Semin Plast Surg. 2010;24:188–97.

41. Chepeha DB, Teknos TN, Fung K, et al. Lateral oromandibular defect: when is it appropriate to use a bridging reconstruction plate combined with a soft tissue revascularized flap? Head Neck. 2008;30:709–17.

42. Danan D, Mukherjee S, Jameson MJ, Shonkda Jr DC. Open reduction internal fixation for midline mandibulotomy: lag screws vs plates. JAMA Otolaryngol Head Neck Surg. 2014;140(12):1884–90.

43. Dubner S, Spiro RH. Median mandibulotomy: a critical assessment. Head Neck. 1991;13:389–93.

44. Amin MR, Deschler DG, Hayden RE. Straight midline mandibulotomy revisited. Laryngoscope. 1999;109(9):1402–5.

45. Shinghal T, Bissada E, Chan HB, Wood RE, Atenafu EG, Brown DH, Gilbert RW, Gullane PJ, Irish JC, Waldron J, Goldstein DP. Medial Mandibulotomies: Is there sufficient space in the midline to allow a mandibulotomy without compromising the dentition? J Otolaryngol Head Neck Surg. 2013;32(1):32.

12

Brief electrical stimulation and synkinesis after facial nerve crush injury

Adrian Mendez[1,3]*, Alex Hopkins[1], Vincent L. Biron[1], Hadi Seikaly[1], Lin Fu Zhu[2] and David W. J. Côté[1]

Abstract

Background: Recent studies have examined the effects of brief electrical stimulation (BES) on nerve regeneration, with some suggesting that BES accelerates facial nerve recovery. However, the facial nerve outcome measurement in these studies has not been precise or accurate. Furthermore, no previous studies have been able to demonstrate the effect of BES on synkinesis. The objective of this study is to examine the effect of brief electrical stimulation (BES) on facial nerve function and synkinesis in a rat model.

Methods: Four groups of six rats underwent a facial nerve injury procedure. Group 1 and 2 underwent a crush injury at the main trunk of the nerve, with group 2 additionally receiving BES for 1 h. Group 3 and 4 underwent a transection injury at the main trunk, with group 4 additionally receiving BES for 1 h. A laser curtain model was used to measure amplitude of whisking at 2, 4, and 6 weeks. Fluorogold and fluororuby neurotracers were additionally injected into each facial nerve to measure synkinesis. Buccal and marginal mandibular branches of the facial nerve were each injected with different neurotracers at 3 months following injury. Based on facial nucleus motoneuron labelling of untreated rats, comparison was made to post-treatment animals to deduce whether synkinesis had taken place. All animals underwent trans-cardiac perfusion with subsequent neural tissue sectioning.

Results: At week two, the amplitude observed for group 1 and 2 was 14.4 and 24.0 degrees, respectively ($p = 0.0004$). Group 4 also demonstrated improved whisking compared to group 3. Fluorescent neuroimaging labelling appear to confirm improved pathway specific regeneration with BES following facial nerve injury.

Conclusions: This is the first study to use an implantable stimulator for serial BES following a crush injury in a validated animal model. Results suggest performing BES after facial nerve injury is associated with accelerated facial nerve function and improved facial nerve specific pathway regeneration in a rat model.

Keywords: Synkinesis, Brief electrical stimulation, Facial nerve, Peripheral nerve regeneration, Regeneration, Peripheral nerve injury, Electrical stimulation

Background

Facial neuromuscular disorders and functional impairment resulting from facial nerve injury are common and can be severe [1]. Aesthetic impairments also impart an affliction leading to social isolation and further emotional distress. Together these can lead to depressive symptoms

and mental health issues, which further exacerbate their functional disabilities [2]. There are several clinical factors that have been identified that further impact recovery of peripheral nerve function following nerve injury including time to repair, type of repair, and the age of the patient [3].

Despite advances in microsurgical technique, functional recovery following facial nerve injury remains suboptimal [4]. Synkinesis, or axonal regeneration from the proximal stump into inappropriate distal pathways, has long been recognized as a significant contributing factor to poor functional recovery [5]. Previous studies have shown that electrical stimulation affects morphological and functional

* Correspondence: amendez@ualberta.ca
[1]Department of Surgery, Division of Otolaryngology – Head and Neck Surgery, University of Alberta, Edmonton, AB, Canada
[3]1E4 Walter C Mackenzie Centre, 8440-112 Street NW, Edmonton, AB T6G 2B7, Canada
Full list of author information is available at the end of the article

properties of neurons including nerve branching, rate and orientation of neurite growth, rapid sprouting, and guidance during axon regeneration [6, 7]. In 2010, Hadlock et al. studied the effect of electrical stimulation on the facial nerve in a rat model using a precise functional outcomes model capable of detecting micrometer movements of rat whisking [2]. The authors were able to demonstrate improvement in facial nerve functional outcome in the first 8 weeks. Similarly, in 2016 our research group published a study looking at the effect of BES on the transected facial nerve shortly after repair. We demonstrated improvement in facial nerve function with BES in the first 2 weeks after injury [8].

It has been hypothesized that the mechanism of action of BES is to induce preferential re-innervation of motor axons over sensory axons, and therefore improve overall function. In 2000, Gordon et al. examined the effect of electrical stimulation on regeneration after nerve transection in a rat sciatic nerve model [4]. The authors were able to demonstrate through retrograde labeling of sciatic nerve motoneurons with fluororuby (FR) and fluorogold (FG), that electrical stimulation dramatically accelerated both axonal regeneration as well as preferentially re-innervated motor nerves over sensory branches. The authors also found short-term, 1 h periods of stimulation were as effective as long-term stimulation lasting days to weeks [4].

Since then, the notion that brief electrical stimulation induces preferential re-innervation of motor axons over sensory axons has been extensively studied and is now well established. However, the effect of BES on reducing the random extension of specific motor axons collaterals to inappropriate distal motor axon branches such as in facial nerve synkinesis, is less clear.

Recently, research groups investigating peripheral nerve injury and regeneration have provided some insight into this question. Angelov and colleagues demonstrated that by using neutralizing antibodies to exogenous neurotrophic factors, including brain-derived neurotrophic factor (BDNF) and glial cell derived neurotrophic factor (GDNF), aberrant and redundant branching of regenerating axons in the facial nerve into inappropriate pathways could be reduced [9]. Furthermore, a separate research group demonstrated that BES is capable of regulation of BDNF expression in motoneurons [10]. Therefore, a possible mechanism of action of BES may be to reduce aberrant branching of regenerating motor axons following peripheral nerve injury by regulation BDNF expression in motoneurons. In regards to facial nerve injury and regeneration, this would potentially imply reduced synkinesis.

Furthermore, in 2005 Brushart et al. demonstrated that BES was capable of promoting the specific reinnervation of sensory pathways by the axotomized dorsal root ganglion

sensory neurons [11]. This finding, which has since been replicated in other experimental designs, seems to indicate that BES is capable of not only preferential motor reinnervation, but overall pathway specific regeneration [12].

There are currently few studies that have examined the effect of BES in improving synkinesis of the facial nerve following injury. The primary objective of this study is to test the hypothesis that BES reduces synkinesis following facial nerve injury. A secondary objective is to examine the effect of BES on facial nerve function following injury.

Methods
Study design
This was a prospective randomized control animal trial conducted at the Surgical Medical Research Institute (SMRI) at the University of Alberta. Twenty-four rats were block randomized into four groups of six. Groups 1 and 2 underwent a crush injury at the main trunk of the nerve, with group 2 additionally receiving BES for 1 h. Groups 3 and 4 underwent a transection injury at the main trunk, with group 4 additionally receiving BES for 1 h. To investigate the effect of BES on synkinesis, the upper and lower main branches (buccal and marginal mandibular) of the facial nerve in all animals were back-labeled with two distinct neurotracers 3 months after injury. The brainstem of all animals was sectioned to identify the motoneurons supplying each of the two main branches. Comparison was made to a control motoneuron labeled brainstem.

To assess the effect of BES on function, facial nerve functional outcome assessment was collected at 2, 4, and 6 weeks post-operatively. A previously validated rat facial nerve model was used [13]. Ethics approval was obtained from the Animal Care and Use Committee (ACUC) overseen by the University Animal Policy and Welfare Committee (UAPWC) at the University of Alberta in Edmonton, Alberta [AUP00000785].

Study subjects
Twenty four female Wistar rats (Charles River Laboratories, Canada) weighing 200–220 g were used as experimental animals for this study. Additional 2 control female Wistar rats were used. Sample size was calculated based on our previous study, which employed a similar outcome measure, powered to detect a difference of 10 degrees in whisking [13]. All rats were housed in pairs at the Health Sciences Laboratory Animal Services (HSLAS) at the University of Alberta. Rats were weighed and handled daily 2 weeks prior to the commencement of the study to reduce animal stress during the study.

Facial nerve functional outcome assessment

The facial nerve functional outcome assessment model employed in this study was based on the model described and validated by Heaton et al. [13]. This model employs a head fixation device, body restraint, and bilateral photoelectric sensors to detect precise whisker movements as an objective measure for facial nerve function. The assessment model was set up and data was acquired using the methodology outlined in Mendez et al., 2016 [8].

Data acquisition

Whisker movement was elicited in each subject by providing a scented stimulus (chocolate milk). The laser micrometers themselves were connected to a 32-Channel Digital I/O Module (NI 9403, National Instruments, Dallas, Tx), which received digital output from the laser micrometers. The I/O module was connected to a PC through a CompactDAQ chassis (cDAQ-9174, National Instruments, Dallas, Tx). The I/O module acquired the laser micrometer signal at a sampling rate of 1 kHz. LabVIEW (LabVIEW Full Development System, National Instruments, Dallas, Tx) software was used as the interface for data acquisition.

Surgical procedure

All non-control subjects underwent both head implantation surgery as well as facial nerve surgery by a single surgeon during the same anesthetic. Groups 2 and 4 additionally received 1 h of BES following nerve injury while remaining anesthetized. All rats were first anesthetized with 3–4% isoflurane. Subjects were then maintained under general anesthesia using 1.5% isoflurane. Hair was then removed from the right side of the face and the top of the head using an electric shaver.

Facial nerve surgery

All facial nerve surgery was completed on the right side of the face on all non-control subjects. A small incision was made just inferior to the right ear bony prominence. Under microscopic visualization, the parotid gland was visualized and everted and retracted out of the surgical field. Distal branches of the facial nerve were identified just inferior to the parotid bed. These were followed proximally until the bifurcation of the buccal and marginal mandibular branches of the facial nerve was identified. Once identified, the area proximal to the bifurcation of the facial nerve was carefully dissected. Groups 1 and 2 received a crush injury to the nerve. A hemostat instrument was applied across the facial nerve proximal to the bifurcation and clamped for a period of 30 s. Groups 3 and 4 received a transection injury to the nerve. A single, sharp transection of the facial nerve proximal to the bifurcation was made using straight microscopic scissors; the cut nerve ends were then immediately repaired using a direct end-to-end technique. Using 9–0 sutures, four simple interrupted sutures were made within the proximal and distal epineural nerve endings. Care was taken to ensure proper nerve alignment.

Brief electrical stimulation

Along with facial nerve crush injury, animals in groups 2 and 4 received brief electrical stimulation. The protocol for stimulation was adapted from that used by Gordon et al. in the sciatic nerve rat model [4]. Two silver Teflon coated wires were bared of insulation for 2–3 mm (AGT0510, W-P Instruments, Inc.). Following nerve repair, the first wire was looped around the proximal stump of the facial nerve. The second wire was imbedded into muscle tissue adjacent to the facial nerve, at a location just proximal to the first wire. The insulated wires were led to a isostim stimulator (A320D, W-P Instruments, Inc.) which delivered a 1.5 mA current in pulses of 100 microseconds in a continuous 20 Hz train for a period of 1 h. The adequacy of stimulation was verified by the presence of a right ear flutter. At the completion of stimulation, the wires were removed from the animal and the incision closed with interrupted 3–0 vicryl sutures.

Head implant surgery

Following the facial nerve procedure, head implant surgery was then completed without reversing the general anesthetic. A small incision was made using a 15-blade scalpel from the anterior to posterior margin of the cranium. Blunt dissection was employed to fully expose the underlying bony cranium. Using an electric drill, 4 holes were made in each quadrant of the skull approximately 15 mm apart from each other. 1.6 mm screws were then placed within each drill site. Dry acrylic resin was then liquefied and placed onto the skull, covering the placed screws. Two larger 5 mm threaded screws were then inverted with the threads directed upwards into the acrylic before it solidified.

Head fixation and body restraint

Two weeks prior to surgery, all animal subjects were handled daily for conditioning. After surgery, all subjects were placed in body restraints daily for a week. At postoperative day 14, whisker measurements were started. Subjects were initially given dose low dose isoflurane and transported to the body restraint apparatus (Fig. 1). Here they underwent head fixation with bolts applied across the exposed threaded screws (Fig. 2). Whisker markers were then placed on either side of the rat's face.

Once this was completed, a scented stimulus was introduced and recording started usually for a period of 5 min. The non-operative left side was used as the control

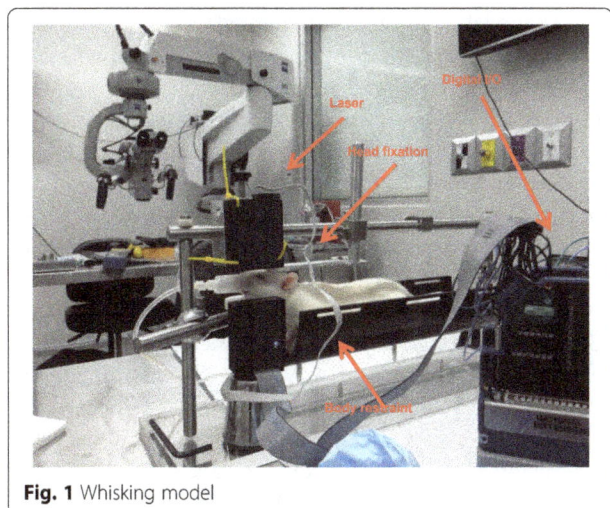

Fig. 1 Whisking model

for each subject. This procedure was completed for each rat at two, four, and 6 weeks post-operatively.

Retrograde labeling of motorneurons

At 3 months postoperatively, the buccal and marginal mandibular branches of the facial nerve were once again carefully dissected and identified. A timeline of 3 months following surgery was chosen as total nerve axonal regeneration is estimated to occur by 10 weeks following injury [4]. The buccal and marginal mandibular branches were then each sharply transected, 5 mm from the bifurcation. Each cut branch was then back-labeled with neurotracers to identify the motorneurons innervating each branch. FG and FR tracers were the neurotracers used, with each individual neurotracer labeling either the upper (buccal) or lower (marginal mandibular) branch.

Each neurotracer was first placed on a small piece of gelfoam. The gelfoam was then placed in contact with the cut end of the nerve branch for a period of 1 h. Each nerve branch was then copiously irrigated with saline.

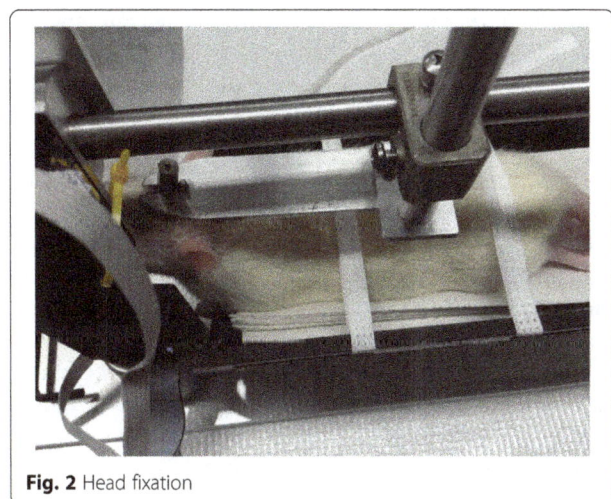

Fig. 2 Head fixation

Care was taken to prevent cross labeling. Animals were kept for 4 days following neurotracer labeling to allow time for each neurotracer to reach the motorneurons in the brainstem.

Tissue fixation by cardiac perfusion

Following neurotracer labeling, all animals underwent transcardiac perfusion in order to perform tissue fixation of the brainstem. Animals first had an intraperitoneal injection of ketamine. An intraabdominal incision was then made to expose the thorax, cardiac ventricles, and descending and ascending aorta. Using an 18 gage catheter, the left ventricle was penetrated and the catheter advanced until the tip was visualized in the ascending aorta. 300 mL of 1 M PBS was then perfused through the catheter. Following the PBS infusion, 400 mL of 4% Paraformaldehyde was then infused through the catheter. The animal was then decapitated and the entire brain exposed and removed. The brain specimen was placed in 4% Paraformaldehyde overnight and then switched over to 30% sucrose for 24 h. The tissue was then frozen in isopentane cooled at - 70 degrees Celsius and stored at - 80 degrees Celsius.

Motoneuron counting

The frozen tissue specimens were removed from storage and sectioned in a cryostat at 20 μm coronal cuts. Sections were mounted on glass slides and dried. The sectioned brainstem cuts were then visualized using a fluorescent microscope with at 10× objective magnification under UV fluorescence at barrier filters of 580 nm for FR and 430 nanameters for FG. All motorneurons labeled with only FR (red), only FG (blue), or both were counted every sixth section. A blinded observer performed all counts and the counting of split cells was corrected for by the method of Abercrombie [14].

Results

All animals tolerated the surgical procedure without perioperative complications. They exhibited normal cage behavior and did not lose weight.

Functional outcome measurements

All experimental animals experienced complete ipsilateral loss of whisking amplitude post-operatively. At week two the average amplitude observed for group 1 (crush, no stimulation) was 14.4 degrees (Table 1). Showing a statistically significant improvement over group 1, the group 2 (crush with BES) average was 24.0 degrees at 2 weeks post-operatively ($p = 0.0004$). Group 3 (transection, no stimulation) and 4 (transection with BES) had average whisking amplitudes of 4.8 and 14.6 degrees, respectively, a statistically significant finding (Table 2). At week four, group 1 showed a minimal amplitude loss,

Table 1 Crush injury. Post-operative whisking amplitudes at week 2, 4, and 6

	Week 2 amplitude (degrees)	Week 4 amplitude (degrees)	Week 6 amplitude (degrees)
NERVE CRUSH (group 1) Right side (operated)	14.4	11.6	17.0
NERVE CRUSH (group 1) Left side (control)	69.7	73.3	67.2
NERVE CRUSH + BES (group 2) Right side (operated)	24.0	23.2	21.8
NERVE CRUSH + BES (group 2) Left side (control)	71.3	68.5	69.7
P value	0.0004	0.0002	0.6328

with an average of 11.6 degrees, while group 2 remained relatively unchanged from week 2 with an average of 23.2 degrees. Group 3 and 4 exhibited average amplitudes of 9.1 and 13.0 degrees at week four, respectively. Group 1 had an average amplitude of 20.3 degrees at 6-weeks from surgery. Group 2 had an average amplitude of 26.7 degrees. There was no statistically significant difference between the two group 1 and 2 at 6 weeks after facial nerve surgery ($p = 0.63$). Group 3 and 4 recorded similar average amplitudes at 6 weeks of 13.4 and 15.2 degrees, respectively.

Overall, BES significantly improved whisking capacity at two and 4 weeks post-injury in the animals that received a crush injury ($p < 0.05$). Similarly, BES significantly improved whisking capacity at 2 weeks post-injury in the animals that received a transection injury ($p < 0.05$). Finally, the BES crush injury animals (group 2) had statistically significant greater whisking capacity than the BES transection injury animals (group 4) at two, four, and 6 weeks post-injury (Fig. 3) ($p < 0.05$).

Table 2 Transection injury. Post-operative whisking amplitudes at week 2, 4, and 6

	Week 2 amplitude (degrees)	Week 4 amplitude (degrees)	Week 6 amplitude (degrees)
NERVE TRANSECTION (group 3) Right side (operated)	4.8	9.1	13.4
NERVE TRANSECTION (group 3) Left side (control)	72.1	66.6	71.8
NERVE TRANSECTION + BES (group 4) Right side (operated)	14.6	13.0	15.2
NERVE TRANSECTION + BES (group 4) Left side (control)	74.9	70.9	67.5
P value	0.0004	0.4715	0.5234

Retrograde labeling of motorneurons

In the non-operated, control animals, a mean of 1388 fluoro-ruby (buccal branch) labeled motorneurons were counted, while a mean of 310 fluorogold (marginal mandibular) labelled motorneurons were observed (Table 3). No double labeled motorneurons were observed in the control animals. Visually, myotopic organization of the motorneurons was observed in the control animals (Fig. 4).

Group 1 and 2 had average counts of 989 (49%) and 934 (46%) double labeled motornuerons, respectively ($p > 0.05$). Group 3 and 4 had an average number of 1299 (68%) and 1222 (62%) double labeled motorneurons, respectively (p > 0.05). Both groups of animals that underwent BES (groups 2 and 4) had, on average, less double labeled motorneurons following facial nerve injury, than their non-stimulated counterpart (groups 1 and 3).

Overall, statistical significantly less double labeled motorneurons were analyzed in groups 1 and 2 (crush injury) as compared to groups 3 and 4 (transection injury) ($p < 0.05$). Groups 1 and 2 also displayed greater myotopic organization as compared to groups 3 and 4 (Figs. 5 and 6).

Discussion

This study sought to evaluate the effect of brief electrical stimulation on synkinesis in a rat model for facial nerve injury. Through the retrograde examination of the facial nerve employing neurotracers, assessment was possible of the distribution of motor neurons in a control rat brainstem whose axons directly innervated either the buccal branch of the facial nerve branch or lower marginal mandibular branch. The buccal branch was labelled with fluroruby (FR) while flurogold (FG) was used to label the marginal mandibular branch of the facial nerve.

In the control animals, myotopic organization of the motorneurons was noted, with each motorneuron single labeled with either FR or FG(Fig. 4). In the experimental animals (groups 1 to 4), there was a significant increase in the number of double-labelled motoneurons (FR + FG) as well as a loss of myotopic organization of the facial motoneurons (Figs. 5 and 6).

These aberrant findings are thought to be caused by two principal processes present during peripheral nerve regeneration. The first process is malfunctioning axonal guidance, where an axon has been misguided along an incorrect fascicle [15]. In this study, this process likely affected the myotopic organization of the facial nucleus in the experimental animals. However, general comparison of the brainstem sections of the animals that had undergone crush injury (group 1, 2) as compared to those with a transection injury (groups 3, 4) revealed improved myotopic organization in the crush injury

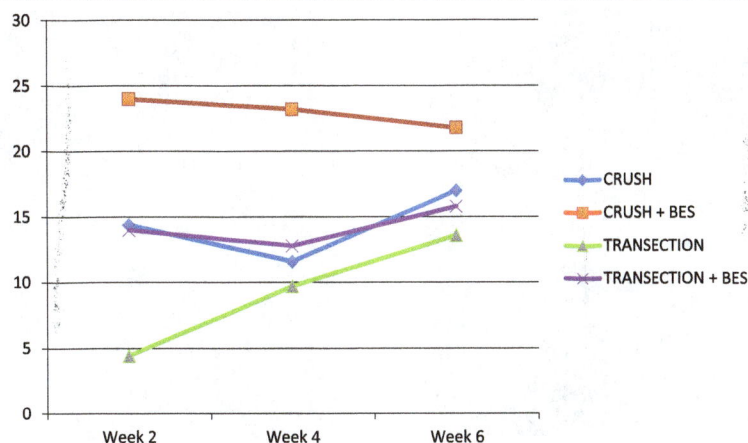

Fig. 3 Whisking amplitude in degrees at 2, 4, and 6 weeks postoperatively. BES = brief electrical stimulation

animals (Figs. 5 and 6). This finding was expected as crush injuries represent Sunderland level two injuries, which do not involve endoneurial disruption, while transection injuries represent a Sunderland level five injury. No appreciable difference in myotopic facial nucleus organization was noted between animals that received BES and those that did not.

The second principal process present during peripheral nerve regeneration is an increase in branches in all transected axons [16]. Because of this, following axonal injury a single motoneuron can send branches through numerous nerve fascicles. In our study, the presence of double-labelled motoneurons is likely due to this process, allowing a single motoneuron to re-innervate both the buccal and marginal mandibular branches, having deleterious effects on synchronized function. As expected, the crush injury animals (groups 1, 2) had significantly less percentage of double-labeled motoneurons as compared to the transection injury animals (groups 3, 4). Interestingly, the animals that received BES also had less percentage of double labelled motoneurons as compared to their non-BES counterparts. Although this finding was not

statistically significant (p value), it does allude to the possibility that BES induces pathway specific regeneration. This would be in keeping with findings from other research groups.

This animal study also directly compared the facial nerve functional outcome in a group of rats receiving brief electrical stimulation following either crush or transection injury versus those not receiving stimulation. The results indicate a significant improvement in whisking amplitude in those animals receiving BES over those with the same injury that did not receive BES in the early weeks following nerve surgery. However, by week four and six post-operatively, no statistically significant difference seen between the two groups receiving transection or crush injuries, respectively. Results of this study are consistent with other reports investigating the effects of electrical stimulation on peripheral nerve regeneration [2, 4, 8]. Based on the neurotracer findings, a potential reason for the improved whisking function in the rats receiving BES is improved pathway specific regeneration of the facial nerve.

Gordon et al. have hypothesized that preferential motor reinnervation in a nerve injury model begins

Table 3 Mean number of retrogradely labeled motorneurons, labeled either as only fluororuby, only fluorogold, or both

	Motorneurons labeled only with FR	Motorneurons labeled only with FG	Motorneurons labeled with FR + FG	Total labeled motorneurons
CONTROL	1488 (82%)	310 (17%)	25 (1%)	1823 (100%)
NERVE CRUSH (group 1)	723 (40%)	198 (11%)	889 (49%)	1810 (100%)
NERVE CRUSH with BES (group 2)	788 (43%)	209 (11%)	834 (46%)	1831 (100%)
NERVE TRANSECTION (group 3)	522 (27%)	88 (5%)	1299 (68%)	1909 (100%)
NERVE TRANSECTION with BES (group 4)	612 (31%)	126 (7%)	1222 (62%)	1960 (100%)

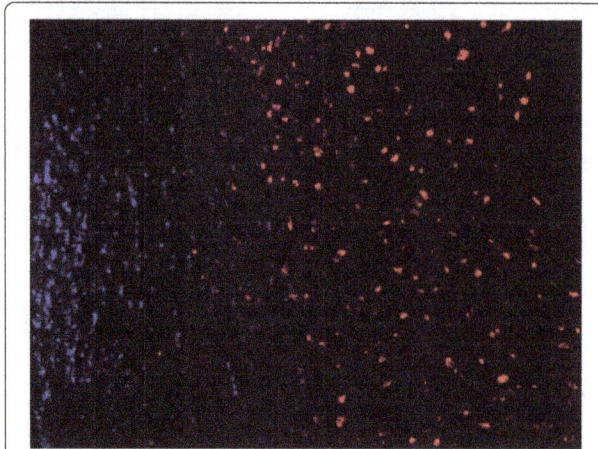

Fig. 4 CONTROL - Facial nucleus after application of FR to the buccal branch and FG to marginal mandibular branch. FR = red, FG = blue. Note the myotopic organization of the nucleus

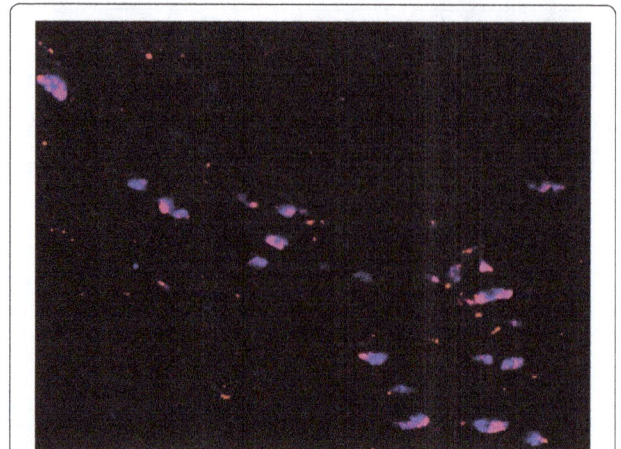

Fig. 6 TRANSECTION - Facial nucleus after application of FR to the buccal branch and FG to marginal mandibular branch. FR = red, FG = blue, double-labeled = pink. Note the increased number of double labelled motorneurons

occurring at approximately 2 to 3 weeks following injury [4]. Up until that time, inappropriate sensory pathways are being created at the same rate as appropriate motor pathways. It appears that electrical stimulation is capable of starting preferential motor reinnervation at an earlier time point compared to non-stimulated nerves.

This is the first animal study incorporating neurotracer retrograde labeling of the facial nerve and brief electrical stimulation. The results of this study taken together with the findings of other researchers indicate the potential for acceleration of facial nerve function with electrical stimulation in animals. Interestingly, BES may also induce pathway specific regeneration of motoneurons following facial nerve injury. Although there are currently no human trials using BES following facial nerve injury,

its application in the human clinical setting appears promising.

Conclusion

This study demonstrates brief electrical stimulation of a rat facial nerve crush injury model is associated with accelerated facial nerve functional outcome. BES may also be capable of inducing pathway specific regeneration of motoneurons following facial nerve injury. This has interesting clinical benefits and potential applications in human facial nerve injuries.

Abbreviations
ACUC: Animal care and use committee; BDNF: Brain-derived neurotrophic factor; BES: Brief electrical stimulation; FG: Fluorogold; FR: Fluororuby; GDNR: Glial cell derived neurotrophic factor; HSLAS: Health sciences laboratory animal services; UAPWC: University animal policy and welfare committee

Acknowledgements
N/A

Funding
Edmonton Civic Employee Grant.

Authors' contributions
AM carried out the rat surgery, whisking testing, study design, data analysis, and drafted the manuscript. AH participated in tissue preparation, imaging, and data analysis. HS participated in the study design and helped revise the manuscript. VB participated in the rat surgery and statistical analysis. LZ participated in rat surgery, animal care, and whisking testing. DC participated in study design, data analysis, and manuscript revision. All authors read and approved the final manuscript.

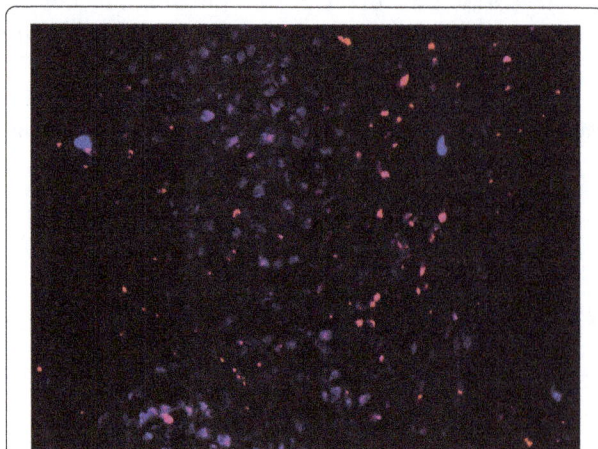

Fig. 5 CRUSH + STIMULATION - Facial nucleus after application of FR to the buccal branch and FG to marginal mandibular branch. FR = red, FG = blue, double-labeled = pink. Note the decreased amount of myotopic organization

Competing interests

The authors declare that they have no competing interests.

Author details

[1]Department of Surgery, Division of Otolaryngology – Head and Neck Surgery, University of Alberta, Edmonton, AB, Canada. [2]Faculty of Medicine and Dentistry, University of Alberta, Edmonton, AB, Canada. [3]1E4 Walter C Mackenzie Centre, 8440-112 Street NW, Edmonton, AB T6G 2B7, Canada.

References

1. Lal D, Hetzler LT, Sharma N, et al. Electrical stimulation facilitates rat facial nerve recovery from a crush injury. Otolaryngol Head Neck Surg. 2008; 139(1):68–73. https://doi.org/10.1016/j.otohns.2008.04.030.
2. Hadlock T, Lindsay R, Edwards C, et al. The effect of electrical and mechanical stimulation on the regenerating rodent facial nerve. Laryngoscope. 2010;120(6):1094–102. https://doi.org/10.1002/lary.20903.
3. Post R, de Boer KS, Malessy MJ. Outcome following nerve repair of high isolated clean sharp injuries of the ulnar nerve. PLoS One. 2012;7(10):e47928. https://doi.org/10.1371/journal.pone.0047928.
4. Al-Majed AA, Neumann CM, Brushart TM, Gordon T. Brief electrical stimulation promotes the speed and accuracy of motor axonal regeneration. J Neurosci. 2000;20(7):2602–8.
5. Sunderland S. Nerve and nerve injuries. London: Churchill Livingstone; 1978.
6. Borgens RB, Roederer E, Cohen MJ. Enhanced spinal cord regeneration in lamprey by applied electric fields. Science. 1981;213(4508):611–7.
7. Borgens RB. Electrically mediated regeneration and guidance of adult mammalian spinal axons into polymeric channels. Neuroscience. 1999;91(1): 251–64.
8. Mendez A, Seikaly H, Biron BL, Zhu LF, Cote DW. Brief electrical stimulation after facial nerve transection and neurorrhaphy: a randomized prospective animal study. J Otolaryngol Head Neck Surg. 2016;1:45. 7
9. Streppel M, Azzolin N, Dohm S, et al. Focal application of neutralizing antibodies to soluble neurotrophic factors reduces collateral axonal branching after peripheral nerve lesion. Eur J Neurosci. 2002;15:1327–42.
10. Al-Majed AA, Brushart TM, Gordon T. Electrical stimulation accelerates and increases expression of BDNF and trkB mRNA in regenerating rat femoral motoneurons. Eur J Neurosci. 2000;12:4381–90.
11. Brushart TM, Jari R, Verge V, Rohde C, Gordon T. Electrical stimulation restores the specificity of sensory axon regeneration. Exp Neurol. 2005;194: 221–9.
12. Geremia NM, Gordon T, Brushart TM, Al-Majed AA, Verge VM. Electrical stimulation promotes sensory neuron regeneration and growth associated gene expression. Exp Neurol. 2007;205:347–59.
13. Heaton JT, Kowaleski JM, Bermejo R, Zeigler HP, Ahlgren DJ, Hadlock TA. A system for studying facial nerve function in rats through simultaneous bilateral monitoring of eyelid and whisker movements. J Neurosci Methods. 2008;171(2):197–206. https://doi.org/10.1016/j.jneumeth.2008.02.023.
14. Abercrombie M. Estimation of nuclear population from microtome sections. Anat Rec. 1946;94:239–47.
15. Brushart TM, Seiler WA. Selective reinnervation of distal motor stumps by peripheral motor axons. Exp Neurol. 1987;97:289–300.
16. Mackinnon SE, Dellon AL, Obrien JP. Changes in nerve fiber diameters distal to a nerve repair in the rat sciatic nerve model. Muscle Nerve. 1991;14: 1116–22. 6

13

The palisade cartilage tympanoplasty technique

Caroline C. Jeffery[1,2], Cameron Shillington[2], Colin Andrews[2] and Allan Ho[1,2*]

Abstract

Background: Tympanoplasty is a common procedure performed by Otolaryngologists. Many types of autologous grafts have been used with variations of techniques with varying results. This is the first systematic review of the literature and meta-analysis with the aim to evaluate the effectiveness of one of the techniques which is gaining popularity, the palisade cartilage tympanoplasty. PubMed, EMBASE, and Cochrane databases were searched for "palisade", "cartilage", "tympanoplasty", "perforation" and their synonyms.

Main body of abstract: In total, 199 articles reporting results of palisade cartilage tympanoplasty were identified. Five articles satisfied the following inclusion criteria: adult patients, minimum 6 months follow-up, hearing and surgical outcomes reported. Studies with patients undergoing combined mastoidectomy, ossicular chain reconstruction, and/or other middle ear surgery were excluded. Perforation closure, rate of complications, and post-operative pure-tone average change were extracted for pooled analysis. Study failure and complication proportions that were used to generate odds ratios were pooled. Fixed effects and random effects weightings were generated. The resulting pooled odds ratios are reported. Palisade cartilage tympanoplasty has an overall take rate of 96% at beyond 6 months and has similar odds of complications compared to temporalis fascia (OR 0. 89, 95% CI 0.62, 1.30). The air-bone gap closure is statistically similar to reported results from temporalis fascia tympanoplasty.

Conclusions: Cartilage palisade tympanoplasty offers excellent graft take rates and good postoperative hearing outcomes for perforations of various sizes and for both primary and revision cases. This technique has predictable, long-term results with low complication rates, similar to temporalis fascia tympanoplasty.

Keywords: Tympanoplasty, Palisade, Cartilage, Type I, Perforation, Tympanic membrane

Background

Tympanoplasty or tympanic membrane (TM) repair is one of the most commonly performed surgeries in Otolaryngology-Head and Neck surgery, with various types of graft and techniques advocated in the literature. The use of cartilage for tympanic membrane repair is well described [1–3] and has reported benefits of long-term graft survival, low recurrence and infection rates, and decreased development of tympanic membrane retraction pockets over time [3–5]. Authors have reported

excellent functional results for small and large perforations [6–8] and often combine tympanoplasty with other middle ear procedures [2]. Cartilage tympanoplasty comprises a heterogeneous group of techniques including that the cartilage-perichondrium composite graft, diced cartilage, butterfly techniques, and palisade cartilage tympanoplasty [9–11].

Tos M. reviewed 23 different cartilage tympanoplasty methods and grouped them into six categories from A to F [10]. The palisade technique is considered a form of Group A cartilage tympanoplasty. The palisade technique specifically involves placement of 0.5 to 3-mm-thick pieces of cartilage placed side by side and often overlapping, under the TM remnant until the defect is

* Correspondence: entalberta@gmail.com
[1]Division of Otolaryngology-Head and Neck Surgery, University of Alberta, Hospital, 8440 112 Street, Edmonton, AB T6G 2B7, Canada
[2]Faculty of Medicine and Dentistry, University of Alberta, Hospital, 8440 112 Street, Edmonton, AB T6G 2B7, Canada

covered [9]. This technique has been used with recurrent perforations, adhesive otitis media or tympanic membrane retractions and other mixed middle ear pathologies [12, 13]. Although several authors have reported success with this technique, we aimed to systematically review the literature on the use of cartilage palisades in Type 1 tympanoplasty and report clinical outcomes of this procedure including hearing and overall graft survival rate.

Methods

Search

A comprehensive search was undertaken using MEDLINE (from 1966), EMBASE (from 1980), CINAHL (from 1982), SCOPUS, and DissAbs in August, 2016. The keywords used were palisade, tympanoplasty, tympanic membrane, tympanic membrane perforation, ear drum, cartilage, and their synonyms. No limitation was placed on date or type of study.

Inclusions/Exclusion

Abstracts of articles obtained from search strategies were independently reviewed by three authors CS, CJ and CA for further assessment. Strict inclusion and exclusion criteria were set *a priori*. English articles and non-English articles with accurate English translation were included. Studies were excluded if they included only pediatric cases, were case reports or reviews or the study design precluded the ability to extract palisade tympanoplasty data. Articles describing the clinical outcomes of palisade cartilage tympanoplasty were then reviewed in full and subjected to further inclusion and exclusion analysis. Studies describing palisade cartilage tympanoplasty performed in conjunction with other middle ear or mastoid surgery (e.g. concurrent ossicular chain reconstruction, mastoidectomy, etc.) were excluded. Specifically, only studies reporting hearing outcomes beyond 6 months were included. In addition to strict inclusion and exclusion criteria, the quality of studies were further assessed by grading their level of evidence based on the Oxford Centre for Evidence-Based Medicine Levels of Evidence for Therapy Studies [13].

Data extraction

Data was then extracted from all articles, including patient demographics, study design, comparison groups, hearing outcomes, perforation closure rates and complications. Two authors extracted the data while a third verified the data extracted. Discrepancies were resolved by consensus. Specific outcomes of interest include graft success with at least 6 months follow-up, closure of the air-bone gap, and complications including middle ear infections, failure of graft survival, persistent perforation or otorrhea.

Data synthesis and meta-analysis

Microsoft Excel (2016) was used to maintain extracted data and articles. Clinical outcomes from studies were pooled to determine rates of failure and complications in the cartilage palisade treatment group versus control. The overall take-rate represents with proportion of studies with complete closure of tympanic membrane perforation at 6 months or beyond. Study-specific odds ratios were calculated to obtain the odds of complications for both treatment and comparator groups. Both random effects and fixed effects models were applied to yield confidence intervals for pooled estimates of odds ratios.

Results

The initial search yielded 199 articles, of which 163 were unique. Through screening of titles and abstracts, 114 were excluded based on initial criteria. The remaining 49 articles were reviewed then screened in detail by examining the full text and 44 more articles were excluded. Specifically, ten of the articles excluded were commentaries or reviews. Another nineteen articles were excluded due to their surgical method; some studies combined results for adult and pediatric patients or patients had concurrent middle ear (e.g. ossicular chain reconstruction) and mastoid surgery. Five more studies were excluded due to the lack of outcome measures or inadequate length of follow up. Ten more articles were excluded due to inability to obtain accurate English translations. This left 5 articles. Figure 1 is a flowchart of literature retrieved, application of inclusion and exclusion criteria, and resulting articles.

Of the included articles, 4 were retrospective studies and one was a prospective study. All articles compared their palisade group to a temporalis fascia group, and one also included patients undergoing repair with tragal perichondrium. Follow-up varied from 6 to 48 months. However, for analytical purposes, the results corresponding to the longest available follow-up time were used. See Table 1 for characteristics and level of evidence of included studies.

Khan et al. [14] included patients with both "small" and "large" perforations and is by far the largest study, with 390 total patients reported. Kazikdas et al. [12], Sishegar et al. [15] and Demirpehlivan et al. [16] only included subtotal perforations, with the defect being described as more than 50% of the area of the whole tympanic membrane. Vashishth et al. [17] selected patients for fascia or palisade group based on various risk factors. Specifically, the authors excluded patients with craniofacial abnormalities, revision tympanoplasties, near-total/total perforations, and persistently discharging ears from the fascia group. However, he did include these difficult to treat patients in the palisade group.

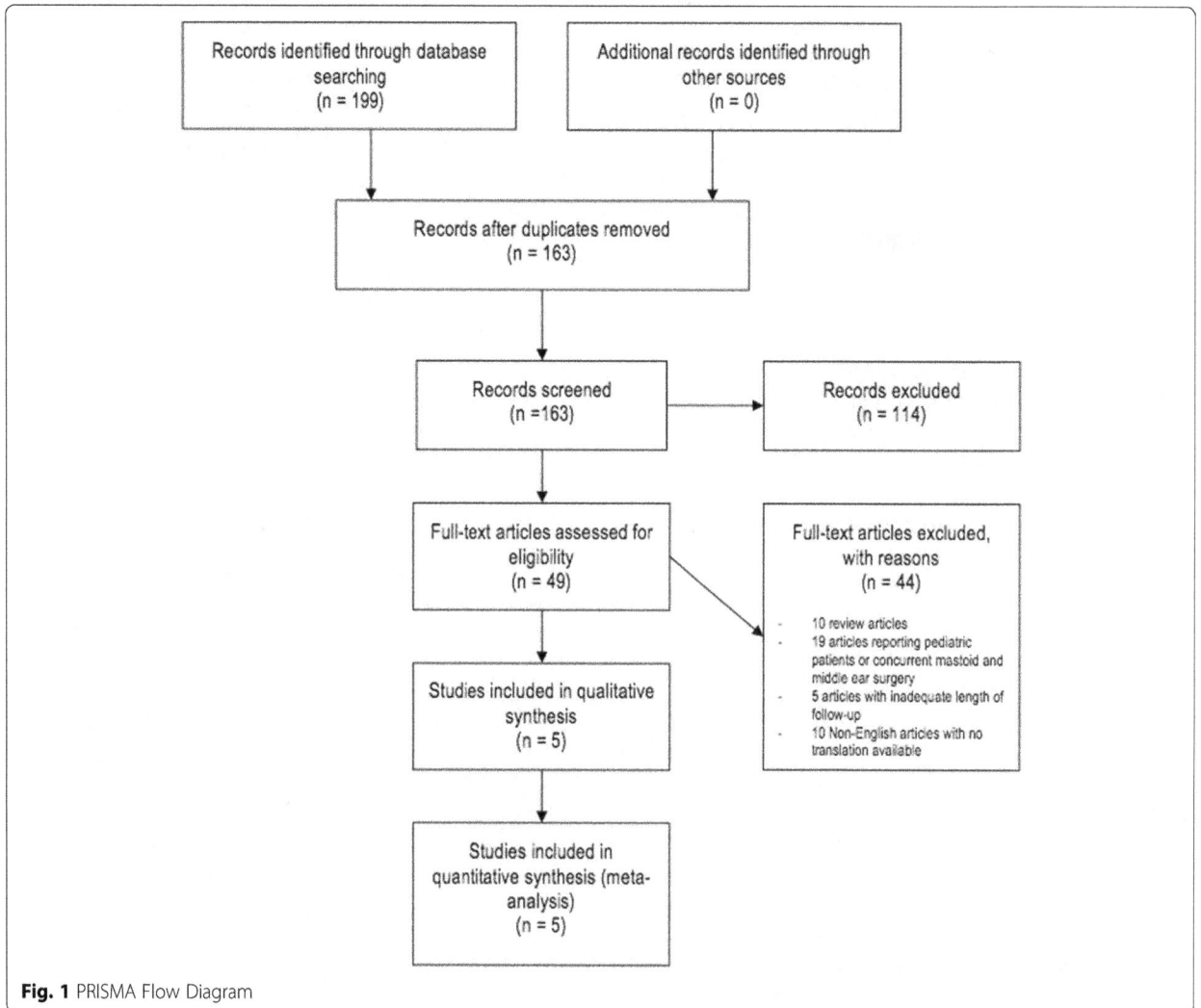

Fig. 1 PRISMA Flow Diagram

Table 1 Summary of included articles

Authors	Type of Article	Number of Patients Total (Palisade)	Comparators	Mean Age (Range)	Follow-up in months (Range)	Level of Evidence (Oxford Scale of Evidence)	Size of Defect
Khan et al. [14]	Retrospective cohort study	390(223)	Temporalis fascia	(11–57)	24 and 48 months	III	Both small and large
Kazikdas et al. [12]	Retrospective cohort study	51(23)	Temporalis fascia	27.6	Mean 18.7 months (7–33)	III	Subtotal perforations (perforation >50% of the whole TM)
Shishegar et al. [15]	Prospective cohort study	54(27)	Temporalis fascia	30	6 months	II	Subtotal perforations
Vashishth et al. [17]	Retrospective cohort study	90(30)	Temporalis fascia	24	12 months	III	Total/near total perforations excluded from fascia group, included in palisade
Demirpehlivan et al. [16]	Retrospective cohort study	120(19)	-Temporalis fascia -Tragal perichondrium	(15–64)	Minimum 12 months	III	Subtotal perforations

Table 2 Individual study results, graft take rates and complication rates for cartilage palisade tympanoplasty compared to temporalis fascia

Authors	Palisade				Temporalis fascia			
	Number of Patients	Overall take rate	Complications	Type of Complications	Number of Patients	Overall take rate	Complications	Types of Complications
Khan et al. [14]	223	97.8%	10.0%	Persistent or recurrent perforation, otorrhea, infection	167	82.6%	17.3%	Persistent or recurrent perforation
Kazikdas et al. [12]	23	95.7%	8.7%	Perforation, otorrhea	28	75.0%	17.4%	Persistent or recurrent perforation
Shishegar et al. [15]	27	100.0%	4.3%	Infection, otorrhea	27	93.0%	25.0%	Persistent or recurrent perforation
Vashishth et al. [17]	30	90.0%	0.0%		60	83.3%	18%	Persistent or recurrent perforation, otorrhea, infection
Demirpehlivan et al. [16]	19	79.0%	10.0%	Persistent or recurrent perforation, infection	67	80.6%	16.7%	Persistent or recurrent perforation
Weighted average (SE)		96.0% (1.1%)	3.1% (1.0%)	Weighted average (SE)		82.5% (2.0%)	17.9% (2.1%)	

SE Standard Error

Individual study results, pooled graft-take rates and complication rates for palisade tympanoplasty versus comparator are found in Table 2. The pre-operative and post-operative air-bone gaps are reported in Table 3 along with average reduction in air-bone gap. The extracted proportion of patients experiencing complications in the palisade tympanoplasty and comparator groups were then used to generated odds ratios (OR). A weighted analysis of pooled ORs indicates no statistical difference in the odds of complications between palisade tympanoplasty and temporalis fascia tympanoplasty (i.e. confidence interval includes 1.0). Using a fixed effects model, which assumes fixed treatment effects, the overall odds ratio was 0.77 (95% CI 0.50, 1.20). Using a random effects model, which accounts for variability of treatment effects between studies, the overall odds ratio was statistically similar at 0.89 (95% CI 0.62, 1.30). Figure 2 demonstrates the forest plot for individual study OR estimates and the final overall estimate obtained by the two weighting methods.

Discussion

The results of this systematic review and meta-analysis are clinically significant. Overall, the palisade cartilage tyampanoplasty technique has excellent functional results for Type 1 tympanoplasty with a 96% take rate at beyond 6 months. The air-bone gap closure is statistically similar to reported results from temporalis fascia tympanoplasty. Complications rates and long-term failure rates appear statistically and clinically comparable to tympanoplasty using temporalis fascia with no difference in the odds ratio of the two groups based on meta-analysis (0.89, 95% CI: 0.62 to 1.30). While this systematic review specifically excluded studies that reported results of palisade cartilage tympanoplasty combined with other procedures, an overall graft take rate of >97% has been reported in patients with who underwent combined palisade tympanoplasty with mastoidectomy for pathologies such as as cholesteatoma, adhesive otitis, and chronic mucosal disease [13, 18]. Our results are consistent with previous

Table 3 Audiologic outcomes of included studies

Authors	Palisade			Temporalis fascia		
	Average Pre-operative ABG	Average Post-operative ABG	Reduction in ABG	Average Pre-operative ABG	Average Post-operative ABG	Reduction in ABG
Khan et al. [14]	30.7	7.1	23.6	32.9	8.1	24.9
Kazikdas et al. [12]	25.6	17.3	8.3	30.7	20.2	10.5
Shishegar et al. [15]	28.5	14.8	13.7	25.4	14.0	11.4
Vashishth et al. [17]	29.0	7.3	21.7	30.4	17.5	12.9
Demirpehlivan et al. [16]	28.0	15.0	13.0	24.5	14.0	10.5
Weighted average (SE)			20.9 (7.5)			17.9 (7.0)

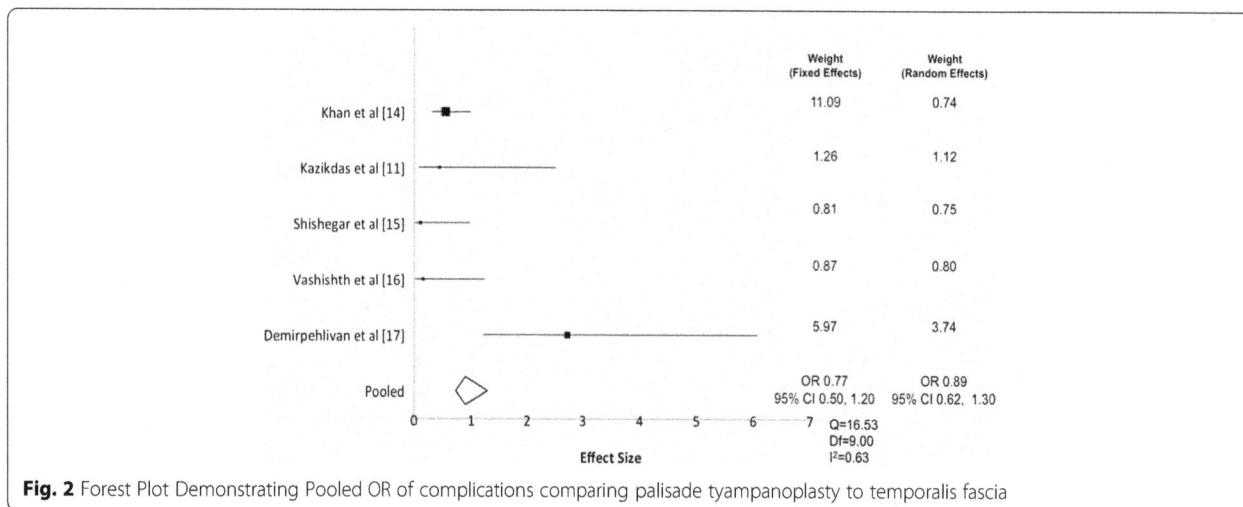

Fig. 2 Forest Plot Demonstrating Pooled OR of complications comparing palisade tyampanoplasty to temporalis fascia

systematic reviews that demonstrate superior graft integration rate with cartilage tympanoplasty compared to temporalis fascia [8, 19]. Those studies did not examine palisade cartilage tympanoplasty alone by subgroup analysis, and thus, our systematic review and meta-analysis offers specific outcomes regarding the clinical effectiveness of this technique, the cartilage palisade tympanoplasty.

There are several limitations to this study. First, with the exception of the study by Khan et al. [14], which reported on 223 patients, the remaining studies had small cohorts of twenty three to thirty patients in the palisade group. These studies represented the results of single surgeons. In addition, there is likely significant publication and reporting bias of positive results. Since these studies are all non-randomized, selection bias remains an issue. In addition, the selection criteria used by authors for using the palisade technique was not consistent. While all the authors stated that operated ears must be dry and free of mucosal disease before surgery, the exact size criteria varied. Khan et al. included ears with "small" perforations, defined as less than 50% of the tympanic membrane and "large" perforations, defined greater than 50% [14]. In contrast, Cabra et al. selected patients with TM perforations >25% [3], while Kazikdas et al. included all primary tympanoplasties with >50% TM perforation [12]. Importantly, authors did not use digitally captured images prior to surgery to evaluate perforation size and there are inherent inaccuracies in the assessment and charting of perforations by subjective clinicians. Thus, future studies with large cohorts of patients need to accurately measure and report perforation size to enhance future comparability amongst surgeons and centers.

In addition to heterogeneity of perforation size, there is considerable heterogeneity in terms of patient age, comorbidities, and other risk factors for graft failure. While the random effects model for pooled odds ratio attempts to address between study variance, we are unable to

explain the drivers of heterogeneity or perform subgroup analysis due to the lack of patient-level data.

Finally, we specifically limited our review to studies of older children and adult patients. To our knowledge, only one study to date specifically examined the use of cartilage palisades in the pediatric population. Vashishth et al. examined outcomes of cartilage palisades over temporalis fascia at 6 months and 1 year in children and adult patients [17]. Although the authors demonstrated excellent results in the palisade group, we were unable to extract data for subgroup analysis (i.e. adult only or pediatric only) and thus excluded their paper from this review. However, given the paucity of literature and lack of consensus regarding pediatric tympanoplasty methods and outcomes, this represents an area in need of better research. Finally, the endoscopic approach to tympanoplasty is gaining popularity in Canada [20], but its adoption for the palisade tympanoplasty technique is unstudied.

Conclusions
There is evidence that cartilage palisade tympanoplasty offers excellent graft take rates and good postoperative hearing outcomes for perforations of various sizes and for both primary and revision cases. This technique has predictable, long-term results with low complication rates, similar to temporalis fascia tympanoplasty.

Abbreviations
OR: Odds ratio; TM: Tympanic membrane

Acknowledgements
None.

Funding
None.

Authors' contributions
CCJ, CS, AH designed the study. CCJ, CS, and CA collected the data and performed data analysis. CCJ and CS prepare the abstract. All authors reviewed the finalized manuscript in preparation for submission. All authors read and approved the final manuscript.

Authors' information
None.

Competing interests
The authors declare that they have no competing interests.

References
1. Dornhoffer J. Cartilage tympanoplasty: indications, techniques, and outcomes in a 1,000-patient series. Laryngoscope. 2003;113:1844–56.
2. Dornhoffer JL. Cartilage tympanoplasty. Otolaryngol Clin North Am. 2006;39:1161–76.
3. Cabra J, Monux A. Efficacy of cartilage palisade tympanoplasty: Randomized controlled trial. Otol Neurotol. 2010;31:589–95.
4. Neumann A, Schultz-Coulon HJ, Jahnke K. Type III tympanoplasty applying the palisade cartilage technique: a study of 61 cases. Otol Neurotol. 2003;24:33–7.
5. Velepic M, Bonifacic M, Manestar D. Cartilage palisade tympanoplasty and diving. Otol Neurotol. 2001;22:430–2.
6. Gerber MJ, Mason JC, Lambert PR. Hearing results after primary cartilage tympanoplasty. Laryngoscope. 2000;110:1994–9.
7. Neumann A, Jahnke K. Reconstruction of the tympanic membrane applying cartilage: indications, techniques and results. HNO. 2005;53:573–84. quiz 585–6.
8. Mohamad SH, Khan I, Hussain SS. Is cartilage tympanoplasty more effective than fascia tympanoplasty? A systematic review. Otol Neurotol. 2012;33:699–705.
9. Tos M. Cartilage tympanoplasty. Stuttgart, New York: Thieme; 2009. in print.
10. Tos M. Cartilage tympanoplasty methods: proposal of a classification. Otolaryngol Head Neck Surg. 2008;139:747–58.
11. Man SC, Nunez DA. Tympanoplasty–conchal cavum approach. J Otolaryngol Head Neck Surg. 2016;45:1.
12. Kazikdas KC, Onal K, Boyraz I, Karabulut E. Palisade cartilage tympanoplasty for management of subtotal perforations: a comparison with the temporalis fascia technique. Eur Arch Otorhinolaryngol. 2007;264:985–9.
13. Neumann A, Hennig A, Schultz-Coulon HJ. Morphological and functional results of Palisade Cartilage Tympanoplasty. HNO. 2002;50:935–9.
14. Khan MM, Parab SR. Comparative study of sliced tragal cartilage and temporalis fascia in type I tympanoplasty. J Laryngol Otol. 2015;129:16–22.
15. Shishegar M, Faramarzi A, Taraghi A. A Short-term Comparison Between Result of Palisade Cartilage Tympanoplasty and Temporalis Fascia Technique. Iran J Otorhinolaryngol. 2012;24:105–12.
16. Demirpehlivan IA, Onal K, Arslanoglu S, Songu M, Ciger E, Can N. Comparison of different tympanic membrane reconstruction techniques in type I tympanoplasty. Eur Arch Otorhinolaryngol. 2011;268:471–4.
17. Vashishth A, Mathur NN, Choudhary SR, Bhardwaj A. Clinical advantages of cartilage palisades over temporalis fascia in type I tympanoplasty. Auris Nasus Larynx. 2014;41:422–7.
18. Uzun C, Cayé-Thomasen P, Andersen J, Tos M. A tympanometric comparison of tympanoplasty with cartilage palisades or fascia after surgery for tensa cholesteatoma in children. Laryngoscope. 2003;113:1751–7.
19. Yang T, Wu X, Peng X, Zhang Y, Xie S, Sun H. Comparison of cartilage graft and fascia in type 1 tympanoplasty: systematic review and meta-analysis. Acta Otolaryngol. 2016;136(11):1085–90. Epub 2016 Jun 16.
20. Yong M, Mijovic T, Lea J. Endoscopic ear surgery in Canada: a cross-sectional study. J Otolaryngol Head Neck Surg. 2016;45:4.

14

IL-5 and IL-6 are increased in the frontal recess of eosinophilic chronic rhinosinusitis patients

Kazunori Kubota[*], Sachio Takeno, Takayuki Taruya, Atsushi Sasaki, Takashi Ishino and Katsuhiro Hirakawa

Abstract

Background: Eosinophilic chronic frontal sinusitis is difficult to treat compared with non-eosinophilic sinusitis because of recurring inflammation and polyp formation in the frontal recess after the post-operative follow-up period. Studying inflammatory mediators in the frontal recess of eosinophilic chronic rhinosinusitis (ECRS) patients and non-eosinophilic chronic rhinosinusitis (non-ECRS) patients may lead to a better understanding of the pathogenesis of chronic frontal sinusitis.

Methods: Homogenates of sinonasal mucosa from 20 non-ECRS patients and 36 ECRS patients were measured for levels of transforming growth factor (TGF)-β, interleukin (IL)-5, IL-6, and inducible nitric oxide synthase (iNOS) using real-time RT-PCR and TaqMan gene expression assays. Sinonasal mucosal specimens were obtained from the frontal recess, ethmoid sinus, and nasal polyp separately.

Results: The expression of IL-5 was significantly elevated in all sinonasal regions tested in the ECRS group, but absent in non-ECRS patients. Furthermore, the ECRS patients showed significantly increased levels of IL-5 in the frontal recess mucosa compared with ethmoid sinus mucosa. IL-6 was also significantly increased in the frontal recess mucosa compared with ethmoid sinus mucosa and nasal polyps in these patients. There were no significant differences in the levels of TGF-β or iNOS between the ECRS and non-ECRS groups in any sinonasal region tested.

Conclusions: This study is the first to characterize the cytokine milieu in the frontal recess of ECRS patients. We should keep these cytokine profiles in mind when we treat ECRS patients with frontal sinusitis.

Keywords: Frontal recess, Eosinophilic chronic rhinosinusitis, IL-5, IL-6

Background

Chronic frontal sinusitis is a complex disease for rhinologists to treat because of the difficulty in complete dissection of frontal recess cells and recurring inflammation. Even if the surgeon could remove all frontal recess cells that compromise the ventilation pathway, damage to the frontal sinus in the operation, such as bone exposure caused by mucosal damage, and a narrow ventilation pathway can lead to the restenosis of the frontal recess. Thus, frontal sinusitis recurs during the post-operative follow-up period [1]. The Modified Lothrop procedure (MLP) or Draf type 3 frontal drillout is often chosen to gain a wider ventilation

pathway to the frontal sinus if the patient is considered at high risk of recurrence [2].

Surgical intervention is therefore essential for the treatment of chronic frontal sinusitis, however, there is a growing evidence base that emphasizes the importance of also understanding the pathophysiology of chronic rhinosinusitis [3].

Eosinophilic chronic rhinosinusitis (ECRS) is a subtype of recalcitrant chronic rhinosinusitis (CRS). Diagnostic criteria were established in 2015 by the Japanese Epidemiological Survey of Refractory Eosinophilic Chronic Rhinosinusitis study (JESREC) in Japan [4]. ECRS is characterized by marked infiltration of eosinophils in the paranasal sinus mucosa. Ostiomeatal complex occlusion may not be a predisposing factor for the development of ECRS, but the degree of mucosal eosinophilic infiltration

* Correspondence: kazunokubota@gmail.com
Department of Otolaryngology, Head and Neck Surgery, Division of Clinical Medical Science, Programs for Applied Biomedicine, Graduate School of Biomedical Sciences, Hiroshima University, 1-2-3 Kasumi, Minami-ku, Hiroshima 734-8551, Japan

and subsequent inflammation is important. Therefore, for the treatment of frontal sinusitis in ECRS patients, it is crucial to know the local cytokine profiles surrounding the frontal recess. The cytokine profile of the ethmoid sinus mucosa and nasal polyps in ECRS or chronic rhinosinusitis with nasal polyp (CRSwNP) patients has been reported previously. Ethmoid sinus mucosa of CRSwNP patients showed significantly increased expression of interleukin (IL)-5, eosinophil-cationic protein, immunoglobulin E (IgE), and *Staphylococcus* enterotoxin (SAE)-IgE compared with chronic rhinosinusitis without nasal polyp (CRSsNP) patients [5, 6]. Ethmoid sinus mucosa of ECRS patients also showed significantly elevated expression of inducible nitric oxide synthase (iNOS) and IL-5 [7, 8]. However, there is no report that investigates the cytokine profile in the frontal sinus mucosa of ECRS patients. In this study, we examined the cytokine profile in the frontal recess of ECRS patients to further elucidate the pathogenesis of the disease. These findings may lead to the prevention of recurrence of inflammation or nasal polyp.

Methods

Patients

Sinonasal mucosa from Japanese patients with ECRS ($n = 36$) and non-ECRS ($n = 20$) was obtained during endoscopic sinus surgery (ESS) at Hiroshima University Hospital from July 2010 to November 2016. Nasal polyps and sinus mucosa from the frontal recess and the ethmoid sinus were harvested separately. Nasal polyps were obtained from the middle meatus, and ethmoid mucosa was obtained mainly from the anterior ethmoid sinuses. Frontal recess mucosa was obtained from as near as possible to the frontal sinus, and included frontal cells and frontal bullar cells. The patients were routinely questioned regarding rhinosinusitis symptoms and received ear, nose and throat examination by flexible endoscopy. Criteria for ECRS from the JESREC study were adopted to distinguish ECRS patients from non-ECRS patients [4]. Computed tomography (CT) scan images of paranasal sinuses were evaluated by the Lund and Mackay scoring system [9]. Peripheral blood samples were obtained from all patients to measure blood eosinophil count and serum IgE levels.. Atopic status was considered positive if the patient had radioallergosorbent test (RAST) scores greater than 2 for any inhaled allergen. These allergens included Japanese cedar, Japanese cypress, house dust mite, common ragweed, orchard grass, and *Aspergillus*. Diagnosis of bronchial asthma was made by a pneumologist based on lung function and challenge tests, where applicable. Patients who received oral or intranasal topical steroids within 4 weeks of the surgery were excluded from the study.

The study protocol was approved by the Institutional Review Board at the Hiroshima University School of Medicine (approval number Hi-136) and written informed consent was obtained from all patients prior to inclusion in the study.

Real-time RT-PCR analysis

Obtained tissue specimens were either minced with scissors immediately after surgery and immersed in RNAlater™ solution (Ambion, Austin, TX, USA) for real time RT-PCR analysis or fixed in 4% paraformaldehyde for immunohistochemistry. We eliminated frontal recess mucosa and nasal polyp specimens which were thought to be too small or damaged by during surgery. In total, we processed 21 frontal recess mucosa, 36 ethmoid mucosa, and 30 nasal polyp samples from 36 ECRS patients and 10 frontal recess mucosa, 20 ethmoid mucosa, and 9 nasal polyp samples from 20 non-ECRS patients.

Cellular RNA was isolated using RNeasy mini kits (Qiagen, Valencia, CA, USA). Total RNA was then reverse-transcribed to cDNA using a High Capacity RNA-to-cDNA kit (Applied Biosystems, Foster City, CA, USA) per the manufacturer's instructions. Gene expression was measured on an ABI Prism 7300 system (Applied Biosystems) using TaqMan Gene Expression Assays. PCR primers specific for TGF-β (Hs99999918_m1), IL-5 (Hs00174200_m1), IL-6 (Hs00985639_m1), iNOS (Hs01075529_m1) and GAPDH (Hs99999905_m1) were used. GAPDH was used as a reference gene. PCR assays were run in triplicate for each sample. Amplifications of the PCR products were quantified by the number of cycles and results were analyzed using the comparative cycle threshold (Ct) method ($2^{-\Delta\Delta Ct}$). The Ct values for target genes were normalized to the value of GAPDH by calculating the change in Ct ($^{\Delta}$Ct). Ct values of 34 or higher were considered as the lowest limit of detection. The quantities of target gene expression are presented relative to the expression of the reference gene (ratio: target gene/GAPDH expression).

Immunohistochemistry

Immunostaining was carried out on 5-μm-thick cryostat sections of mucosal specimens. The anti-human IL-5 rabbit polyclonal antibody was from Acris (Rockville, MD, USA) and IL-6 rabbit polyclonal antibody was from GeneTex (Irvine, CA, USA). For antigen retrieval, sections were immersed in Histo VT One (Nacalai Tesque, Kyoto, Japan) at 70 °C for 40 min. The sections were then incubated overnight at 4 °C in the presence of the primary antibodies. Color development was performed using the streptavidin-biotin amplification technique (ChemMate En Vision kit, Dako, Glostrup, Denmark). Control specimens developed without the primary antibody were used to verify the absence of nonspecific binding. Consecutive sections were stained with hematoxylin-eosin (HE) to view the mucosal pathology and assess the degree of eosinophil infiltration.

Statistical analysis

Statistical analyses were performed using Excel Statistics 2010 (Shakai Jouhou Corp., Tokyo, Japan). Baseline characteristics were compared with the Mann-Whitney U test between the non-ECRS and ECRS patients. Data are expressed as the mean and range. For the RT-PCR analysis, the Mann-Whitney U test was used to compare the groups. A value of $p < 0.05$ was considered statistically significant for all measurements.

Results

Comparison of clinical characteristics of ECRS and non-ECRS patients

The clinical characteristics of patients in this study are shown in Table 1. The average age of the ECRS patients was significantly younger than the non-ECRS patients. The atopic status and serum IgE levels did not show a significant difference between the non-ECRS and ECRS groups, whereas the peripheral blood eosinophil count was significantly higher in the ECRS group as expected. Sinonasal findings including bilateral lesion, nasal polyps, and predominant opacification of the ethmoid sinus were significantly worse in the ECRS patients. CT scores of the ethmoid and frontal sinuses were significantly higher in the ECRS patients. A significantly higher frequency of comorbid asthma was reported in ECRS patients.

Table 1 Baseline characteristics of the study population

	non-ECRS	ECRS	P value
Number of patients	20	36	-
Age(years old; range)	64.7 (39–76)	56.1 (23–74)	0.009
Female/male	5/15	11/25	N.S.
Atopic status(over class 2)	9/20	20/36	N.S.
Serum IgE(IU/ml)	424.5 (13–3767)	441.4 (8.6–3700)	N.S.
Peripheral blood eosinophil count(%)	3.0 (0.6–8.5)	8.5 (1.8–21.7)	<0.001
Bilateral lesion	10/20	35/36	<0.001
Nasal polyps	11/20	34/36	<0.001
Predoninant opacification of the ethmoid sinus	1/20	27/36	<0.001
Mean ethmoid score	1.23 (0–4)	3.02 (1–4)	<0.001
Mean frontal score	1.20 (0–3)	2.28 (0–4)	0.012
Comorbidity of Asthma	1/20	13/36	0.010
Comorbidity of otitis media	0/20	5/36	N.S.

Data are shown as the mean with ranges in parentheses. The level of significance was obtained by the Mann-Whitney U test

IL-5 and IL-6 expression are increased in the frontal recess mucosa of ECRS patients

Immunohistological staining showing the distribution of IL-5 and IL-6 positive cells in the frontal recess mucosa, with corresponding H&E staining is shown in Fig. 1. The ECRS patients demonstrated greater accumulation of eosinophils in the submucosal layer as compared with the non-ECRS patients (Fig. 1a, b). The frontal recess mucosa of the ECRS patients also tended to show stronger staining for IL-5 (Fig. 1c, d) and IL-6 (Fig. 1e, d) in the epithelial cell cytoplasm and submucosal gland cell cytoplasm as compared with the non-ECRS patients.

Messenger RNA (mRNA) levels of TGF-β, IL-5, IL-6, and iNOS in the frontal recess, ethmoid mucosa and nasal polyps were assessed by quantitative RT-PCR analysis (Figs. 2, 3, 4, 5, 6 and 7). There was no significant difference in mRNA levels of TGF-β (Fig. 2), IL-6 (Fig. 4) and iNOS (Fig. 5) between the two groups in any sinonasal region; frontal recess mucosa, ethmoid sinus mucosa, or nasal polyps. However, ECRS patients showed significant upregulation of IL-5 mRNA compared with non-ECRS patients in all sinonasal regions, with the increase being more prominent in the frontal recess and nasal polyps (Fig. 3). Moreover, in ECRS patients, frontal recess mucosa showed significantly higher levels of IL-5 mRNA compared with ethmoid sinus mucosa. Additionally, frontal recess mucosa showed significantly higher levels of IL-6 compared with ethmoid sinus mucosa and nasal polyp (Fig. 7). In non-ECRS patients, no such specific profile of cytokine expression was observed among sinonasal regions (Fig. 6).

Discussion

There is growing evidence that not all CRS is a simple disease treated by medication and ESS [3]. Notably, the number of CRS patients who have recurrence of nasal polyposis after the initial ESS and need revision surgery is increasing [2]. Based on this background, a scoring systems for refractory chronic rhinosinusitis, also called ECRS in Japan, was established in 2015. This system enabled us to easily classify CRS patients into two groups and to compare various clinical parameters between them [4].

ECRS is characterized by high eosinophil counts, significant inflammation in the ethmoid sinus, and inflammatory lesions that also includes the frontal recess. Findings such as higher eosinophil counts and predominant ethmoid inflammatory disease are not surprising in ECRS patients as they are part of the diagnostic criteria [4]. MLP or Draf type 3 frontal drillout have become popular in treating recalcitrant frontal sinusitis. However, post-operative frontal ostium restenosis associated with accumulation of eosinophilic mucin is sometimes inevitable in ECRS patients [10].

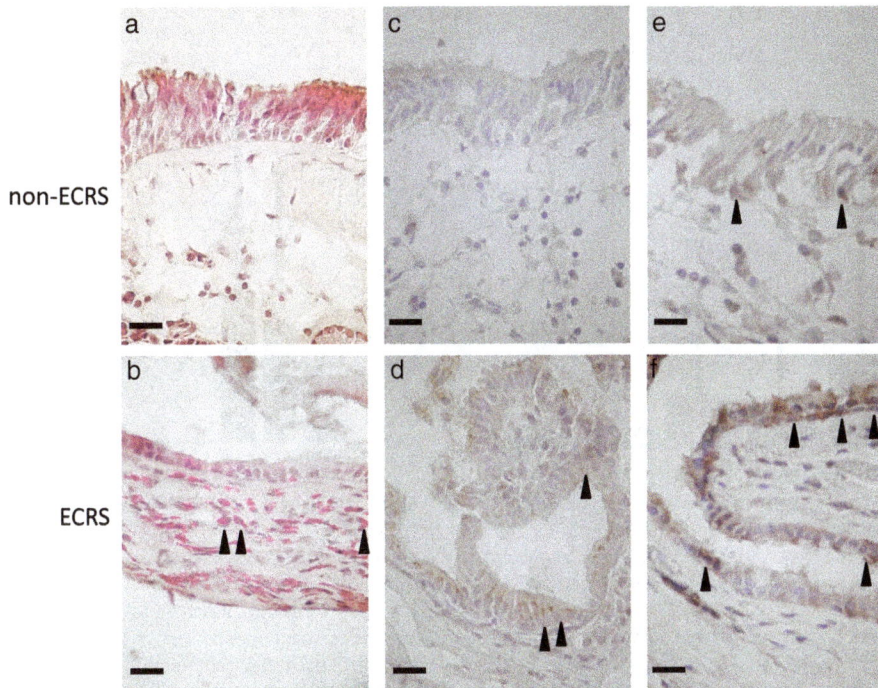

Fig. 1 Histopathological features and cytokine expression in the frontal recess of ECRS and non-ECRS patients. Histopathological findings of frontal recess mucosa from non-ECRS patients (**a**, **c** and **e**) and ECRS patients (**b**, **d** and **f**). Hematoxylin-eosin staining (**a** and **b**), and immunohistochemistry (**c** and **d** show IL-5 positive cells, E and F show IL-6 positive cells) of patient samples. *Arrow heads* point to positive cells. Scale bars: 20 μm. Magnification: ×400

We previously investigated the relationship between the prevalence of frontal sinusitis and the radiological features of frontal recess cells [11]. In the present study, we have extended this to examine the cytokine profile of frontal recess mucosa that underlies the prolonged

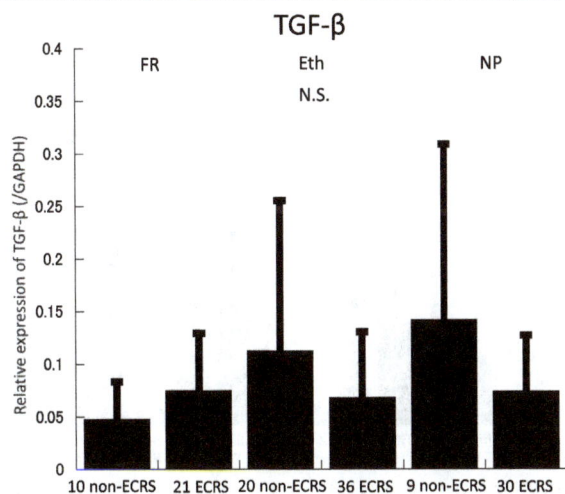

Fig. 2 Measurement of TGF-β in 20 non-eosinophilic chronic rhinosinusitis (non-ECRS) patients and 36 eosinophilic chronic rhinosinusitis (ECRS) patients by RT-PCR. Data are presented as the mean values and error bars indicate standard deviation. FR = frontal recess; Eth = ethmoid sinus; NP = nasal polyp; N.S. = not significant

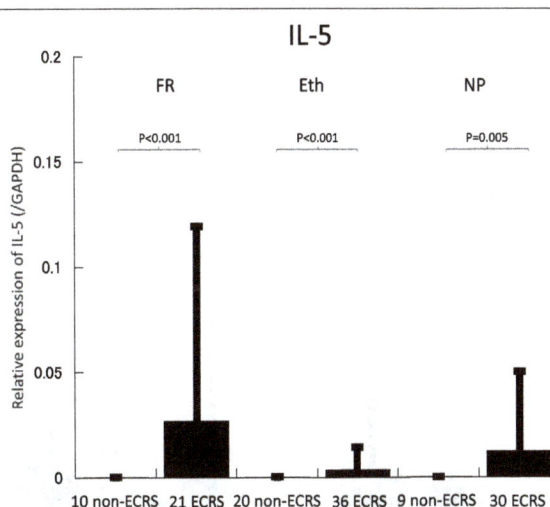

Fig. 3 Measurement of IL-5 in 20 non-eosinophilic chronic rhinosinusitis (non-ECRS) patients and 36 eosinophilic chronic rhinosinusitis (ECRS) patients by RT-PCR. IL-5 is significantly increased in the frontal recess, ethmoid sinus and nasal polyp of patients with ECRS compared with non-ECRS. Data are presented as the mean values and error bars indicate standard deviation. FR = frontal recess; Eth = ethmoid sinus; NP = nasal polyp

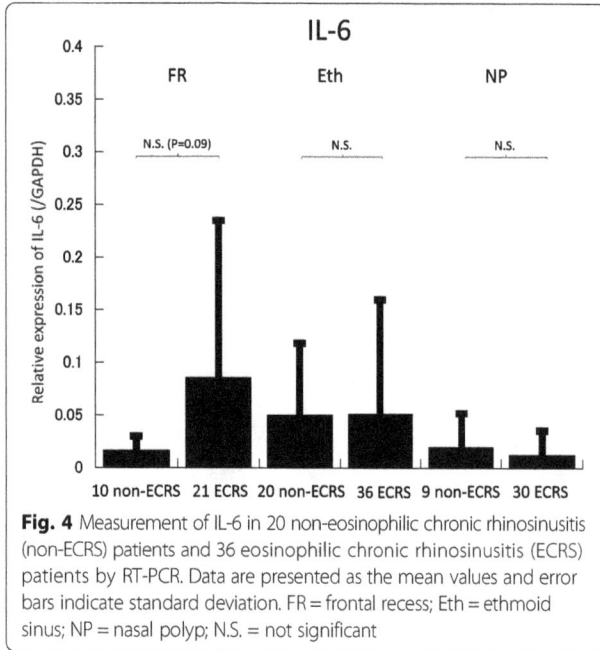

Fig. 4 Measurement of IL-6 in 20 non-eosinophilic chronic rhinosinusitis (non-ECRS) patients and 36 eosinophilic chronic rhinosinusitis (ECRS) patients by RT-PCR. Data are presented as the mean values and error bars indicate standard deviation. FR = frontal recess; Eth = ethmoid sinus; NP = nasal polyp; N.S. = not significant

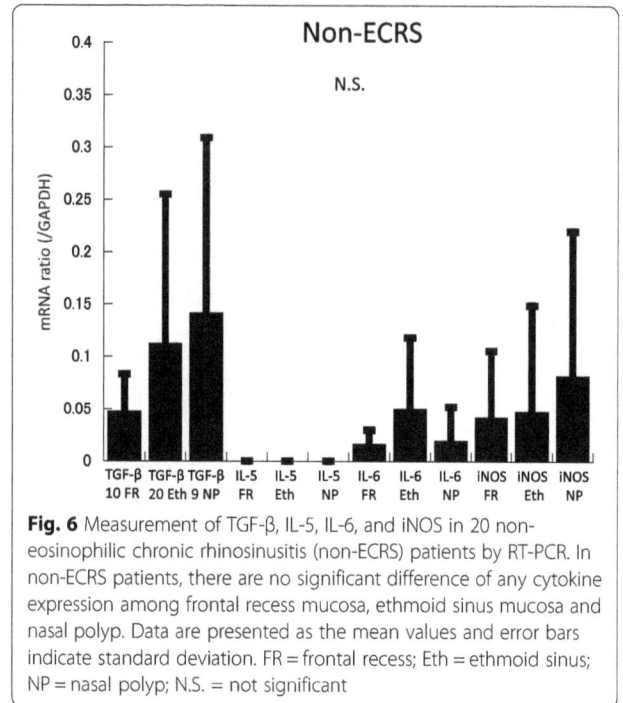

Fig. 6 Measurement of TGF-β, IL-5, IL-6, and iNOS in 20 non-eosinophilic chronic rhinosinusitis (non-ECRS) patients by RT-PCR. In non-ECRS patients, there are no significant difference of any cytokine expression among frontal recess mucosa, ethmoid sinus mucosa and nasal polyp. Data are presented as the mean values and error bars indicate standard deviation. FR = frontal recess; Eth = ethmoid sinus; NP = nasal polyp; N.S. = not significant

inflammatory processes. For this purpose, we selected three representative cytokines (TGF-β, IL-5, IL-6) and one enzyme (iNOS) that may discriminate between the pathophysiology of ECRS and non-ECRS.

It is widely accepted that the cytokine expression in the paranasal mucosa of CRSwNP patients differs from that of CRSsNP patients [6, 12, 13]. In fact, nasal polyp tissue, when compared with adjacent inflammatory nasal mucosa, was shown to express higher levels of IL-5 and lower levels of TGF-β mRNA. These data suggest that local

upregulation of IL-5 may lead to nasal polyp formation at specific sites in the face of diffuse mucosal inflammation.

TGF-β, present in high amounts in regenerating epithelial cells, plays an essential role in the tissue remodeling process by regulating structural or inflammatory cell activation, proliferation and differentiation, and the deposition of extracellular matrix proteins [14, 15]. Many previous papers in western countries have reported that patients with CRSsNP showed higher levels of TGF-β

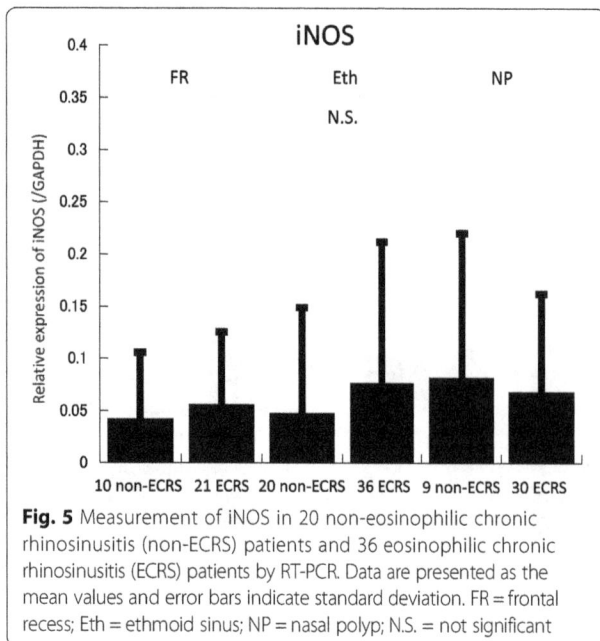

Fig. 5 Measurement of iNOS in 20 non-eosinophilic chronic rhinosinusitis (non-ECRS) patients and 36 eosinophilic chronic rhinosinusitis (ECRS) patients by RT-PCR. Data are presented as the mean values and error bars indicate standard deviation. FR = frontal recess; Eth = ethmoid sinus; NP = nasal polyp; N.S. = not significant

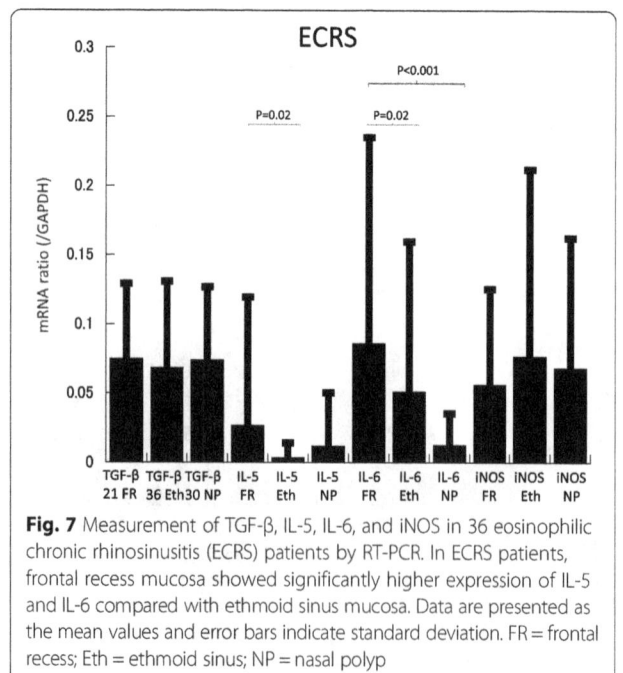

Fig. 7 Measurement of TGF-β, IL-5, IL-6, and iNOS in 36 eosinophilic chronic rhinosinusitis (ECRS) patients by RT-PCR. In ECRS patients, frontal recess mucosa showed significantly higher expression of IL-5 and IL-6 compared with ethmoid sinus mucosa. Data are presented as the mean values and error bars indicate standard deviation. FR = frontal recess; Eth = ethmoid sinus; NP = nasal polyp

expression, whereas those with CRSwNP showed lower TGF-β expression levels compared with the control subjects [6, 14, 16, 17]. However, there was no significant difference in TGF-β between our ECRS and non-ECRS groups. Thus, TGF-β may not be a suitable biomarker for classification of CRS patients.

Paranasal sinus mucosa from the ECRS patients demonstrated increased IL-5 expression in all harvested sites as compared with those from non-ECRS patients. In addition, the frontal recess mucosa of ECRS patients showed a significant increase in IL-5 compared with ethmoid sinus mucosa of ECRS patients. This result is quite innovative because significant ethmoid sinus eosinophilic inflammation is characteristic of ECRS patients and predominant opacification of the ethmoid sinus is one of the criteria of ECRS. IL-5 is pivotal for the recruitment and survival of eosinophils [14]. Thus, the frontal recess mucosa of the ECRS group is likely to be immensely influenced by persistent eosinophilic inflammation, to the same or greater extent as the ethmoid sinus. Therefore, the finding provides us with a rationale for the development of treatment strategies targeting eosinophilic inflammatory responses in the frontal sinus of ECRS patients.

Increased levels of IL-5 mRNA expression or protein production has been previously reported in the paranasal sinus mucosa of CRSwNP patients [6, 13, 18, 19]. Although our results in the frontal recess cannot be directly compared with the previous reports, both CRSwNP and ECRS are characterized by severe eosinophilic inflammation and may be based on similar pathogenic mechanisms.

IL-6 is a proinflammatory Th2 type cytokine that stimulates fibroblast proliferation and collagen synthesis. IL-6 is produced by a variety of cells including T and B lymphocytes, macrophages, eosinophils, epithelial cells, and fibroblasts [20]. In this study, a significant increase in IL-6 expression was noted in the frontal recess mucosa in the ECRS group as compared with the ethmoid sinus mucosa and nasal polyp in the ECRS group. In contrast, IL-6 expression in the frontal recess mucosa was not significantly different compared with the ethmoid sinus mucosa and nasal polyp in non-ECRS group. Thus, IL-6 expression may be associated with the pathophysiology of frontal sinusitis in ECRS patients and mechanisms of frontal eosinophilic sinusitis that differ from non-ECRS patients.

Exhaled NO measurements have become a standardized, reliable, and objective tool in the diagnosis and management of airway eosinophilic inflammation [21]. Interestingly, the human paranasal sinuses are a sizable source of intrinsic NO production, although the origin of nasal NO measured from human nasal airways has been a matter of debate [22]. We have previously reported that higher nasal NO levels in ECRS patients were closely correlated with augmented iNOS expression in response to proinflammatory cytokines and were also accompanied by the excretion of NO metabolites into the sinus mucosa [3].

In this study, the frontal recess and ethmoid sinus mucosa in the ECRS patients did not show a significant difference in iNOS expression as compared with the non-ECRS patients. This result may be due to the patient selection and sample size, or may reflect unimpaired ciliary clearance function in the non-ECRS patients with a sizable NO production. Further evidence, including local NO measurements for each paranasal sinus, is needed for a better understanding of the regulatory mechanisms of NO in ECRS.

Conclusions

This study revealed that the cytokine expression profiles in the frontal recess mucosa in ECRS and non-ECRS patients are distinct. We therefore need to keep in mind the underlying eosinophilic inflammation that may cause intractable aggravation of mucosal diseases in the postoperative follow-up period when we treat frontal sinusitis in ECRS patients.

Abbreviations
CRS: Chronic rhinosinusitis; CRSsNP: Chronic rhinosinusitis without nasal polyp; CRSwNP: Chronic rhinosinusitis with nasal polyp; CT: Computed tomography; ECRS: Eosinophilic chronic rhinosinusitis; ESS: Endoscopic sinus surgery; HE: Hematoxylin-eosin; IgE: Immunoglobulin E; IL-5: Interleukin-5; iNOS: Inducible nitric oxide synthase; JESREC: Japanese Epidemiological Survey of Refractory Eosinophilic Chronic Rhinosinusitis study; MLP: Modified Lothrop procedure; mRNA: messenger RNA; RAST: Radioallergosorbent test; SAE: Staphylococcus enterotoxin; TGF-β: Transforming growth factor-β

Acknowledgements
The authors thank Ms. Ai Kashima for technical assistance.

Funding
This study was supported in part by a Hiroshima University Ryokufukai grant, a Japan Society for the Promotion of Science KAKENHI grant, and a grant from the Practical Research Project for Rare/Intractable Diseases by the Japan Agency for Medical Research and Development.

Authors' contributions
KK carried out the real-time RT-PCR analysis, immunohistochemistry and drafted the manuscript. ST participated in the design of the study and helped to draft the manuscript. TT, AS, and TI participated in ESS and collected mucosal samples. HW conceived the study and participated in its design and coordination. All authors read and approved the final manuscript.

Authors' information
KK: Graduate student at Hiroshima University. ST: Associate Professor at Hiroshima University. TT: Medical Doctor at Hiroshima University. AS: Graduate student at Hiroshima University. TI: Research associate at Hiroshima University. KH: Professor at Hiroshima University.

Competing interests
The authors declare that they have no competing interests.

References

1. Han JK, Ghanem T, Lee B, Gross CW. Various causes for frontal sinus obstruction. Am J Otolaryngol. 2009;30:80–2.
2. Bassiouni A, Wolmald PJ. Role of frontal sinus surgery in nasal polyp recurrence. Laryngoscope. 2013;123:36–41.
3. Snidvongs K, Chin D, Sachs R, Earls P, Harvey RJ. Eosinophilic rhinosinusitis is not a disease of ostiomeatal occlusion. Laryngoscope. 2013;123:1070–4.
4. Tokunaga T, Sakashita M, Haruna T, Asaka D, Takeno S, Ikeda H, et al. Novel scoring system and algorithm for classifying chronic rhinosinusitis: the JESREC Study. Allergy. 2015;70:995–1003.
5. Shi LL, Xiong P, Zhang L, Cao PP, Liao B, Lu X, et al. Features of airway remodeling in different types of Chinese chronic rhinosinusitis are associated with inflammation patterns. Allergy. 2013;68:101–9.
6. Sejima T, Holtappels G, Kikuchi H, Imayoshi S, Ichimura K, Bachert C. Cytokine profiles in Japanese patients with chronic rhinosinusitis. Allergol Int. 2012;61:115–22.
7. Taruya T, Takeno S, Kubota K, Sasaki A, Ishino T, Hirakawa K. Comparison of arginase isoform expression in patients with different subtypes of chronic rhinosinusitis. J Laryngol Otol. 2015;129:1194–200.
8. Takeno S, Taruya T, Ueda T, Noda N, Hirakawa K. Increased exhaled nitric oxide and its oxidation metabolism in eosinophilic chronic rhinosinusitis. Auris Nasus Larynx. 2013;40:458–64.
9. Lund VJ, Mackay IS. Staging in rhinosinusitis. Rhinology. 1993;31:183–4.
10. Tran KN, Beule AG, Singal D, Wormald PJ. Frontal ostium restenosis after the endoscopic modified Lothrop procedure. Laryngoscope. 2007;117:1457–62.
11. Kubota K, Takeno S, Hirakawa K. Frontal recess anatomy in Japanese subjects and its effect on the development of frontal sinusitis: computed tomography analysis. J Otolaryngol Head Neck Surg. 2015;44:21.
12. Van Zele T, Claeys S, Gevaert P, Van Maele G, Holtappels G, Van Cauwenberge P, et al. Differentiation of chronic sinus diseases by measurement of inflammatory mediators. Allergy. 2006;61:1280–9.
13. Cao PP, Li HB, Wang BF, Wang SB, You XJ, Cui YH, et al. Distinct immunopathologic characteristics of various types of chronic rhinosinusitis in adult Chinese. J Allergy Clin Immunol. 2009;124:478–84.
14. Otto BA, Wenzel SE. The role of cytokines in chronic rhinosinusitis with nasal polyps. Curr Opin Otolaryngol Head Neck Surg. 2008;16:270–4.
15. Watelet JB, Claeys C, Perez-Novo C, Gevaert P, Van Cauwenberge P, Bachert C. Transforming growth factor β1 in nasal remodeling: differences between chronic rhinosinusitis and nasal polyposis. Am J Rhinol. 2004;18:267–72.
16. Pezato R, Balsalobre L, Lima M, Bezerra TFP, Voegels RL, Gregorio LC, et al. Convergence of two major pathophysiologic mechanisms in nasal polyposis: immune response to staphylococcus aureus. J Otolaryngol Head Neck Surg. 2013;42:27.
17. Kou W, Hu GH, Yao HB, Wang XQ, Shen Y, Kang HY, et al. Regulation of transforming growth factor-β1 activation and expression in the tissue remodeling involved in chronic rhinosinusitis. ORL J Otorhinolaryngol Relat Spec. 2012;74:172–8.
18. Ba L, Du J, Liu F, Yang F, Han M, Liu S, et al. Distinct inflammatory profiles in atopic and nonatopic patients with chronic rhinosinusitis accompanied by nasal polyps in western China. Allergy Asthma Immunol Res. 2015;7:346–58.
19. Hamilos DL, Leung DY, Wood R, Cunningham L, Bean DK, Yasruel Z, et al. Evidence for distinct cytokine expression in allergic versus nonallergic chronic sinusitis. J Allergy Clin Immunol. 1995;96:537–44.
20. Ghaffer O, Lavigne F, Kamil A, Renzi P, Hamid Q. Interleukin-6 expression in chronic sinusitis: colonization of gene transcripts to eosinophils, macrophages, T lymphocytes, and mast cells. Otolaryngol Head Neck Surg. 1998;118:504–11.
21. Taylor DR, Pijnenburg MW, Smith AD, DeJongste JC. Exhaled nitric oxide measurements: clinical application and interpretation. Thorax. 2006;61:817–27.
22. Ragab SM, Lund VJ, Saleh HA, Scadding G. Nasal nitric oxide in objective evaluation of chronic rhinosinusitis therapy. Allergy. 2006;61:717–24.

15

Cochlear implants and 1.5 T MRI scans: the effect of diametrically bipolar magnets and screw fixation on pain

Ingo Todt[1*], Grit Rademacher[2], Gloria Grupe[1], Andreas Stratmann[1], Arne Ernst[1], Sven Mutze[2] and Philipp Mittmann[1]

Abstract

Background: The probability that a patient will need an MRI scan at least once in a lifetime is high. However, MRI scanning in cochlear implantees is associated with side effects. Moreover, MRI scan-related artifacts, dislodging magnets, and pain are often the most frequent complications. The aim of this study was to evaluate the occurrence of pain in patients with cochlear implant systems using 1.5T MRI scans.

Methods: In a prospective case study of 10 implantees, an MRI scan was performed and the degree of pain was evaluated by a visual analog scale. Scans were performed firstly with and depending on the degree of discomfort/pain, without a headband. Four of the cochlear implants contained a screw fixation. Six cochlear implants contained an internal diametrically bipolar magnet. MRI observations were performed with a 1.5 T scanner.

Results: MRI scans were performed on all patients without causing any degree of pain, even without the use of a headband.

Conclusion: Patients undergoing 1.5 T MRIs with devices including a diametrically bipolar magnet or a rigid implant screw fixation, experienced no pain, even without headbands.

Keywords: MRI, Cochlear implant, Complication, Pain, Diametrically bipolar magnet, Screw fixation

Background

Cochlear implantation is the treatment of choice for patients with severe hearing loss, and those who have profound hearing loss (deafness affecting one or both ears). So far, about 400,000 patients have been provided with a cochlear implant.

MRI observations in cochlear implantees are a long-term problem. Because the fixation of the implant audio processor is magnet-based, MRI scans need special modifications to circumvent possible inaccuracy. On the other hand, previous trials with magnet-free implant systems did not lead to significant acceptance [1].

The internal cochlear implant magnet leads to a number of testing difficulties. The magnet generates significant artifacts, leading to the inability to assess specific ipsilateral

structures [2]. Magnet dislocations can occur, cause pain, and act as a source of infections [3]. Depending on the sequencing used and the position of the implant, the visibility of the scan can be modified to allow an assessment of the cochlea and the internal auditory canal [4, 5]. With specific headbands, the number of magnet dislocations described are rare [6]. However, the occurrence of pain during the scan is a frequent complication even in cases where a dislocation did not occur [6, 7]. Often MRI scans cannot be performed because of the related pain [7].

Concerning how specific devices measure rates of pain, Grupe et al. [6] described an overall pain/ discomfort rate of 70% including Advanced Bionics 90 K, 90 K Advance devices, Cochlear 512, 422, 24 RCA and MEDEL Concerto systems.

Kim observed pain/discomfort in 7 out of 19 cases without performed general anesthesia [7] for the scanning. Causing devices were Nucleus 24 RCA, 22 M, Advanced Bionics 90 k and CII. Crane [8] described a

* Correspondence: todt@gmx.net
[1]Department of Otolaryngology, Head and Neck Surgery, Unfallkrankenhaus Berlin, Warenerstr.7, 12683 Berlin, Germany
Full list of author information is available at the end of the article

general mild sedation protocol, but in two out of 22 scans (Nucleus, 90 k) pain-related problems occurred. Carlson found in two out of 34 scans the occurrence of pain, which did not allow a regular completion of the scan [9] with Nucleus 24 devices.

Therefore, the use of an MRI in a cochlear implantee warrants special consideration. Because all of these side effects are well-known, manufacturers (Cochlear Corp., Sydney, Australia; Advanced Bionics, Stäfa, Switzerland; Medel, Innsbruck, Austria; Oticon, Valaudaris, France) recommend head bandages for safety reasons for 1.5T (Cochlear 24, 422, 512, 522, 532; Advanced Bionics 90 k, 90 k Advance, Ultra; MEDEL Concerto, Synchrony; Oticon ZTI), or magnet removal at 3T (Cochlear 24, 422, 512, 522, 532; Oticon ZTI) or headbands for 3T (Medel Synchro-ny). Generally different from other systems are two MRI-relevant device specifications. One option is to use screws to anchor the implant (Neuro ZTI, Oticon, Valaudaris, France), and the other is to incorporate a diametrically bipolar magnet (Synchrony, Medel, Innsbruck, Austria) to decrease the force on the implant and therefore prevent magnet dislocations, demagnetization and pain.

The aim of this study was to evaluate the occurrence of pain in patients with cochlear implant systems using 1.5T MRI scans.

Methods

The study was approved by the institutional review board of the Unfallkrankenhaus Berlin, Germany (IRB-ukb-HNO-2016/01). Patients gave their written informed consent for the use of their clinical records in this prospective study.

In this prospective case study, from 2014 through 2016, 10 patients under-went a 1.5T MRI observation provided in a tertial referral center with varying cochlear implant types. Six patients were implanted with a Medel Synchrony implant (Medel, Innsbruck, Austria) and a bipolar magnet. The implant was intraoperatively anchored with a absorbable suture. An implant bed was drilled for these cases. Four patients were implanted with an Oticon Neuro ZTI implant (Oticon, Vallauris, France). The implant was only fixed with two selftaping screws. An implant bed was not drilled.

All examinations were performed in a 1.5 Tesla MR imaging unit (Ingenia, Philips Medical Systems, Best, NL) using an 8-channel array head coil. All patients underwent two MRI scans. First the patient was introduced into the MRI scanner with a headband. The headband consists of a tight self-taping wrap with a hard plain piece to prevent dislodging of the magnet. After the evaluation of pain and inspection of the implant area, the patient was introduced into the scanner without a headband a second time.

The evaluation of pain was performed with a visual analog scale (VAS) scoring from 0 to 10. Zero indicated the non-occurrence of pain and discomfort. Ten indicated a pain-related interruption during the scan. The questionnaire was used directly after the first and directly after the second scan. Magnet strength was subjectively evaluated by the attraction force of the antenna coil. Magnet displacement was evaluated by the digital control of the implant magnet area.

Scanning parameters:

TSE T2 2D: TR: 3300 ms, TE 120 ms, slice thickness 1.5 mm, reconstruction resolution of 0.55 × 0.55 × 1.5 mm, F0 V 120 × 120. 12 slices.

TSE T1 2D: TR: 550 ms, TE 20 ms, slice thickness 3 mm, reconstruction resolution of 0.23 × 0.23 × 3 mm, F0 V 120 × 120. 20 slices, matrix size: 400 × 318.

Results

In all patients, two MRI scans at 1.5T were performed without complications, in terms of magnet dislocation and pain. One scan with the headband and one scan without the headband were performed. In all cases, a headband was not necessary to prevent pain or magnet dislocation. The mean VAS with and without head-band, in terms of pain, was 0. The evaluation was performed directly after the scan. Individual data are given (Table 1). A change of the magnet strength or polarization was not observed for either implant.

Discussion

MRI observations are frequently necessary in cochlear implantees for head-related reasons (exclusion of tumor, unclear vertigo, exclusion of infarction) or non-head-related reasons. The probability for an MRI once in a lifetime has been described to be 50–75% [10]. 1.5T MRI scans for cochlear implantees are associated with artifacts [8] and magnet dislocations [5],

Table 1 Patients individual MRI data

Name	sex	age	implant	VAS for MRI with headband	VAS for MRI without headband
Pat.1	f	45	MEDEL Synchrony	0	0
Pat.2	m	56	MEDEL Synchrony	0	0
Pat.3	f	72	MEDEL Synchrony	0	0
Pat.4	f	43	MEDEL Synchrony	0	0
Pat.5	f	43	MEDEL Synchrony	0	0
Pat.6	f	35	MEDEL Synchrony	0	0
Pat.7	f	65	Oticon ZTI	0	0
Pat.8	m	67	Oticon ZTI	0	0
Pat.9	f	45	Oticon ZTI	0	0
Pat.10	f	70	Oticon ZTI	0	0

and, as a most frequent topic, pain [6]. At 3T additional demagnetization has been described [2].

While manufacturers recommend a headband during the MRI scan to prevent pain and magnet dislocation, it has been shown to be ineffective [6] in many cases. Pain is often the reason not to scan. The complication rate of MRI scans due to pain or discomfort is between 70% [6], 2 out of 22 [8], 7 out of 19 [7] and 2 non-tolerated cases out of 34 cases of MRI scans experience pain or discomfort [9]. All studies, to date, have used implants that contain magnets in silicon pockets or rigid incorporated magnets with a non-fixed implant body. Out of the experience with the two observed implant specifications in terms of pain, it can be assumed that the movement of the implant magnet out of the silicon pocket (Nucleus 24 to 512, Advanced Bionics 90 k) or the implant itself (Advanced Bionics CII, Medel Concerto) causes pain during scanning.

It can be assumed that the mechanism of pain occurrence is related to the magnet movement inside the MRI magnet field which results in a hard-to-contact signal between magnet,periostium and inner skin layer.

Clinically the effectiveness of a diametrically bipolar magnet and screwing fixed implant modification to prevent this complication is unknown and therefore the first description of this topic.

Medel Synchrony implant includes a diametrically bipolar magnet, which directs itself in the magnetic field of an MRI scanner. This direction was assumed to prevent demagnetization at 3T. The effect on pain prevention is so far unclear. We were able to show that the implant magnet configuration even prevents the occurrence of pain. A magnet dislocation was not observed.

The second implant (Oticon Neuro ZTI) includes a rigid implant corpus with a magnet to screw in and out of the corpus. The implant itself is fixed with screws on the skull. This anchor seems to prevent a torsion of implant and magnet to press on the periost and skin. Magnet dislocation could not be observed.

The prevention of pain and magnet dislocation is of high importance because these two factors are the most frequent and relevant in the clinical routine.

The ability to perform an MRI scan without pain or the risk of magnet dislocation offers the clinician and the radiologist the field to perform 1,5T MRI scans routinely with only some limitations (e.g., artifact relevant limitations, Tesla strength limitations, demagnetization for ZTI Implant at 3 T).

Conclusion

Patients undergoing 1.5 T MRIs with devices including a diametrically bipolar magnet or a rigid implant screw fixation have no pain, even without headbands.

All procedures performed in studies involving human participants were in accordance with the ethical standards of the institutional and/or national research committee and with the 1964 Helsinki declaration and its later amendments or comparable ethical standards.

Abbreviations
CI: Cochlear implant; MRI: Magnet resonance imaging; T: Tesla; VAS: Visual analog scale

Acknowledgements
None

Funding
No

Authors' contributions
IT- idea, writer. GR- performing scans. AS- patient acquisition. GG- patient acquisition. SM- helping in manuscript writing. AE- helping in manuscript writing. PM-analyzing data, scans. All authors read and approved the final manuscript.

Authors' information
IT- head of implant division.
GR-head of MR group.
AS- junior resident.
GG- junior resident.
SM- head of radiology department.
AE- head of department.
PM- resident.

Competing interests
The authors declare that they have no competing interests.

Author details
[1]Department of Otolaryngology, Head and Neck Surgery, Unfallkrankenhaus Berlin, Warenerstr.7, 12683 Berlin, Germany. [2]Department of Radiology, Unfallkrankenhaus Berlin, Berlin, Germany.

References
1. Weber BP, Neuburger J, Lenarz T. Development and clinical testing of a non-magneticcochlear implant. Preliminary experimental studies and surgical concept. Results in the first 10 patients. Laryngorhinootologie. 1998 Jul;77(7):376–81.
2. Majdani O, Rau TS, Götz F, Zimmerling M, Lenarz M, Lenarz T, Labadie R, Leinung M. Artifacts caused by cochlear implants with non-removable magnets in 3T MRI: phantom and cadaveric studies. Eur Arch Otorhinolaryngol. 2009;266(12):1885–90.
3. Hassepass F, Stabenau V, Maier W, Arndt S, Laszig R, Beck R, Aschendorff A. Revision surgery due to magnet dislocation in cochlear implant patients: an emerging complication. Otol Neurotol. 2014;35(1):29–34.

4. Walton J, Donnelly NP, Chuen Tam Y, Joubert I, Durie-Gair J, Jackson C, Mannion RA, Tysome JR, Axon PR, Scoffings DJ. MRI without magnet removal in Neurofibromatosis type 2 patients with Cochlear and auditory brainstem implants. Otol Neurotol. 2014;35:821–5.

5. Todt I, Rademacher G, Mittmann P, Wagner J, Mutze S, Ernst A. MRI Artifacts and Cochlear Implant Positioning at 3 T In Vivo.Otol Neurotol. 2015 (b)Jul;36(6):972–6.

6. Grupe G, Wagner J, Hofmann S, Stratmann A, Mittmann P, Ernst A, Todt I Prevalence and Complications of MRI Scans of Cochlear Implant Patients. HNO 2016, Feb 17 (epub ahead of print).

7. Kim BG, Kim JW, Park JJ, Kim SH, Kim HN, Choi JY. Adverse events and discomfort during magnetic resonance imaging in cochlear implant recipients. JAMA Otolaryngol Head Neck Surg. 2015;141(1):45–52.

8. Crane BT, Gottschalk B, Kraut M, Aygun N, Niparko JK. Magnetic resonance imaging at 1.5 T after cochlear implantation. Otol Neurotol. 2010 Oct;31(8):1215–20.

9. Carlson ML, Neff BA, Link MJ, Lane LI, Watson RE, McGee KP, Bernstein MA, Driscoll CLW. Magnetic resonance imaging with Cochlear implant magnet in place: safety and imaging quality. Otol Neurotol. 2015;36:965–71.

10. Kalin R, Stanton MS. Current clinical issues for MRI scanning of pacemaker and defibrillator patients. Pacing Clin Electrophysiol. 2005;28:326–8.

16

Development and validation of an administrative data algorithm to identify adults who have endoscopic sinus surgery for chronic rhinosinusitis

Kristian I. Macdonald[1*], Shaun J. Kilty[1] and Carl van Walraven[2]

Abstract

Background: This was a diagnostic accuracy study to develop an algorithm based on administrative database codes that identifies patients with Chronic Rhinosinusitis (CRS) who have endoscopic sinus surgery (ESS).

Methods: From January 1st, 2011 to December 31st, 2012, a chart review was performed for all hospital-identified ESS surgical encounters. The reference standard was developed as follows: cases were assigned to encounters in which ESS was performed for Otolaryngologist-diagnosed CRS; all other chart review encounters, and all other hospital surgical encounters during the timeframe were controls. Algorithm development was based on International Classification of Diseases, version 10 (ICD-10) diagnostic codes and Canadian Classification of Health Interventions (CCI) procedural codes. Internal model validation was performed with a similar chart review for all model-identified cases and 200 randomly selected controls during the following year.

Results: During the study period, 347 cases and 185,007 controls were identified. The predictive model assigned cases to all encounters that contained at least one CRS ICD-10 diagnostic code and at least one ESS CCI procedural code. Compared to the reference standard, the algorithm was very accurate: sensitivity 96.0% (95%CI 93.2–97.7), specificity 100% (95% CI 99.9–100), and positive predictive value 95.4% (95%CI 92.5–97.3). Internal validation using chart review for the following year revealed similar accuracy: sensitivity 98.9% (95%CI 95.8–99.8), specificity 97.1% (95%CI 93.4–98.8), and positive predictive value 96.9% (95%CI 93.0–99.8).

Conclusion: A simple model based on administrative database codes accurately identified ESS-CRS encounters. This model can be used in population-based cohorts to study longitudinal outcomes for the ESS-CRS population.

Keywords: Chronic rhinosinusitis, Administrative database research, Endoscopic sinus surgery, Diagnostic codes

Background

Chronic Rhinosinusitis (CRS) is a common and debilitating inflammatory disease of the sinonasal cavities. CRS is associated with significant resource utilization and burden on health care expenditures [1]. The prevalence of CRS has been quoted as between 5 and 15% of the population [1, 2], and appears to be rising [3]. Patients with CRS self-report their overall health status at a level similar to those with other chronic diseases including current or previous cancer, asthma, migraine, arthritis and epilepsy [4].

Much of the epidemiological data that forms our understanding of CRS is based on studies that identify CRS within large administrative databases and health surveys. We recently published a systematic review of studies that determined the accuracy of these methods to identify CRS [5], and found three studies that compared CRS identification (ascertained from diagnostic codes and self-reporting) to a reference standard (including clinician-performed chart review, nasal endoscopy, and Otolaryngologist-based CRS clinical diagnosis), with moderate to good accuracy.

* Correspondence: krmacdonald@toh.on.ca
[1]MD FRCSC, Department of Otolaryngology – Head & Neck Surgery, University of Ottawa, Ottawa, ON, Canada
Full list of author information is available at the end of the article

Health administrative (HA) data may provide the best research modality to develop reliable population-based statistics for CRS patients. HA data have great potential to answer important research questions because of their low cost (since the data are already collected), wide external validity (since the data can cover all people within a particular health care system), and large numbers of patients to provide statistical power [6].

Administrative databases are not built for research purposes, and HA research *"creates risks that can make them uninterpretable or bias their results"* [7]. Within HA data, diseases and procedures are represented with codes. The validity of using HA data to answer research questions is dependent on the accuracy of these codes for the entity they are supposed to represent. Inaccuracies via coding errors that occur in defining the initial cohort, the exposure, or the outcome in an administrative data project can result in biased conclusions. Despite the importance of establishing the accuracy of administrative database codes, such validation is performed in less than 20% of administrative database studies [8]. One of the core (and arguably most important) requirements for using ADs for research involves validation of the codes that serve as proxies of a defined population [9, 10].

Our objective was to identify a model that that would accurately identify CRS patients within HA data. The single physician diagnostic CRS code "473.x" (Version 9 of the International Classification of Disease (ICD-9)) is one such model for identifying CRS cases. However, the aforementioned systematic review identified one study in which this code had just a 34% positive predictive value (PPV). A more feasible solution to meet our objective of capturing a CRS cohort within HA data was to examine CRS patients who had ESS. CRS patients who fail medical therapy are potential surgical candidates, and this subgroup therefore represents patients with medically refractory CRS [11].

We first created a chart review-based reference standard cohort of patients who had ESS for CRS, and then derived a model based on health administrative data to identify this population within a surgical cohort. The final objective was a model that, when applied to all surgical encounters, accurately identified ESS-CRS encounters.

Methods

This was a validation study of diagnostic test accuracy using several measures of accuracy including sensitivity, specificity and predictive values. To achieve current standards in performing studies of diagnostic accuracy, we adhered to the Standards for Reporting of Diagnostic Accuracy Studies (STARD, 2015 version [12], Appendix). This study received institutional research ethics board approval (OHSN-REB 20140164).

Databases used

The Ottawa Hospital Data Warehouse (OHDW) contains data from several source systems of patient data dating back as far as 1996 for patients treated at the Ottawa Hospital (TOH), a 1000-bed tertiary care hospital serving over 1.2 million patients and affiliated with the University of Ottawa. Several groups of variables are recorded for each patient encounter including unique identifiers, patient demographics, encounter type, diagnoses, and services rendered (including surgeries). We used the surgery dataset, an online computerized charting and scheduling system for all operations that occur at TOH back to April 2008, having several checklists in place to ensure the correct surgery for the correct indication is recorded (such as the surgeon completing and submitting the paperwork for the surgery, the actual procedure(s) that was (were) performed during the operation), all of which is confirmed by the surgeon at the end of the case.

While the OHDW contains data for TOH patients, the Institute for Clinical Evaluative Sciences (ICES) maintains administrative data for over 13 million people covered by the publically funded health plan. Patients treated at TOH can be identified and linked through both databases with unique identifiers.

Identifying patients undergoing ESS for CRS at TOH

We obtained a cohort of all TOH surgical encounters that were recorded as Otolaryngologist-performed ESS procedures between January 1st, 2011 and December 31st, 2012 for patients ≥18 years old. The encounters selected for the chart review were identified as follows: because ESS is only performed by Otolaryngologists, we first identified all surgical encounters performed by this type of surgeon. We then selected all encounters that listed ESS as at least a minor component of the surgery performed during that encounter.

The extracted cohort therefore included all ESS surgeries performed by TOH Otolaryngologists, meaning that all other surgeries conducted at TOH during this time period (all by non Otolaryngologists) were not ESS.

Chart review: determine whether ESS was conducted for CRS

A chart review was performed of all Otolaryngologist-performed ESS cases to identify those in which ESS was the predominant surgery performed (as opposed to other procedures such as open sinus approaches), and in which ESS was performed for Otolaryngologist-diagnosed CRS (as opposed to other indications such as benign tumours, cerebrospinal fluid leaks, encephaloceles, trauma, foreign bodies, and invasive fungal sinusitis) [13–15]. The chart review was performed by a single author (KM), and involved analysis of primary care physician referrals, clinic notes, operative notes, and sinus CT imaging. We used Otolaryngologist-diagnosed CRS as opposed to a retrospective chart review to identify symptoms and objective findings meeting CRS diagnostic criteria [11], because the latter approach would more likely result in incomplete data collection and misclassification. If the listed diagnosis was recurrent sinusitis, a more detailed chart review was performed to determine if the patient had coexisting CRS. This included clinic notes, preoperative imaging, and prior OR reports. If the patient had associated CRS, the encounter was labeled as a case, otherwise a control.

Patient encounters in which the chart review confirmed ESS for CRS were categorized as cases. All other encounters were categorized as controls.

Linkage to population-based datasets at ICES

This dataset was linked to ICES via unique identifiers that were encrypted to maintain patient confidentiality. This linked dataset with assigned ESS-CRS cases and controls then provided the reference standard from which the predictive model was created.

Derivation and internal validation of model to identify ESS for CRS encounters

The same clinician (KM) who performed the chart review created the model. Model development was based on an *a*

priori identification of codes that could differentiate cases and controls. Table 1 lists the ICD-10 (International classification of diseases, version 10 [16]) diagnostic codes for CRS and CCI (Canadian Classification of Health Interventions, version 2015 [17]) codes for ESS that were identified from this process.

Model variations were developed in a trial and error approach. We considered several variable types for model inclusion, including hospital length of stay (as most ESS is day surgery), age and major comorbidities (because ESS for CRS is usually an elective surgery that may be performed in younger and healthier people compared to other major surgeries), and the CCI and ICD-10 codes listed in Table 1. Our aim was to develop a simple model that used as few codes and variable types as possible, but that made clinical sense. We theorized that each ESS-CRS surgical encounter should contain some variation of ICD-10 CRS and CCI ESS codes, and so we determined to use at least these two variable types in our model. The model was built and adjusted based on comparing the accuracy of model case ascertainment to the reference standard.

The final model accuracy was displayed in a 2x2 table comparing the case status of the model output to the reference standard. Validation statistics with 95% confidence intervals (95% CI) were calculated, using SAS version 9.3 for UNIX (SAS Institute, Inc., USA).

Table 1 Administrative database codes used in predictive model

Chronic Rhinosinusitis			Endoscopic sinus surgery	
Diagnosis	ICD-10 code*	ICD-09 code*	Procedure	CCI code*
Chronic sinusitis	J32	473	Therapeutic Interventions on the Ethmoidal Sinus	1.EU.^^.^^
Chronic maxillary sinusitis	J32.0	473.0	Drainage, ethmoidal sinus	1.EU.52.^^
Chronic frontal sinusitis	J32.1	473.1	Excision partial, ethmoidal sinus	1.EU.87.^^
Chronic ethmoidal sinusitis	J32.2	473.2	Therapeutic Interventions on the Sphenoidal Sinus	1.EV.^^.^^
Chronic sphenoidal sinusitis	J32.3	473.3	Drainage, sphenoidal sinus	1.EV.52.^^
Chronic pansinusitis	J32.4	N/A	Excision partial, sphenoidal sinus	1.EV.87.^^
Other chronic sinusitis	J32.8	473.8	Therapeutic Interventions on the Maxillary Sinus	1.EW.^^.^^
Chronic sinusitis, unspecified	J32.9	473.9	Excision partial, sphenoidal sinus	1.EV.87.^^
Nasal polyp	J33	471	Therapeutic Interventions on the Maxillary Sinus	1.EW.^^.^^
Polyp of nasal cavity	J33.0	471.0	Drainage, maxillary sinus	1.EW.52.^^
Polypoid sinus degeneration	J33.1	471.1	Therapeutic Interventions on the Frontal Sinus	1.EX.^^
Other polyp of sinus	J33.8	471.8	Drainage, frontal sinus	1.EX.52.^^
Nasal polyp, unspecified	J33.9	471.9	Destruction, frontal sinus	1.EX.59.^^
			Repair, frontal sinus	1.EX.80.^^
			Excision partial, frontal sinus	1.EX.87.^^
			Therapeutic Interventions on the Paranasal Sinuses	1.EY.^^.^^
			Excision partial, paranasal sinuses	1.EY.87.^^
			Excision radical, paranasal sinuses	1.EY.91.^^

Codes used in predictive model to identify patients who had endoscopic sinus surgery for chronic rhinosinusitis, with a chart review as a reference standard
International Classification of Diseases, version 10; *CCI* Canadian Classification of Health Interventions

Internal validation was then performed to determine model accuracy within another TOH cohort from a different time-period. Using model criteria, all TOH patient encounters identified by the model as cases and 200 randomly selected controls between Jan. 1st, 2013 and Dec. 31st, 2013 were retrieved. A chart review was performed of the approximate 400 encounters to determine reference standard case status, by the same clinician, (KM) blinded to the model-predicted case status. Once the chart review was completed, model case status was revealed, and another 2x2 table and set of validation statistics were created to determine internal validation of the model.

Results

Chart review

From Jan. 1st 2011, to Dec. 31st, 2012, 411 TOH surgical encounters were identified as having ESS (Fig. 1). Of these, 17 were excluded after the chart review revealed that the major surgery was one other than ESS, leaving 394 encounters that included at least endoscopic antrostomy and ethmoidectomy. Another 37 encounters were excluded because the procedures were for diagnoses other than chronic sinusitis, including 18 sinonasal tumours and 8 with recurrent sinusitis with no evidence of associated CRS. The OR report (with the surgery and indication) for the specified surgical encounter was sufficient to establish case status in all but the 8 patients with recurrent sinusitis. For these 8 patients, no satisfactory evidence of associated CRS could be determined

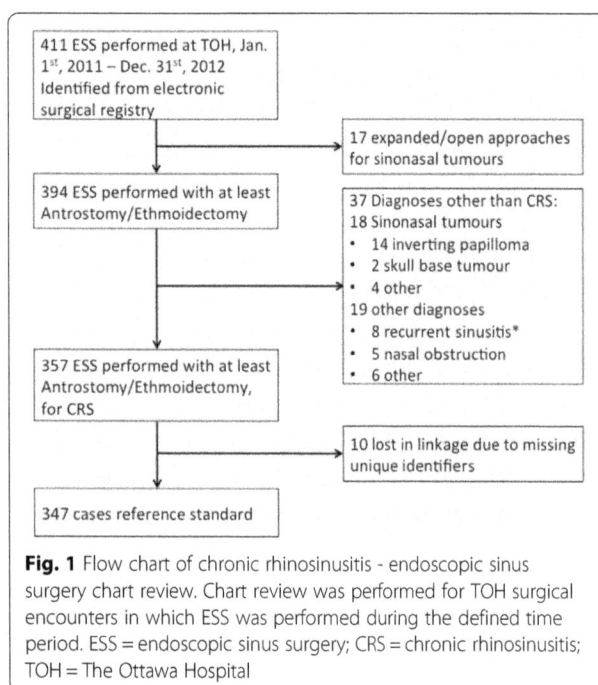

Fig. 1 Flow chart of chronic rhinosinusitis - endoscopic sinus surgery chart review. Chart review was performed for TOH surgical encounters in which ESS was performed during the defined time period. ESS = endoscopic sinus surgery; CRS = chronic rhinosinusitis; TOH = The Ottawa Hospital

from the chart review. This resulted in 357 ESS-CRS cases during the study period.

Linkage of chart review data to ICES dataset

Patient encounters within the TOH chart review cohort and ICES dataset were linked via encrypted unique identifiers. Thirteen patients (ten cases and three controls) were lost in the linkage due to missing unique identifiers. The linked dataset contained 185,354 hospital encounters representing all surgeries performed at TOH from Jan. 1st, 2011, to Dec. 31st, 2012. This linked dataset, with 347 cases and 185,007 controls, (case prevalence = 0.19) was used to develop the predictive model.

Model development

The model was created through a trial and error approach, using variables within the linked dataset. It was evident from analyzing the variable types and values that each case encounter contained commonly assigned CRS diagnostic and ESS procedural codes. The first model assigned cases if an encounter listed any of the ICD-10 CRS diagnostic codes listed in Table 1. Compared to the reference standard case ascertainment, this model had excellent validation statistics: sensitivity 96.5% (95% CI 93.9–98.1) and positive predictive value (PPV) 93.3% (95% CI 90.1–95.6).

The second model was based on procedural ESS codes only. Cases were assigned if an encounter listed any one of the CCI ESS procedural codes listed in Table 1. Compared to the reference standard case ascertainment, this model had similarly high validation statistics: sensitivity 96.8% (95%CI 94.2–98.3) and PPV 93.3% (95%CI 90.1–95.6).

The third and final model combined features from the first two models, resulting in a slightly improved PPV. Encounters were classified by the final model as ESS for CRS if they had been coded with any of the ICD-10 CRS diagnostic codes listed in Table 1 along with any of the CCI ESS surgical codes listed in Table 1. All encounters not meeting these criteria were classified as controls (i.e. not ESS for CRS). Table 2 compares validation statistics of the three model variations. Specificity for all three models was 100%.

Table 3 displays a 2x2 table comparing the final model output to the reference standard, with validation statistics including sensitivity 96.0% (95%CI 93.2–97.7), specificity 100% (95%CI 99.9–100), positive predictive value 95.4% (95%CI 92.5–97.3), positive likelihood ratio 11,096 (95%CI 6,794–18,120), and negative likelihood ratio 0.04 (95%CI 0.02–0.07). Fig. 2 displays a graphical overview of the final model.

Further examination of the 16 false positives (encounters identified as cases by the model but were controls

Table 2 Comparison of validation statistics of three models to predict CRS-ESS encounters

Model version	Sensitivity % (95%CI)	Specificity % (95%CI)	PPV % (95%CI)
#1: Any CRS diagnostic ICD-10 code	96.5 (93.9–98.1)	100 (99.9–100)	93.3 (90.1–95.6)
#2: Any ESS procedural CCI code	96.8 (94.2–98.3)	100 (99.9–100)	93.3 (90.1–95.6)
#3: #1 AND #2	96.0 (93.2–97.7)	100 (99.9–100)	95.4 (92.5–97.2)

Comparison of three different model versions to predict CRS-ESS status, compared to the reference standard
CI confidence interval, *CRS* Chronic rhinosinusitis, *ESS* Endoscopic sinus surgery, *PPV* positive predictive value

by the reference standard), revealed that eight were patients with recurrent sinusitis according to the reference standard.

Internal validation of model

Using criteria from the final model, we retrieved a hospital cohort of all cases and 200 randomly selected controls from year following the derivation cohort, Jan. 1st, 2013 to Dec. 31st, 2013. A chart review, blinded to model output case status, was then performed to determine reference standard case status. The OR report for the selected surgical encounter was sufficient to determine case status in all encounters. After the model output case status was revealed, a 2x2 table was again created with excellent accuracy: sensitivity 98.9% (95%CI 95.8–99.8) specificity 97.1% (95%CI 93.4–98.8), positive predictive value 96.9% (95%CI 93.0–98.7) positive likelihood ratio 33.6 (95%CI 15.3–74.0), and negative likelihood ratio of 0.01 (95%CI 0.00–0.04). (Table 4)

Discussion

We developed an internally validated model that accurately identified patient encounters in which endoscopic sinus surgery was performed for chronic rhinosinusitis at the Ottawa Hospital over a 3-year period. This model is simple and includes readily available administrative data to accurately differentiate between ESS-CRS cases and controls within a surgical cohort. The criteria for a case (at least one ICD-10 CRS diagnostic code and at least one CCI ESS procedural code) were not created *a priori*, but instead through a trial and error process with the observations and variables contained within the dataset, with knowledge of the chart review data.

Table 3 Predictive model vs reference standard for ESS-CRS status

Model output	Reference standard		Total
	Case	Control	
Case	333	16	349
Control	14	184,991	185,005
Total	347	185,007	185,354

Predictive model based on administrative database codes
CCI Canadian Classification of Health Interventions, *CRS* Chronic rhinosinusitis, *ESS* Endoscopic sinus surgery, *ICD-10* International Classification of Disease, version 10

However, we argue that this model has face validity for Otolaryngologic epidemiology research.

Despite the importance of validation studies for AD codes, the lack of code validation is hardly unique to CRS: a 2011 review of a random Medline sample of 115 AD research studies found that only 14 (12.1%) "measured or referenced the association of the code with the entity is supposedly represented", and "of five studies reporting code sensitivity and specificity, the estimated probability of code-related condition in code-positive patients was less than 50% in two" [8]. Therefore, "people with a code frequently do not have the condition it represents". Applying this to our population, it is incorrect to assume ESS and CRS codes are accurate without measuring the ability of a code to differentiate between a case and a control, with an acceptable reference standard.

Validation studies like this one are essential for future AD research using specific codes. As one example, a recent publication used a similar chart review method used to validate National Surgical Quality Improvement Program 30-day readmission codes [18].

Conducting such health administrative database research in Ontario is aided by the fact that ESS is a

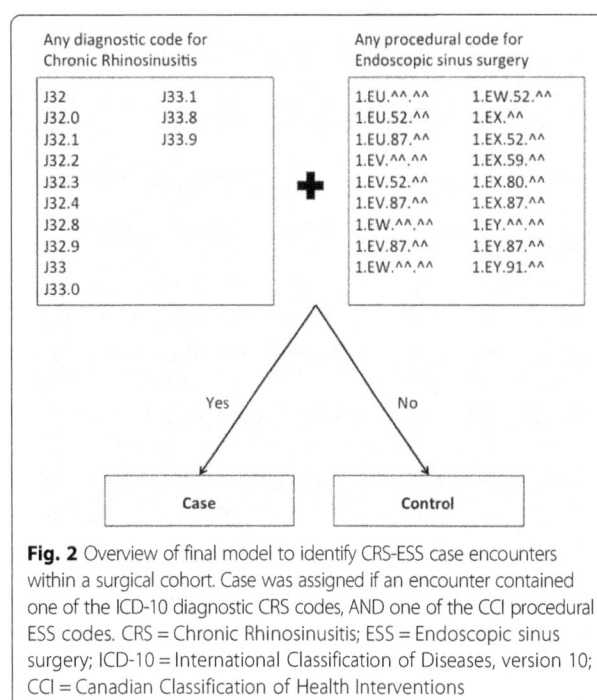

Fig. 2 Overview of final model to identify CRS-ESS case encounters within a surgical cohort. Case was assigned if an encounter contained one of the ICD-10 diagnostic CRS codes, AND one of the CCI procedural ESS codes. CRS = Chronic Rhinosinusitis; ESS = Endoscopic sinus surgery; ICD-10 = International Classification of Diseases, version 10; CCI = Canadian Classification of Health Interventions

Table 4 Internal validation of predictive model of ESS-CRS status

Model output	Reference standard		Total
	Case	Control	
Case	186	6	192
Control	2	198	200
Total	188	204	392

The ESS-CRS predictive model was applied to all TOH surgical patients in 2013. Sensitivity 98.9% specificity 97.1%, positive predictive value 96.9%
CRS Chronic rhinosinusitis, *ESS* Endoscopic sinus surgery, *TOH* The Ottawa Hospital

publically funded procedure. As a result, all ESS performed in Ontario should be captured within these databases. Advantages of this population-based method to identify patients undergoing ESS for CRS include: 1) minimal cost, as most work for this research is at the computer and through a chart review; 2) large numbers of patients from a population-based database allow complete analyses without sampling; and 3) if externally validated, this model can be used to study longitudinal outcomes for ESS as an intervention in CRS patients.

Others have identified ESS procedures (for all indications, not just CRS) in HA databases using similar procedural codes for ESS (similar CCI codes in Alberta [19], and Common Procedural Terminology codes in the US [20]). In these studies, the authors did not attempt to determine code accuracy to determine if patients identified by these methods actually had ESS. Our chart review revealed that 17/411 (4%) patients who were identified as having ESS actually had a more invasive open procedure, and 37/394 (9.4%) patients who had at least endoscopic antrostomy/ethmoidectomy did not have CRS. Combined, 54/411 (13.1%) patients who were coded at TOH as having ESS did not truly have ESS or CRS. However, despite these potential inadequacies in code accuracy, a model based only on ESS codes achieved almost the same accuracy in identifying ESS-CRS cases as our final model (sensitivity 96.8% (95%CI 94.2–98.3), specificity 100% (95%CI 99.9–100), PPV 93.3% (95%CI 90.1–95.6)), giving validity to previous authors' work. In an analysis similar to ours (although again without an attempt at code validation), Benninnger et al. identified ESS-CRS patients within a cohort of 35.5 million patients enrolled in the Market Scan Commercial Claims and Encounter database in 2010 [21]. They used analogous codes: sinus surgery codes (CPT-4 31254-31288 [Common Procedure Terminology, 4th Ed]), and ICD-9 CRS diagnostic codes (473.X), and identified 2,833 ESS-CRS patients. Our results provide argument that these methods of identifying ESS procedures may be accurate – this statement would be further supported if our model was externally validated or if other authors carried out similar validation projects.

We found that eight of the false positives identified by the final model were encounters in which ESS was performed for recurrent sinusitis with no coexisting CRS. This misclassification reflects a potential inability of administrative database codes to differentiate between these two conditions. Although this did not greatly affect our validation statistics, it could affect external validity, for example in centres where a greater proportion of ESS is performed for recurrent sinusitis.

Several assumptions must be made that could be interpreted as study weaknesses. First, development of the reference standard, predictive model, and internal validation were all performed by the one clinician. This bias could influence case ascertainment in the reference standard and internal validation, as well as variable selection for the final model, falsely elevating the model accuracy. Second, we used Otolaryngologist-diagnosed CRS for reference standard case ascertainment. This infers that the Otolaryngologist correctly diagnosed CRS. It is possible that strict diagnostic criteria were not applied. We considered establishing a guideline-based CRS diagnosis as the reference standard through a retrospective chart review of the patient charts (including clinic notes and imaging) but this would have been exposed to recall and selection bias. Third, we must also assume that patient encounters are correctly recorded in the surgical database, and specifically that ESS encounters were correctly identified for the chart review.

Future direction

Our future direction includes external validation at other tertiary care centres, similar to the methods used in internal validation. An externally validated model can then be used to study longitudinal outcomes and health services research of this population. Other centres may be encouraged to perform their own external validation based on our model criteria, with the overarching objective of producing much needed accurate CRS epidemiological data.

Conclusions

A simple model based on administrative database codes accurately identified surgical encounters in which endoscopic sinus surgery was performed for chronic rhinosinusitis (CRS) at a tertiary care centre. Compared to a reference standard including a chart review and Otolaryngologist-diagnosed CRS, this model achieved excellent validation statistics: sensitivity 96.0% (95%CI 93.2–97.7), specificity 100%, and positive predictive value 95.4% (95%CI 92.5–97.3). Internal validation was achieved with similarly high validation statistics.

This model has potential for large population-based cohorts to study longitudinal outcomes of patients who have endoscopic sinus surgery for chronic rhinosinusitis.

Appendix

Table 5 Standards for reporting diagnostic accuracy studies checklist [12] (2015 version)

Section & Topic	No	Item	On page & line
Title or Abstract	1	Identification as a study of diagnostic accuracy using at least one measure of accuracy (such as sensitivity, specificity, predictive values, or AUC)	P6 L2
Abstract	2	Structured summary of study design, methods, results, and conclusions	P2
Introduction	3	Scientific and clinical background, including the intended use and clinical role of the index test	P4
	4	Study objectives and hypotheses	P5 L9
Methods			
Study design	5	Whether data collection was planned before the index test and reference standard were performed (prospective study) or after (retrospective study)	P7 L5
Participants	6	Eligibility criteria	P7 L5
	7	On what basis potentially eligible participants were identified (such as symptoms, results from previous tests, inclusion in registry)	P7 L5
	8	Where and when potentially eligible participants were identified (setting, location and dates)	P7 L5
	9	Whether participants formed a consecutive, random or convenience series	P7 L5
Test methods Analysis	10a	Index test, in sufficient detail to allow replication	P8 L13
	10b	Reference standard, in sufficient detail to allow replication	P7 L10
	11	Rationale for choosing the reference standard (if alternatives exist)	P8 L13
	12a	Definition of and rationale for test positivity cut-offs or result categories of the index test, distinguishing pre-specified from exploratory	P8 19
	12b	Definition of and rationale for test positivity cut-offs or result categories of the reference standard, distinguishing pre-specified from exploratory	P8 L19
	13a	Whether clinical information and reference standard results were available to the performers/readers of the index test	P8 L19
	13b	Whether clinical information and index test results were available to the assessors of the reference standard	P8 L20
	14	Methods for estimating or comparing measures of diagnostic accuracy	P9 L3
	15	How indeterminate index test or reference standard results were handled	N/A
	16	How missing data on the index test and reference standard were handled	N/A
	17	Any analyses of variability in diagnostic accuracy, distinguishing pre-specified from exploratory	N/A
	18	Intended sample size and how it was determined	N/A
Results			
Participants	19	Flow of participants, using a diagram	Fig. 1
	20	Baseline demographic and clinical characteristics of participants	N/A
	21a	Distribution of severity of disease in those with the target condition	N/A
	21b	Distribution of alternative diagnoses in those without the target condition	P11 L21
	22	Time interval and any clinical interventions between index test and reference standard	N/A
Test results	23	Cross tabulation of the index test results (or their distribution) by the results of the reference standard	Tables 3 & 4
	24	Estimates of diagnostic accuracy and their precision (such as 95% confidence intervals)	Tables 3 & 4
	25	Any adverse events from performing the index test or the reference standard	
Discussion			
	26	Study limitations, including sources of potential bias, statistical uncertainty, and generalisability	P15 L19
	27	Implications for practice, including the intended use and clinical role of the index test	P17 L3
Other Information	28	Registration number and name of registry	N/A
	29	Where the full study protocol can be accessed	P17 L8
	30	Sources of funding and other support; role of funders	P17 L8

Acknowledgments

The Ottawa Hospital Academic Medical Organization supported this project. The full study protocol can be obtained by contacting the lead author at krmacdonald@toh.on.ca.

Funding

The Ottawa Health Sciences Network Research Ethics Board approved this project (OHSN-REB 20140164). They had no access to data or any steps relating to manuscript preparation.

Authors' contributions

KM was the lead author, and was responsible for the study design, research-ethics board application, Institute for Clinical Evaluative Sciences (ICES) application, chart review, model development and internal valid- ation, statistical analysis, and writing and preparation of the thesis. CvW was the last author, and provided intellectual expertise, guidance, and thoroughly reviewed and revised all content. SK was the second reviewer and reviewed and provided feedback. All authors read and approved the final manuscript.

Competing interests

The authors declare that they have no competing interests.

Author details

[1]MD FRCSC, Department of Otolaryngology – Head & Neck Surgery, University of Ottawa, Ottawa, ON, Canada. [2]MD MSc FRCPC, Department of Medicine, Ottawa Hospital Research Institute, University of Ottawa, Ottawa, ON, Canada.

References

1. Ray NF, Baraniuk JN, Thamer M, et al. Healthcare expenditures for sinusitis in 1996: Contributions of asthma, rhinitis, and other airway disorders. J Allergy Clin Immunol. 1999;103(3):408–14.
2. Chen Y, Dales R, Lin M. The epidemiology of chronic rhinosinusitis in Canadians. Laryngoscope. 2003;113(7):1199–205.
3. Kilty S. Canadian guidelines for rhinosinusitis: practical tools for the busy clinician. BMC Ear Nose Throat Disord. 2012;12:1.
4. Macdonald KI, McNally JD, Massoud E. The health and resource utilization of Canadians with chronic rhinosinusitis. Laryngoscope. 2009;119(1):184–9.
5. Macdonald KI, Kilty SJ, van Walraven C. Chronic rhinosinusitis identification in administrative databases and health surveys: A systematic review. Laryngoscope 2015; Dec 9; epub ahead of print doi:10.1002/lary.25804.
6. McIsaac DI, Gershon A, Wijeysundera D, et al. Identifying Obstructive Sleep Apnea in Administrative Data: A Study of Diagnostic Accuracy. Anesthesiology. 2015;123:253–63.
7. van Walraven C, Austin P. Administrative database research has unique characteristics that can risk biased results. J Clin Epidemiol. 2012;65:126–31.
8. van Walraven C, Bennett C, Forster AJ. Administrative database research infrequently used validated diagnostic or procedural codes. J Clin Epidemiol. 2011;64:1054–9.
9. Pisesky A, Benchimol EI, Wong CA et al. Incidence of Hospitalization for Respiratory Syncytial Virus Infection amongst Children in Ontario, Canada: A Population-Based Study Using Validated Health Administrative Data. PLoS ONE 2016 Mar 9;11(3):e0150416. doi: 10.1371/journal.pone.0150416.
10. Benchimol EI, Manual DG, To T, et al. Development and use of reporting guidelines for assessing the quality of validation studies of health administrative data. J Clin Epi. 2011;64(8):821–29.
11. Desrosiers M, Evans GA, Keith PK, et al. Canadian clinical practice guidelines for acute and chronic rhinosinusitis. J Otolaryngol Head Neck Surg. 2011;40 Suppl 2:S99–193.
12. Bossuyt PM, Reitsma JB, Bruns DE, et al. STARD 2015: An Updated List of Essential Items for Reporting Diagnostic Accuracy Studies. Radiology. 2015; 277:826–32.
13. Harvey RJ, Parmar P, Sacks R, et al. Endoscopic skull base reconstruction of large dural defects: A Systematic Review of Published Evidence. Laryngoscope. 2010;122:452–9.
14. Gotlib T, Krzeski A, Held-Ziółkowska M, et al. Endoscopic transnasal management of inverted papilloma involving frontal sinuses. Videosurg Miniinv. 2010;4:299–303.
15. Woodworth BA, Bhargave GA, Palmer JN, et al. Clinical outcomes of endoscopic and endoscopic-assisted resection of inverted papillomas: A 15-year experience. Am J Rhinol. 2007;21:591–600.
16. World Health Organization. The ICD-10 classification of mental and behavioural disorders: clinical descriptions and diagnostic guidelines. Geneva: World Health Organization; 1992.
17. Canadian Institute for Health Information. Canadian Classification of Health Interventions, Version 2015. Ottawa, ON: CIHI; 2015.
18. Sellers MM, Merkow RP, Halverson et al. Validation of new readmission data in the American College of Surgeons National Surgical Quality Improvement Program. J Am Coll Surg 2013; 216, 420–427.
19. Rudmik L, Holy CE, Smith TL. Geographic variation of endoscopic sinus surgery in the United States. Laryngoscope. 2015;125:1772–8.
20. Psaltis AJ, Soler ZM, Nguyen SA, et al. Changing trends in sinus and septal surgery, 2007 to 2009. Int Forum Allergy Rhinol. 2012;2:357–36.
21. Benninger MS, Sindwani R, Holy CE, et al. Early versus Delayed Endoscopic Sinus Surgery in Patients with Chronic Rhinosinusitis: Impact on Health Care Utilization. Otolaryngol - Head Neck Surg. 2015;152:546–52.

17

Laryngeal recurrence sites in patients previously treated with transoral laser microsurgery for squamous cell carcinoma

P. Horwich[1]* (iD), M. H. Rigby[1], C. MacKay[1], J. Melong[1], B. Williams[1], M. Bullock[2], R. Hart[1], J. Trites[1] and S. M. Taylor[1]

Abstract

Background: The laryngeal framework provides a natural barrier preventing tumour spread to extralaryngeal structures. Transoral laser microsurgery (TLM) for laryngeal squamous cell carcinoma (SCC) may violate these boundaries, altering the pathways of tumor spread for potential recurrences. Our project objective is to describe laryngeal SCC recurrence patterns and overall survival in patients requiring total laryngectomy (TL) after TLM.

Methods: Patients undergoing TLM for laryngeal SCC requiring salvage TL were identified from a prospective CO2 laser database containing all patients undergoing TLM for head and neck malignancies at the QEII Health Sciences Center in Halifax, Nova Scotia between March 2002 – May 2014. Surgical pathology reports were analyzed for tumor characteristics, extent of recurrence and invasion of local structures. Kaplan-Meier analyses were performed to evaluate overall survival, disease specific survival (DSS) and locoregional control.

Results: Fifteen patients were identified from the database as receiving salvage TL for recurrent disease after initial TLM resection for laryngeal SCC. Final pathology reports demonstrated that 67% (10/15) of patients had thyroid cartilage involvement while 53% (9/15) of patients had cricoid cartilage involvement on salvage TL pathology. 33% (5/15) of patients had perineural invasion and 27% (4/15) had lymphovascular invasion. Mean and median follow-up times were 36.7 months and 26.8 months respectively (range 3.9–112.6). The Kaplan-Meier estimate for overall survival at 36 months was 40% post TL with a standard error (SE) of 13.6%. DSS was 47% (SE 14.2%), and locoregional control was 55% (SE 14.5%) post TL.

Conclusions: Laryngeal recurrence sites following TLM seem to be consistent with historical data at known laryngeal sites of vulnerability. Treatment with TLM does not predispose patients to a lower rate of locoregional control and overall survival after total laryngectomy and salvage outcomes are consistent with literature values.

Keywords: Laryngeal Recurrence, Transoral Laser Microsurgery, Squamous Cell Carcinoma

Background

Treatment for laryngeal squamous cell carcinoma (SCC), even for advanced disease, has shifted from radical laryngectomies in favour of organ preservation therapies. Transoral laser microsurgery (TLM) is an example of one such organ preserving technique. TLM involves resecting the tumour in pieces as opposed to en bloc tumour resection, thereby allowing for preservation of

surrounding structures. TLM has been shown to be an effective alternative to open surgical techniques with comparable or even superior local control for both supraglottic and glottic SCC primary tumours [1, 2]. Dalhousie University has a well-established TLM program, and we have published multiple studies on laryngeal SCC outcomes and cost-effectiveness of TLM treatment [1–4]. Locoregional control at 2 years for early glottic cancer treated with TLM has been shown to be 95% [3]. TLM has become the treatment modality of choice for all early, and some advanced cases of laryngeal SCC at our center. However, there are concerns that TLM and other minimally invasive techniques may alter the

* Correspondence: Peter.Horwich@dal.ca

[1]Department of Surgery, Division of Otolaryngology–Head and Neck Surgery, Queen Elizabeth II Health Science Centre and Dalhousie University, 3rd Floor Dickson Building, VG Site, 5820 University Avenue, Halifax, NS B3H 2Y9, Canada

Full list of author information is available at the end of the article

natural laryngeal framework, predisposing patients to future recurrences and atypical tumour spread.

The laryngeal framework contains various cartilaginous and ligamentous structures, such as the conus elasticus, that provide natural anatomic barriers to tumour spread. Initially published by Kirchner in 1976, these framework studies also mapped out paths of least resistance for tumour spread, such as through the pre-epiglottic space and paraglottic spaces. This allows clinicians to have a sense of predictability for tumour spread and is the basis of both modern tumour staging guidelines and oncologic surveillance for recurrent disease.

The violation or compromise of these natural anatomic barriers of the laryngeal framework may lead to atypical tumour spread through perichondrial defects potentially facilitating early extralaryngeal spread and ultimately impacting patient survival. It is unclear from the literature if previous treatment with TLM alters the pathways for tumour spread in the larynx.

The purpose of this study is to determine if TLM of laryngeal SCC alters the natural barriers of the larynx leading to atypical sites of recurrence and to evaluate if TLM predisposes patients to lower rates of locoregional control and survival.

Methods

This is a case series based on a center specific CO2 laser database containing all patients undergoing TLM for head and neck malignancies at the QEII Health Sciences Center in Halifax, Nova Scotia. Our TLM database is prospectively maintained and contains over 300 patients up to the publication date. All patients undergoing salvage total laryngectomy with a previous history of TLM treatment from April 2002 – March 2014 were identified. Baseline patient characteristics, pre-operative tumour stage, pathology report information and follow-up data were collected from the database proper. Pathology reports were all signed off by our local head and neck pathologist (MB). Our standardized, center specific pathological reporting for total laryngectomy specimens was followed that includes data on laryngeal subsites, areas of cartilage or bone involvement and areas of extra-laryngeal extension. Ethics approval for the study was obtained from the Nova Scotia Health Authority Research Ethics Board (ROMEO #1020643).

Kaplan-Meier 36-month survival analyses were performed using SPSS for the following endpoints: overall survival (OS) post TL, disease-specific survival post TL, and locoregional control post TL.

Results

From the database, 15 patients were identified to have biopsy confirmed SCC of the larynx initially treated with TLM who required salvage TL for recurrent disease. Five out of 15 patients were found to have two TLM

Table 1 Baseline Patient Characteristics

Patient Characteristics	Value
Male	14/15 (93%)
Mean Age (range)	66.5 (48–94)
History of Smoking	6/15 (40%)
Radiation Prior to TL	9/15 (60%)
Initial Laser to TL in Months (range)	19.6 (2–87)
TLM with Salvage Radiation	9/15 (60%)

treatments prior to proceeding to total laryngectomy. The majority of patients were male (93%) with a mean age of 66 (range 48–64). Baseline patient characteristics are illustrated in Table 1.

Thirteen patients had a glottic primary site while two patients had a supraglottic primary site. Both supraglottic primaries were centered on the left arytenoid cartilage with extension to the infra-hyoid epiglottis. Tumour stage on initial presentation varied from T1a (7%) to T3 (47%) (Table 2).

Lymphovascular and perineural invasion was found in 27% (4/15) and 33% (5/15) of patients respectively. Cricoid cartilage invasion was found in 60% (9/15) of specimens while thyroid cartilage invasion was found in 67% (10/15) of specimens. (Fig. 1).

Extra-laryngeal extension was present in 53% (8/15) of patients. Of those with extra-laryngeal extension, 62% (5/8) had tumour penetration through the thyroid cartilage and similarly 62% (5/8) had thyroid gland invasion. Tracheal involvement was found in 12% (1/8) of patients, while strap muscle involvement and cricothyroid membrane penetration were found in 37% (3/8) of patients. (Fig. 2).

Mean and median follow-up times were 36.7 months and 26.8 months respectively (range 3.9–112.6). The Kaplan-Meier estimate for OS was 40% (SE 13.6%) at 36 months post TL. The Kaplan-Meier estimate for disease specific survival (DSS) was 47% (SE 14.2%) at 36 months post TL. The Kaplan-Meier estimate for locoregional control was 55% (SE 14.5%) at 36 months post TL.

Discussion

Previous anatomical studies have demonstrated that the natural laryngeal framework provides a predictable pathway for tumour spread [5–9]. Physical barriers to tumour spread in the larynx include the conus elasticus, and the

Table 2 TNM Staging on Initial Presentation

Tumor Stage	Value
T1AN0M0	1/15 (7%)
T2N0M0	7/15 (47%)
T3N0M0	6/15 (40%)
T3N1M0	1/15 (7%)

Tumor Characteristics on TL (N=15)

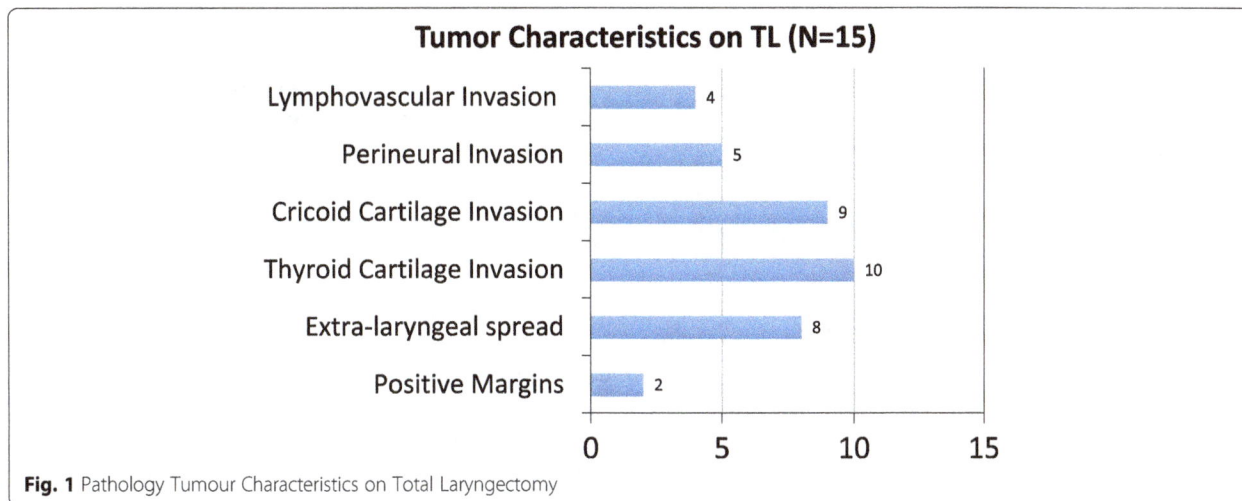

Fig. 1 Pathology Tumour Characteristics on Total Laryngectomy

perichondrium of the thyroid cartilage. With the introduction of minimally invasive techniques such as TLM, there are concerns that this natural framework may be altered, increasing the risk of atypical tumour spread and ultimately tumour recurrence. Our current study is the first in the literature to address this issue, by reviewing the pathology of tumour spread in patients who required a salvage TL after initial TLM resection.

Our study demonstrated that despite initial TLM resection, patients who developed a laryngeal recurrence did so in a similar predictable manner as demonstrated in previous anatomical studies [5–9]. The pre-epiglottic space and paraglottic spaces are known to contain fibrofatty tissue and multiple lymphatic channels, providing a path of least resistance for tumour spread [5]. The pre-epiglottic space is bound by the epiglottis posteriorly, the thyroepiglottic ligament inferiorly and the hyoepiglottic ligament superiorly. The pre-epiglottic space communicates with the bilateral paraglottic spaces, which are bound laterally by the perichondrium of the thyroid cartilage, posteriorly by the mucosa of the pyriform sinus and medially by either

the quadrangular membrane superior, or the conus elasticus inferior to the laryngeal ventricle.

Tumour spread after TLM in our study occurred most frequently by paraglottic extension into the cricoid and thyroid cartilage. Similarly, among patients with extra-laryngeal extension, tumour spread occurred most commonly through the thyroid cartilage (Fig. 3) and cricothyroid membrane, in keeping with known laryngeal framework vulnerabilities and tumour spread patterns described by Kirschner. The perichondrium of the thyroid cartilage is an important barrier to prevent direct extralaryngeal extension [6, 7]. As shown in Fig. 4, the medial perichondrium and thyroid cartilage have been invaded however the anterior perichondrial layer remains intact.

Interestingly, 5/15 (33%) patients had direct thyroid gland involvement on pathology review in our study – this is significantly higher than literature values. A recent systematic review and meta-analysis including 1180 patients by Kumar et al. noted a thyroid gland involvement rate of 10.7% in patients undergoing total laryngectomy [10]. A 2015 publication from Mourad et al. reported thyroid

Extralaryngeal Locations (N=8)

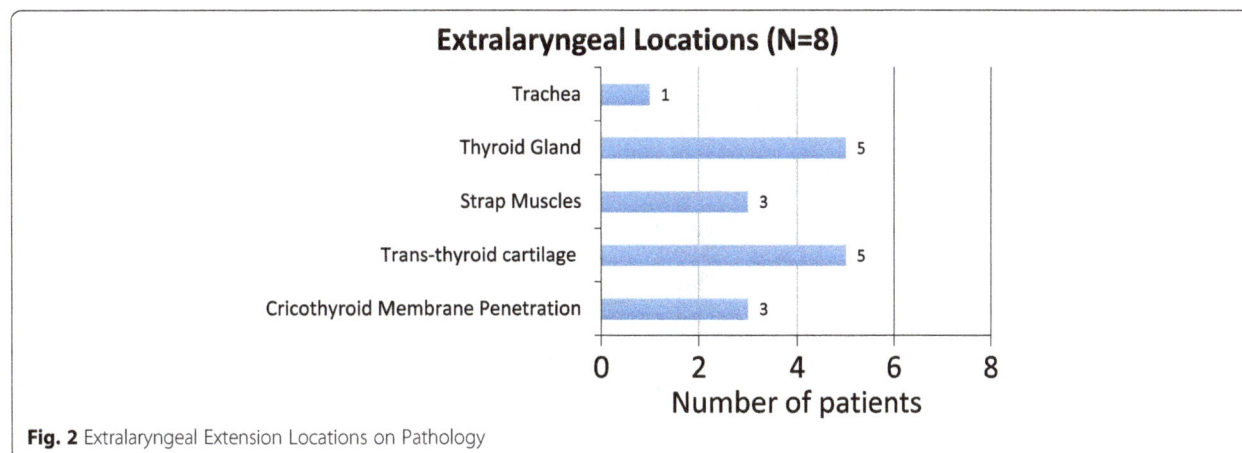

Number of patients

Fig. 2 Extralaryngeal Extension Locations on Pathology

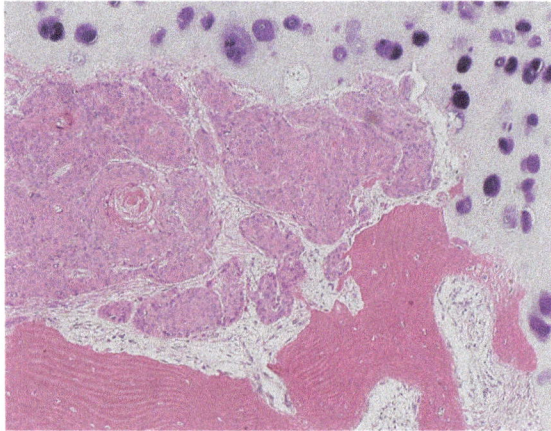

Fig. 3 Squamous cell carcinoma recurrence infiltrating thyroid cartilage at top of slide

gland involvement in 2.7% of 343 patients undergoing primary or salvage total laryngectomy [11]. Our results may indicate that previous TLM treatment may be an indication for thyroidectomy during total laryngectomy however with such a small sample size further study on this subject is required.

Our study also demonstrates that patients who undergo initial TLM resection for laryngeal SCC are not at an increased risk of locoregional recurrence or have a decrease in DSS after salvage TL when compared to patients undergoing primary TL. At 36 months, our patient population's DSS was found to be 47% — similar to previous studies reporting DSS between 50 and 60% for laryngeal SCC treated with primary TL [9, 12, 13].

Previous studies have demonstrated that radiation may induce changes to the laryngeal framework at the molecular level, possibly increasing the risk of tumour invasion [14, 15]. Five patients received primary RT prior to

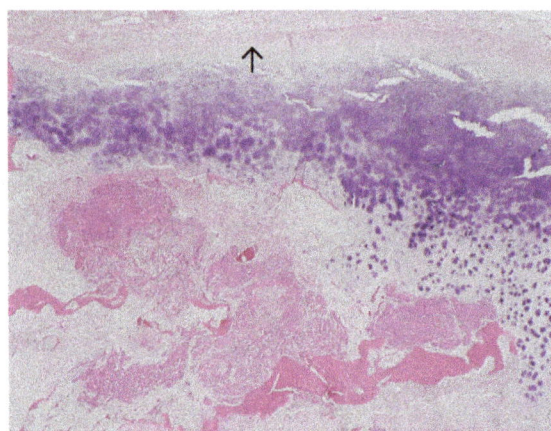

Fig. 4 Squamous cell carcinoma invading medial thyroid perichondrium, thyroid cartilage. Anterior perichondrium intact, indicated by arrow

TLM and subsequent TL. In the current study, 10 patients (66%) had postoperative radiation therapy (after TLM), prior to salvage TL. As a result, postoperative radiation may have caused changes to the laryngeal framework demonstrated in the final pathology. Zbaren et al. demonstrated that patients with primary radiation failures requiring salvage TL had statistically increased tumor multifocality versus concentric growth patterns found in primary laryngeal cancers treated with total laryngectomy [15]. Given our study had maintained predicted laryngeal patterns of tumour spread, it is unlikely that radiation therapy had a significant impact on our results.

Our study is not without limitations. One of the major limitations of our study is the relatively small sample size. In order for tumour spread after TLM to be adequately characterized, pathology of the entire larynx needed reviewing. This limited our inclusion criteria to only those patients who underwent a salvage TL for locoregional recurrence after initial TLM resection. Previous studies have also demonstrated that different subsite involvement can affect tumour spread and extralaryngeal involvement [5–8]. With our limited sample size, it is difficult for us to draw overall conclusions with respect to this.

Conclusion
Laryngeal recurrence sites following TLM seem to be consistent with historical data at known laryngeal sites of vulnerability. Treatment with TLM does not predispose patients to a lower rate of locoregional control and overall survival is consistent with literature values.

Abbreviations
DSS: Disease Specific Survival; OS: Overall Survival; RT: Radiation Treatment; SCC: Squamous Cell Carcinoma; SE: Standard Error; TL: Total Laryngectomy; TLM: Transoral Laser Microsurgery

Acknowledgements
No applicable further acknowledgements.

Funding
No sources of funding were used for this research.

Authors' contributions
PH is the corresponding author and was involved in data acquisition, analysis and interpretation, and drafting of the manuscript. MHR and CM was involved in data acquisition, statistical analysis and interpretation and assisted with preparation and revision of the manuscript. JM and BW assisted in interpretation and manuscript preparation. MB was involved in tumour pathology characterization and assisted with revision of the manuscript. RH and JT participated in data acquisition and assisted with revision of the manuscript. SMT was the research supervisor and assisted with primary data acquisition, analysis and interpretation, and assisted with preparation and revision of the manuscript. All authors have read and approved the final manuscript.

Competing interests

The authors declare that they have no competing interests.

Author details

[1]Department of Surgery, Division of Otolaryngology–Head and Neck Surgery, Queen Elizabeth II Health Science Centre and Dalhousie University, 3rd Floor Dickson Building, VG Site, 5820 University Avenue, Halifax, NS B3H 2Y9, Canada. [2]Department of Pathology, Division of Anatomical Pathology, Queen Elizabeth II Health Science Centre and Dalhousie University, Halifax, NS, Canada.

References

1. Butler A, Rigby MH, Scott J, Trites J, Hart R, Taylor SM. A retrospective review in the management of T3 laryngeal squamous cell carcinoma: an expanding indication for transoral laser microsurgery. J Otolaryngol Head Neck Surg. 2016;45(1):34.
2. Reynolds LF, Rigby MH, Trites J, Hart R, Taylor SM. Outcomes of transoral laser microsurgery for recurrent head and neck cancer. J Laryngol Otol. 2013;127(10):982–6.
3. Taylor SM, Kerr P, Fung K, Aneeshkumar MK, Wilke D, Jiang Y, Scott J, Hart RD, Trites JR, Rigby MH. Treatment of T1b glottic SCC: laser vs. radiation–a Canadian multicenter study. J Otolaryngol Head Neck Surg. 2013;42:22.
4. Phillips TJ, Sader C, Brown T, Bullock M, Wilke D, Trites JR, Hart RD, Murphy M, Taylor SM. Transoral laser microsurgery versus radiation therapy for early glottic cancer in Canada: cost analysis. J Otolaryngol Head Neck Surg. 2009; 38(6):619–23.
5. Buckley JG, MacLennan K. Cancer spread in the larynx: a pathologic basis for conservation surgery. Head Neck. 2000;22(3):265–74.
6. Blitzer A. Mechanisms of spread of laryngeal carcinoma. Bull N Y Acad Med. 1979;55(9):813–21.
7. Kirchner JA. Two hundred laryngeal cancers: patterns of growth and spread as seen in serial section. 1977. Laryngoscope. 2015;125(2):281.
8. Lam KH. Extralaryngeal spread of cancer of the larynx: a study with whole-organ sections. Head Neck Surg. 1983;5(5):410–24.
9. Leong SC, Kartha SS, Kathan C, Sharp J, Mortimore S. Outcomes following total laryngectomy for squamous cell carcinoma: one centre experience. Eur Ann Otorhinolaryngol Head Neck Dis. 2012 Dec;129(6):302–7.
10. Kumar R, Drinnan M, Robinson M, Meikle D, Stafford F, Welch A, et al. Thyroid gland invasion in total laryngectomy and total laryngopharyngectomy: a systematic review and meta-analysis of the English literature. Clin Otolaryngol. 2013;38(5):372–8.
11. Mourad M, Saman M, Sawhney R, Ducic Y. Management of the thyroid gland during total laryngectomy in patients with laryngeal squamous cell carcinoma. Laryngoscope. 2015;125(8):1835–8.
12. Papadas TA, Alexopoulos EC, Mallis A, Jelastopulu E, Mastronikolis NS, Goumas P. Survival after laryngectomy: a review of 133 patients with laryngeal carcinoma. Eur Arch Otorhinolaryngol. 2010 Jul;267(7):1095–101.
13. Stankovic M, Milisavljevic D, Zivic M, Stojanov D, Stankovic P. Primary and salvage total laryngectomy. Influential factors, complications, and survival. J BUON. 2015;20(2):527–39.
14. Dyess CL, Carter D, Kirchner JA, Baron RE. A morphometric comparison of the changes in the laryngeal skeleton associated with invasion by tumor and by external-beam radiation. Cancer. 1987;59(6):1117–22.
15. Zbären P, Nuyens M, Curschmann J, Stauffer E. Histologic characteristics and tumor spread of recurrent glottic carcinoma: analysis on whole-organ sections and comparison with tumor spread of primary glottic carcinomas. Head Neck. 2007;29(1):26–32.

18

Usage of the HINTS exam and neuroimaging in the assessment of peripheral vertigo in the emergency department

Alexandra E. Quimby[1]*[iD], Edmund S. H. Kwok[2], Daniel Lelli[3], Peter Johns[4] and Darren Tse[5]

Abstract

Background: Dizziness is a common presenting symptom in the emergency department (ED). The HINTS exam, a battery of bedside clinical tests, has been shown to have greater sensitivity than neuroimaging in ruling out stroke in patients presenting with acute vertigo. The present study sought to assess practice patterns in the assessment of patients in the ED with peripherally-originating vertigo with respect to utilization of HINTS and neuroimaging.

Methods: A retrospective cohort study was performed using data pertaining to 500 randomly selected ED visits at a tertiary care centre with a final diagnostic code related to peripherally-originating vertigo between January 1, 2010 - December 31, 2014.

Results: A total of 380 patients met inclusion criteria. Of patients presenting to the ED with dizziness and vertigo and a final diagnosis of non-central vertigo, 139 (36.6%) received neuroimaging in the form of CT, CT angiography, or MRI. Of patients who did not undergo neuroimaging, 17 (7.1%) had a bedside HINTS exam performed. Almost half (44%) of documented HINTS interpretations consisted of the ambiguous usage of "HINTS negative" as opposed to the terminology suggested in the literature ("HINTS central" or "HINTS peripheral").

Conclusions: In this single-centre retrospective review, we have demonstrated that the HINTS exam is under-utilized in the ED as compared to neuroimaging in the assessment of patients with peripheral vertigo. This finding suggests that there is room for improvement in ED physicians' application and interpretation of the HINTS exam.

Keywords: HINTS, Head impulse, Neuroimaging, Vertigo, Dizziness

Background

Dizziness is a common presenting symptom in the emergency department (ED), accounting for 2–3% of all US ED visits [1, 2]. In Canada, data from one large tertiary care centre, The Ottawa Hospital (TOH), demonstrated that from 2009 to 2014 dizziness represented almost 2% of all ED visits. Acute vertigo presents a particular challenge to ED physicians, who must differentiate vertigo caused by central nervous system pathology (eg. cerebellar stroke) from that caused by disorders of the peripheral vestibular

end organs (eg. vestibular neuritis). Several multicentre studies have cited the prevalence of centrally-originating vertigo among the ED patient population to range between 3.2–12.5% [2–5]. Potential consequences of a missed diagnosis of cerebellar stroke are high, including increased patient mortality [6, 7]. As a result, neuroimaging (computed tomography [CT], and magnetic resonance imaging [MRI] of the brain) is commonly used in the diagnostic work-up of acutely dizzy patients presenting to the ED [8]. In the same data collected from 2009 to 2014, almost 30% of patients presenting to ED with a final diagnosis relating to acute dizziness (a total of 3559 patients) had either CT or MRI of the brain. This neuroimaging cost the hospital an estimated $1.6 million dollars over that

* Correspondence: Aquim047@uottawa.ca

[1]Department of Otolaryngology- Head and Neck Surgery, University of Ottawa, S3, 501 Smyth Road, Ottawa, ON K1H 8L6, Canada

Full list of author information is available at the end of the article

period (Le A, Tse D: The cost of dizziness: a cost analysis of overall costs of dizziness at a tertiary care hospital, forthcoming). This figure does not take into account additional costs associated with extended ED stays, or the total amount of cranial ionizing radiation to which patients were exposed.

The HINTS exam was developed as a means of assessing patients with the acute vestibular syndrome (AVS), defined as acute onset and persistent vertigo, gait instability, nausea/vomiting, nystagmus, and head motion intolerance [9]. This battery of bedside clinical tests consists of three examinations: the head impulse test (HI-), characterization of spontaneous nystagmus (-N-), and test of skew (-TS) [10]. Each of the three components of the HINTS exam is analyzed separately, and a finding in keeping with central vertigo on any one component of the test indicates the need for neuroimaging. The HINTS exam has been shown to have greater sensitivity than neuroimaging in ruling out stroke in patients presenting with AVS, and to outperform other commonly used stroke risk stratification rules [9, 11]. The exam can be performed at the bedside in approximately 1 min and requires no extra equipment or tools.

A recent study demonstrated that despite its ease of use, the head impulse test (HIT) is greatly under-utilized in the ED [12]. Possible reasons for this include a lack of awareness of the test, knowledge of the evidence of its efficacy, and physician confidence in correctly performing or interpreting the exam. Practice patterns in the use of the testing battery of the HINTS exam in the ED have not been previously studied.

The current study sought to assess practice patterns in the assessment of patients with peripherally-originating vertigo presenting to the ED at one large Canadian tertiary care centre. Specifically, we sought to determine relative proportions of HINTS exams and neuroimaging performed on patients presenting with vertigo and dizziness with a final diagnosis of peripheral vertigo, and to better characterize the use of the HINTS exam in examining patients with peripheral vertigo in the ED.

Methods

Design
A retrospective cohort study was performed using data obtained over a 5-year period.

Study objective
The objective of our study was to describe current ED practice patterns in the assessment of acutely vertiginous patients with a final diagnosis of peripheral vertigo. We sought to demonstrate relative proportions of HINTS exams and neuroimaging performed in the assessment of these patients. We also aimed to further characterize ED practice patterns in the use of the HINTS exam, including its interpretation, relative proportions of the exam

performed by learners as compared to staff ED physicians, and changes in the use of the HINTS exam over time.

Setting
The study was performed using data collected prospectively at two campuses of The Ottawa Hospital (TOH), a Canadian academic tertiary care centre. TOH consists of three hospital campuses, two of which have emergency departments. There are > 170,000 ED visits annually at TOH [13].

Data sources
Patient data was retrieved from The Ottawa Hospital Data Warehouse (TOHDW). TOHDW is a data repository that contains routinely-generated information relevant to all patient visits at TOH. All patient registration, admission, and discharge information, as well as health records data using standardized coding of diagnoses (International Classification of Diseases, 10th revision [ICD-10]) and procedures (Canadian Classification of Interventions) are captured.

Patient population and data acquisition
We reviewed data pertaining to all patients who presented to TOH ED between January 1, 2010- December 31, 2014 who received one of the following final diagnostic codes (ICD-10): Meniere's disease (H810), Benign paroxysmal vertigo (H811), Other peripheral vertigo (H813), Dizziness and Giddiness (R42). Data retrieved included patient age, date of presentation, presenting complaint, imaging procedures ordered, referrals made, and final diagnosis codes.

In order to audit the use of the HINTS examination in the emergency department for patients presenting with dizziness, 100 patients were randomly selected who presented each year from 2010-2014, for a total of 500 patients.

Patient unique identifier numbers were retrieved from TOHDW and used to link this sample of 500 patients with patient electronic medical records (EMRs) in order to abstract final charted diagnoses, and whether any bedside test of vertigo (HINTS exam or other) was performed in ED. We also extracted from patient EMRs whether or not the patient was assessed by a trainee (medical student or resident) or a staff ED physician.

Following data extraction from EMRs, we excluded any patients who were captured in our cohort by included ICD-10 codes but whose final charted diagnosis was unrelated to vertigo or dizziness. Examples included diagnoses of pre-syncope, syncope, and other cardiac diagnoses which had been assigned one of our four included ICD-10 diagnostic codes. We also excluded any patients whose EMR indicated that they had left the ED before being assessed by an emergency physician.

Outcomes of interest
Primary outcomes of interest were: 1) was neuroimaging (CT or MRI of the brain) ordered in the ED, and, 2) was

the HINTS exam performed in the ED. Secondary outcomes of interest were: 3) were other bedside tests of vertigo performed (eg. Dix-Hallpike, Romberg, or any single component of the HINTS exam alone), 4) were patients assessed by ED staff physicians or trainees (ie. resident physicians or medical students), and, 5) how were HINTS exam findings charted and interpreted.

When analyzing charted HINTS exam interpretations, we considered the literature citing proper interpretation of the exam. A correct interpretation of the HINTS exam should take into account the results of each of the three components of the test: 1) Head impulse testing: considered abnormal or "positive" when rapid rotation of the head results in loss of fixation of the eyes with a corresponding refixation saccade, which occurs mostly in cases of peripheral vertigo (ie. in vestibular neuritis). In patients with central vertigo, the head impulse test will usually appear to be normal, or "negative", in that the vestibuloocular reflex remains intact, and the patient's eyes remain fixed on the target. 2) Examination of patients' nystagmus: direction-fixed horizontal jerk nystagmus that obeys Alexander's law, beating away from the affected side, occurs in cases of peripheral vertigo. 3) Vertical skew deviation: absent in cases of peripheral vertigo, with its presence typically indicating a central cause. If any portion of the test is in keeping with a central etiology of vertigo, the HINTS is considered "central", indicating the need for further investigation (in the form of neuroimaging) (Table 1) [14].

Data analysis

As our primary and secondary outcomes of interest were descriptive in nature, we performed qualitative data analysis.

IRB approval

Our study was approved by our hospital REB (Ottawa Health Science Network Research Ethics Board [OHSN-REB], protocol no. 20160726-01H).

Results

Data pertaining to a total of 10,348 patients who presented to the ED with a final diagnosis related to dizziness or peripheral vertigo between January 1, 2010 and December 31, 2014 was retrieved. Demographic data from this cohort is presented in Table 2. Analyzed encounters were evenly distributed across the 5 years. The majority of discharge diagnoses were represented by the broad ICD-10 diagnostic code of dizziness and giddiness (68%), followed by benign paroxysmal vertigo (15.6%), other peripheral vertigo (14.2%), and Meniere's disease (1.9%).

Analysis of the EMRs of our sample of 500 patients from this cohort revealed that 120 of them (24%) had a final charted diagnosis unrelated to dizziness or vertigo (eg. syncope, pre-syncope) ($n = 82$, 68%), or did not receive a final diagnosis due to having left ED before being assessed by an emergency physician ($n = 38$, 32%). This left 380 patients with a final charted diagnosis related to dizziness or vertigo.

Of the 380 patients remaining in our sample who had a final charted diagnosis related to dizziness or vertigo, a total of 139 (36.6%) received neuroimaging in the form of CT, CT angiography (CT-A), or MRI of the head/ brain. Of these, 137 (36%) had non-contrast CT heads, 5 patients (1.3%) had an MRI, and 15 patients (4%) had CT-A. Of these 139 patients who received neuroimaging, 8 (5.8%) had a documented HINTS exam performed at bedside by

Table 1 Interpretation of the HINTS exam

HINTS exam component	Peripheral Vertigo	Central vertigo
Head Impulse Test (HIT)	Loss of eye fixation with head impulse; "positive" or "abnormal"	Intact vestibulo-ocular reflex; "negative" or "normal"
Nystagmus (N)	None or horizontal unidirectional	Vertical, rotatory, or horizontal bidirectional
Test of Skew (TS)	No skew; "negative"	Skew; "positive"

Table 2 Cohort Demographics

Variable		Total Cohort N (%)	Sample N (%)
Age (Mean)		55	56
Year Presented to ED	2010	1863 (18.0)	100 (20.0)
	2011	1922 (18.6)	100 (20.0)
	2012	2095 (20.2)	100 (20.0)
	2013	2171 (21.1)	100 (20.0)
	2014	2292 (22.1)	100 (20.0)
Presenting Complaint	Dizziness/Vertigo	6314 (61.0)	310 (62.0)
	Syncope/Pre-syncope	1096 (10.6)	50 (10.0)
	General Weakness	544 (5.3)	28 (5.6)
	Nausea and/or vomiting	485 (4.7)	31 (6.2)
	Headache	311 (3.0)	19 (3.8)
	Symptoms of CVA	143 (1.4)	5 (1.0)
	Palpitations/Irregular Heart Rate	105 (1.0)	0 (0)
	Sensory Loss/ Paresthesias	35 (0.3)	1 (0.2)
	Gait Disturbance/Ataxia	20 (0.2)	0 (0)
	Other	1295 (12.5)	56 (11.2)
ED Discharge Diagnosis	Dizziness and Giddiness	7036 (68.0)	329 (65.8)
	Benign paroxysmal vertigo	1613 (15.6)	81 (16.2)
	Other Peripheral Vertigo	1473 (14.2)	68 (13.6)
	Meniére's disease	195 (1.9)	17 (3.4)
Patients who had CT/MRI head		3012(29.1)	139 (27.8)
Total		10,348	500

an ED physician or trainee. Fifty-seven patients (41%) who underwent CT did not have a HINTS exam performed, but did have another bedside test of vertigo performed (any combination of the Romberg test ($n = 24$), the Dix-Hallpike test ($n = 35$), or the head impulse test (HIT) ($n = 1$) or vestibulo-ocular reflex (VOR) testing not otherwise specified (n = 2)). The remainder of patients who had neuroimaging ($n = 74$, 53.2%) did not undergo any bedside testing of vertigo. As anticipated, the total number of reported positive findings on CT/ MRI/CT-A in these patients was 0 (Fig. 1).

Of patients who did not undergo neuroimaging ($n = 241$), 17 (7.1%) had a bedside HINTS exam performed. Ninety-eight patients (40.7%) did not have a HINTS exam performed, but had some other bedside test of vertigo performed (varying combinations of Romberg, $n = 40$; Dix-Hallpike test, $n = 65$; HIT, $n = 5$). The remaining 126 patients (52.3%) who did not undergo CT did not have the HINTS exam or any other bedside test of vertigo performed. Final charted diagnoses of patients who did not undergo neuroimaging or any bedside tests of vertigo included diagnoses such as "dizziness NYD", "vertigo NYD", "benign vertigo", "peripheral vertigo", "Meniere's", and "BPPV".

Relative proportions of patients receiving neuroimaging, HINTS exams, and other bedside tests of vertigo are displayed in Fig. 2.

Analysis of the number of HINTS exams performed each year over our 5-year study period revealed a trend of increasing numbers of HINTS exams over time, which was statistically significant ($p < 0.005$) (Fig. 3). In particular, an increase in the number of HINTS exams was noted between the years 2012 and 2013. Dr. Newman-Toker, the originator of the HINTS exam, presented at Emergency Department rounds at TOH on the utility of the HINTS exam in October 2012.

Of the 26 HINTS exams performed on patients in our sample, 7 (27%) of these were performed by trainees – either resident physicians or medical students – and 19 (73%) by staff ED physicians.

Analysis of the charted interpretations of the HINTS exams performed in our sample revealed that almost half of the time, the exam was charted as "HINTS negative" ($n = 11$, 44%). Of these 11 "HINTS negative" patients, 4 (36.3%) underwent CT. For patients on whom the exam was charted with the results of its three separate components, neuroimaging was appropriately ordered in 50% of the cases. There were 11 patients (44%) for whom charted interpretations of the HINTS examination would suggest HINTS central (ie. any one component of the exam positive OR no nystagmus present), indicating the need for neuroimaging. Of these 11 patients, neuroimaging was subsequently ordered in 4 (36.3%) (Table 3).

Discussion

The HINTS exam is a well-validated tool to rule out stroke in patients presenting with AVS, with greater sensitivity than neuroimaging [9, 11]. However, the exam has previously been shown to be under-utilized in the ED [12]. Our study expands upon the existing literature by qualitatively characterizing practice patterns in the use of the HINTS exam and neuroimaging for the assessment of patients with peripheral vertigo in the ED.

We have demonstrated that of patients presenting to ED with dizziness or vertigo and a final diagnosis of peripheral vertigo, a high proportion (36%) undergo neuroimaging, and the HINTS examination is relatively under-utilized in this population in comparison (7%). Furthermore, when the HINTS exam was used in our ED cohort, it was often applied inappropriately, with neuroimaging still ordered in cases of HINTS peripheral.

Our demonstration of a low overall proportion of HINTS exams performed on vertiginous patients in whom neuroimaging was ordered may be a result of several factors. First, awareness of the HINTS exam may be low among ED physicians. This is supported by our demonstration that use of the HINTS exam at our centre increased over time, especially since Dr. Newman-Toker's presentation of the examination in 2012. Similarly, publications citing evidence for the efficacy of the HINTS exam only first appeared 2009, and have increased in number since.

Second, ED physicians and trainees may be uncomfortable or unfamiliar with the HINTS exam technique and interpretation. In the published literature, the accuracy of the HINTS exam has been demonstrated in the setting of being performed by specialist physicians, including neurologists, neuro-ophthalmologists, and expert-trained emergency room physicians [14]. This may lead ED physicians to avoid the exam altogether, or not trust the reliability of the results they obtain. In our sample, almost 50% of patients who underwent the HINTS exam had their results charted as "HINTS negative". Of these patients, approximately one third (36%) underwent subsequent neuroimaging, with the remainder receiving no further testing. As well, of patients on whom ED charting of HINTS exam results corresponded to HINTS central ($n = 11$ or 44% of patients on whom the exam was performed), indicating the need for subsequent neuroimaging, only 36% went on to have CT or MRI. In many of these cases, even though the HINTS exam was fully documented, it was inappropriately interpreted as peripheral in 28.5% of patients who had no nystagmus present. These findings suggest ambiguity in ED physicians' interpretation of the HINTS exam. Extensive use of neuroimaging may stem from practitioners' lack of self-confidence in their technique and interpretation of the exam. It is possible that with adequate training on technique and interpretation of the exam, the number of HINTS exams performed and

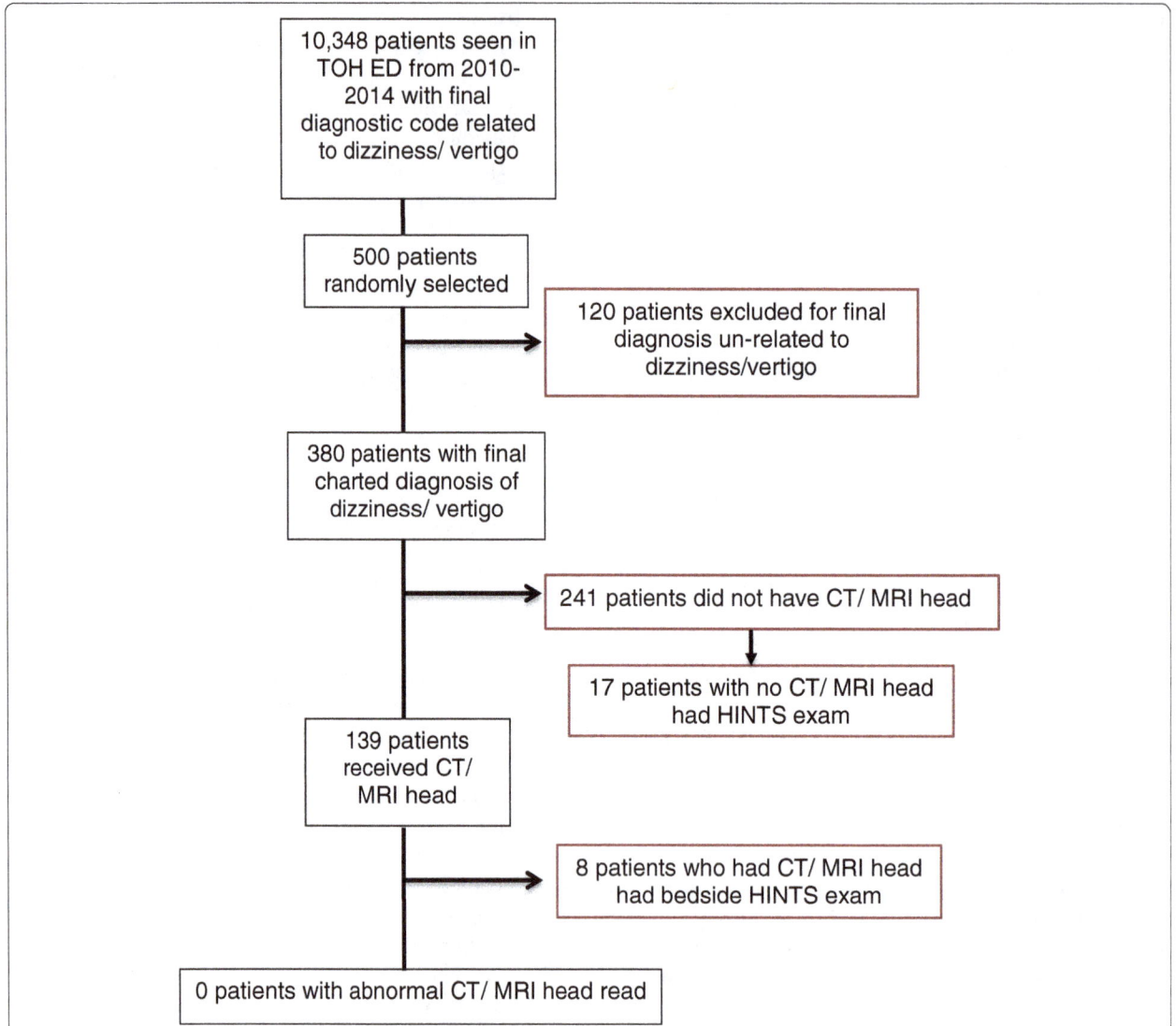

Fig. 1 Flow diagram of the use of HINTS and neuroimaging in assessment of patients presenting to ED with dizziness/ vertigo, 2010–2014

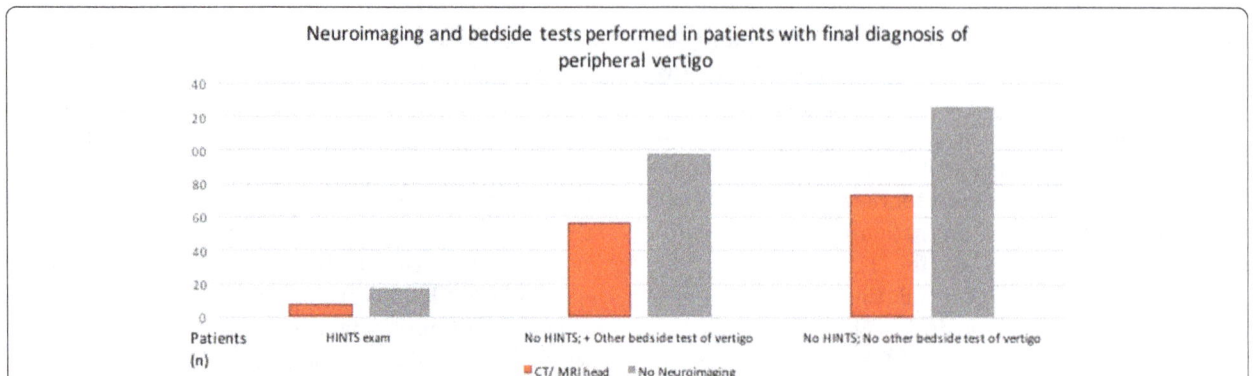

Fig. 2 Relative proportions of patients receiving neuroimaging, HINTS exams, and other bedside tests of vertigo

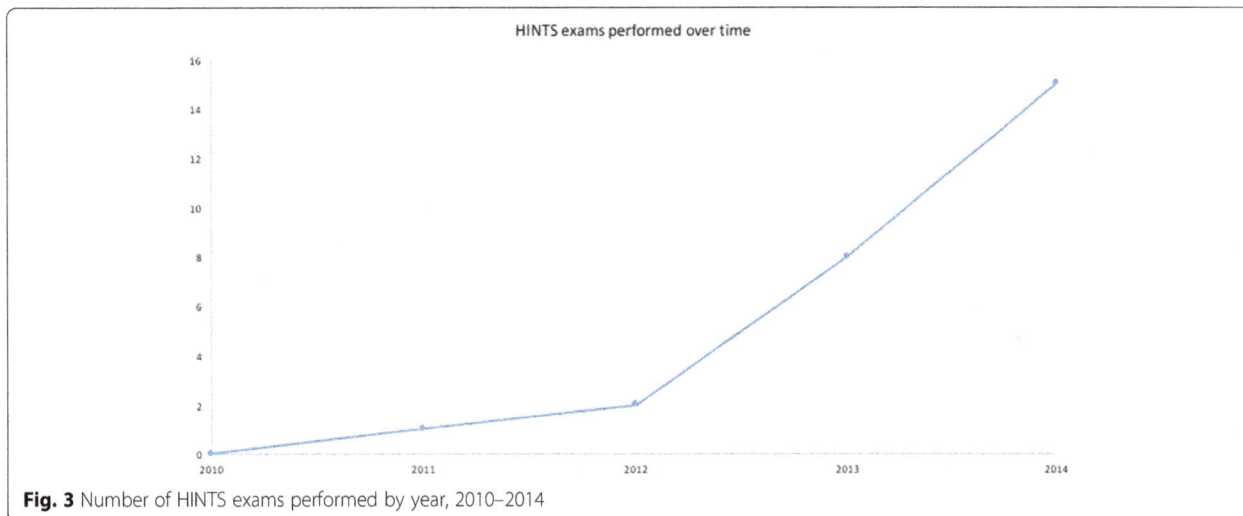

Fig. 3 Number of HINTS exams performed by year, 2010–2014

properly interpreted in the ED would increase, and the use of neuroimaging would decrease. Our demonstration of a relatively larger proportion of HINTS exams being performed by staff ED physicians (73%) as compared to residents and medical students (27%) also suggests the possibility for improvement in use of the exam with teaching targeted to various levels of medical training.

Possible implications of broadening usage of the HINTS exam in the ED are improved patient care outcomes, decreased ED wait-times for neuroimaging, and decreased exposure to ionizing radiation. Improved patient satisfaction is likely to result. Decreasing the use of neuroimaging will also result in healthcare cost savings.

Our study expands upon existing literature demonstrating HINTS under-utilization in the ED. We have quantitatively

Table 3 Charted ED interpretations of HINTS exams, and neuroimaging ordered

Charted Interpretation of HINTS exam		Charted Interpretation corresponds to HINTS Central, or HINTS Peripheral?	Neuroimaging Indicated?	Patients with charted interpretation (n)	CT performed? (n)	CT positive findings?
"HINTS negative" (n = 11)		NA	NA	11	Yes (4)	No
Results of each of 3 components of exam charted (n = 14)	HIT +ve, Nystagmus right, Test of skew –ve	Peripheral	No	1	No (0)	\
	HIT normal, nystagmus none, test of skew normal	Central	Yes	3	Yes (2)	No
	HI = + lag, Nystagmus = N, TS = N	Peripheral	No	1	No (0)	\
	HIT abnormal, Nystagmus horizontal, Test of skew normal	Peripheral	No	1	No (0)	\
	No lag on head impulse, unilateral nystagmus, lateral skew	Central	Yes	1	Yes (1)	No
	Head impulse abnormal, Nystagmus vertical, no skew	Central	Yes	1	Yes (1)	No
	HINTS = peripheral cause	Peripheral	No	1	No (0)	\
	Symptoms reproducible with quick head turn to the right, no nystagmus, no skew	Peripheral	No	1	No (0)	\
	Head impulse abnormal, Nystagmus bilateral, Test of skew positive	Central	Yes	1	No (0)	\
	HIT –ve, N –ve, TS –ve	Central	Yes	1	No (0)	\
	Head impulse +, no skew, no nystagmus	Peripheral	No	1	No (0)	\
	HI + ve, N –ve, T –ve	Peripheral	No	1	No (0)	\

demonstrated proportions of HINTS exams and neuroimaging performed in the ED assessment of patients with peripheral vertigo, as well as qualitatively shed light on these practices. Though an overall small number of HINTS exams were performed, we have qualitatively demonstrated charted ED interpretations of these HINTS exam, relative proportions of the exam performed by trainees as compared to staff physicians, and changes in practice patterns over time. By depicting the impact of teaching on the HINTS exam– that is, how HINTS ED usage increased at our centre following demonstration of the exam by Newman-Toker – we have shown that these practice patterns are amenable to change with appropriate educational initiatives.

Several important factors must be taken into consideration when interpreting our results. The HINTS examination should only be used in patients with AVS: that is, acute onset and persistent vertigo, gait instability, nausea/ vomiting, nystagmus, and head motion intolerance. Of our sample of 380 patients with coded diagnoses of dizziness or vertigo, it is likely that a proportion of these did not meet the criteria for AVS, making the use of a HINTS examination inappropriate. Indeed, in some patients in our cohort with a final charted diagnosis of BPPV, a HINTS exam and neuroimaging were still performed. It is difficult to ascertain which patients truly met criteria for AVS on the basis of charted ED notes. Therefore, the calculation of 7% ($n = 25$) of patients with dizziness/ vertigo who underwent a HINTS exam is likely an under-estimate of the percentage of patients who appropriately underwent HINTS testing. However, of 139 vertiginous patients who underwent neuroimaging (CT or MRI head), only 6% of these ($n = 8$) underwent a HINTS exam in advance, indicating the HINTS exam is under-utilized in patients in whom ED physicians are concerned about central vertigo. Other limitations of our study include its retrospective design and our reliance on charted ED diagnoses. Data used in our sample was retrieved on the basis of ICD-10 diagnostic codes, which are dependent on both accurate charting by physicians and coding of charted diagnoses by non-clinical clerks. We also cannot comment on the sensitivity nor specificity of the HINTS exam when used by ED physicians, since we only analyzed patients with a final diagnosis of peripheral vertigo. However, by analyzing trends in charted interpretations of the HINTS exam performed by ED physicians, we were able to show that ambiguity regarding the proper interpretation of the test exists in this population, and that there is therefore room for improvement with additional training of the proper technique and interpretation of the HINTS exam.

Given the findings of this qualitative analysis, future directions include implementing an educational campaign within our centre's ED with the goals of increasing awareness, proper technique, documentation, and interpretation of the HINTS exam. By doing this, we would hope to institute a measurable change in practice, with increased use of the HINTS examination and decreased use of neuroimaging in the assessment of acutely vertiginous patients in the ED. If use of the HINTS exam in the ED could be increased and a more robust dataset curated, this information could be used to develop an algorithm for the assessment of acutely dizzy patients in the ED. Though a single centre study, we believe that the observed trends in the use of neuroimaging in our patient population are likely consistent with ED practices more generally, as is suggested by concordance of our results with other studies [12, 15]. Through implementing measurable change in the utilization of the HINTS exam at our own centre, our hope would be to confer a generalizable shift in practice patterns.

Conclusion

Dizziness is a common presenting complaint in the emergency department, and can be challenging for ED physicians who must exclude potentially life-threatening central causes of vertigo. The HINTS examination, designed to differentiate peripheral and central vertigo, is significantly under-utilized compared to neuroimaging in the ED assessment of patients with peripheral vertigo. We have demonstrated that there is room for improvement in the application and interpretation of the HINTS exam in the ED, creating the potential for both improved patient care outcomes and healthcare cost-savings.

Authors' contributions

AEQ participated in the design of the study, acquired and extracted data, drafted, and edited the manuscript. ESHK participated in the design of the study and edited the manuscript. DL participated in the design of the study and edited the manuscript. PJ participated in the design of the study and edited the manuscript. DT conceived of the study, participated in the design of the study, and edited the manuscript. All authors read and approved the final manuscript.

Competing interests

The authors declares that they have no competing interests.

Author details

[1]Department of Otolaryngology- Head and Neck Surgery, University of Ottawa, S3, 501 Smyth Road, Ottawa, ON K1H 8L6, Canada. [2]Department of Emergency Medicine, University of Ottawa, 501 Smyth Rd, Ottawa, ON K1H 8L6, Canada. [3]Department of Medicine, Division of Neurology, University of Ottawa, 501 Smyth Rd, Ottawa, ON K1H 8L6, Canada. [4]Department of Emergency Medicine, University of Ottawa, 501 Smyth Rd, Ottawa, ON K1H 8L6, Canada. [5]Department of Otolaryngology- Head and Neck Surgery, University of Ottawa, 501 Smyth Rd, Ottawa, ON K1H 8L6, Canada.

References

1. Newman-Toker DE, Hsieh YH, Camargo CA Jr, et al. Spectrum of dizziness visits to US emergency departments: cross-sectional analysis from a nationally representative sample. Mayo Clin Proc. 2008;83:765–75.
2. Kerber KA, Meurer WJ, West BT, Fendrick M. Dizziness presentations in U.S. emergency departments, 1995-2004. Aca Emerg Med. 2008;15(8):744–50.
3. Kerber KA, Brown DL, Lisabeth LD, Smith MA, Morgenstern LB. Stroke among patients with dizziness, vertigo, and imbalance in the emergency department: a population-based study. Stroke. 2006;37:2484–7.
4. Schneiderman N, Bies C, Chan SB, Garcia C. Vertigo, ataxia, and strokes: an emergency department study. Ann Emerg Med. 2015;66(4):S84.
5. Ozono Y, Kitahara T, Fukushima M, Michiba T, Imai R, et al. Differential diagnosis of vertigo and dizziness in the emergency department. Acta Otolaryngol. 2014;134:140–5.
6. Savitz SI, Caplan LR, Edlow JA. Pitfalls in the diagnosis of cerebellar infarction. Acad Emerg Med. 2007;14:63–8.
7. Tohgi H, Takahashi S, Chiba K, et al. Tohoku cerebellar infarction study group. Cerebellar infarction. Clinical and neuroimaging analysis in 293 patients. Stroke. 1993;24:1697–701.
8. Tarnutzer AA, Berkowit AL, Robinson KA, Hsieh Y, Newman-Toker DE. Does my dizzy patient have a stroke? A systematic review of bedside diagnosis in acute vestibular syndrome. CMAJ. 2011;183(9):E571–92.
9. Kattah JC, Talkand AV, Zang DZ, Hsieh YH, Newman-Toker DE. HINTS to diagnose stroke in the acute vestibular syndrome: three-step bedside oculomotor examination more sensitive than early MRI diffusion-weighted imaging. Stroke. 2009;40:3504–10.
10. Newman-Toker, David E. 3-Step HINTS Battery Video 200-4. Neuro-Ophthalmology Virtual Education Library: NOVEL Web Site [online]. Available at: http://www.kaltura.com/index.php/extwidget/preview/partner_id/797802/uiconf_id/27472092/entry_id/0_b9t6s0wh/embed/auto. Accessed 22 Nov 2017.
11. Newman-Toker DE, Kerber KA, Hsieh YH, Pula JH, Omron R, et al. HINTS outperforms ABCD2 to screen for stroke in acute continuous vertigo and dizziness. Aca Emerg Med. 2013;20(10):987–96.
12. McDowell T, Moore F. The under-utilization of the head impulse test in the emergency department. Can J Neurol Sci. 2016;43(3):398–401.
13. "Statistics." The Ottawa Hospital. The Ottawa Hospital, 2017. Web. 3 July 2017.
14. Thomas DB, Newman-Toker DE. Avoiding "HINTS Positive/ Negative" to minimize diagnostic confusion in acute vertigo and dizziness. J Acute Care Phys Ther. 2016;00(00):1–3.
15. Ammar H, Govindu R, Fouda R, Zohdy W, Supsupin E. Dizziness in a community hospital: central neurological causes, clinical predictors, and diagnostic yield and cost of neuroimaging studies. J Community Hosp Intern Med Perspect. 2017;7(2):73–8.

19

Smartphone adapters for flexible Nasolaryngoscopy

A. E. Quimby[1*†], S. Kohlert[1†], L. Caulley[2] and M. Bromwich[3]

Abstract

Background: Flexible nasolaryngoscopy is an essential component of the otolaryngological physical exam. Historically, the ability to create and share video recordings of these endoscopic exams has been limited by poor mobility of fixed endoscopy towers. The advent of smartphone endoscope adapters has allowed physicians to create and share video recordings of endoscopy in a wide variety of locations that would not have previously been feasible. This paper sought to review the literature on the effect of smartphone endoscope adapters on patient care, patient satisfaction, and resident learning.

Methods: This systematic review was conducted according to PRISMA guidelines. A systematic literature search was performed for all relevant English language studies (1946–2017) using Ovid MEDLINE, PubMed, and EMBASE. The study protocol was registered with the PROSPERO database.

Results: A total of 91 abstracts were identified and screened by two independent reviewers. Based on inclusion and exclusion criteria, three studies were selected and subjected to full-text extraction as well as quality assessment. These studies demonstrated high diagnostic accuracy and quality of smartphone adapter-recorded videos, and a benefit of these devices on resident education. Due to the heterogeneity of included studies' methods and measures, a meta-analysis was not possible, so a qualitative synthesis of the literature results was performed.

Conclusion: Despite a paucity of data on the subject, the present study provided a comprehensive review of the literature, and suggested overall high diagnostic accuracy, quality, and enhancement of resident education with the use of smartphone endoscope adapters for flexible nasolaryngoscopy.

Keywords: Smartphone endoscope adapters, Flexible nasolaryngoscopy, Laryngoscopy, FNL

Background

Flexible nasolaryngoscopy (FNL) provides invaluable insight to the practicing Otolaryngologist and can be used to diagnose a wide variety of pathology. It is an essential skill that must be mastered by all trainees in Otolaryngology - Head and Neck Surgery (OTOHNS).

While FNL is not technically challenging to the experienced otolaryngologist, there are many subtleties to its use and interpretation that may not be immediately appreciated by junior learners. As such, senior residents and attending physicians are often required to be present during the endoscopic exam to verify the junior trainee's findings. As endoscopy towers are expensive and stationary, they are not conducive to remote locations such as emergency departments or patient wards, where patients commonly undergo FNL. Historically, FNL performed in these locations were not recorded and patients were then subjected to repeat examination, leading to redundancy and additional discomfort.

Smartphone endoscope adapters are a relatively new technology which provide a mechanism to record flexible nasolaryngoscopy examinations performed in remote locations using portable scopes. In doing so, they allow attending physicians to remotely provide opinion and advice following a single assessment performed with a portable scope. Recorded videos obtained in this

* Correspondence: Aquim047@uottawa.ca

†Equal contributors

[1]Department of Otolaryngology - Head and Neck Surgery, University of Ottawa, 501 Smyth Rd, Module S, Room M2566, Box 216, Ottawa, ON K1H 8L6, Canada

Full list of author information is available at the end of the article

manner may additionally be retained for educational or research purposes.

Since their introduction, there have been few articles examining the use of smartphone endoscope adapters. The purpose of this study was to perform a systematic review of the literature on the use of these devices. Specifically, we sought to assess the effect of smartphone endoscope adapters on video recording quality, patient satisfaction and care, and trainee educational experience. We also present our own institution's experience with the use of smartphone endoscope adapters.

Methods

A systematic review of the literature based on the Cochrane handbook and the Preferred Reporting Items for Systematic reviews and Meta-analyses (PRISMA) guidelines was performed [1, 2]. The study protocol was registered with the PROSPERO database.

Eligibility criteria

Studies were selected using Population, Intervention, Comparator, Outcome, Study Design (PICOS) guidelines. We included all studies from 1946 to September 2017 published in English language in peer-reviewed journals.

Information sources and search strategy

With the help of an experienced librarian, we conducted a literature search using the following databases: Ovid MEDLINE, PubMed, and EMBASE. A MeSH terms and keywords search was conducted using truncation and adjacency operator and Boolean operators. MeSH terms were: endoscop*, otorhinolaryngologic diseases; otolaryngology; otorhinolaryngologic surgical procedures; nose; nasal; larynx*; laryngoscopy; laryngoscopes; nasolaryngoscop*; smart phone*; iphone*; andrid*, adaptor*, or adapter. We also performed a hand search of citations from relevant articles.

Study selection

Study inclusion and exclusion criteria were clearly defined, and are illustrated in Table 1.

Data collection and extraction

Data was extracted from the studies using a pre-written data entry form. Titles and abstracts were independently screened by two reviewers (A.Q., L.C) to assess for initial relevance. Titles or abstracts that were deemed relevant by either reviewer were obtained in full document or PDF form. Papers were then screened to determine if they met eligibility criteria, and if so, data was extracted accordingly. Data extraction was completed by two reviewers (A.Q., L.C.) and included important clinical

Table 1 Inclusion and Exclusion Criteria

Inclusion Criteria	
Population	○ Endoscopy performed by Otolaryngology residents/ physicians ○ Adult or pediatric patients
Intervention	○ Use of smartphone adapters for flexible nasolaryngoscopy
Comparator	○ Endoscopy tower video recordings of flexible nasolaryngoscopy, or no recording
Outcome	○ Patient satisfaction ○ Patient care ○ Trainee learning ○ Video quality ○ Diagnostic accuracy
Study Design	○ Randomized and non-randomized comparative studies, retrospective and prospective cohort studies, case series ○ Published in English language
Exclusion Criteria	
Population	○ Non-Otolaryngology-trained residents/ physicians
Intervention	○ Endoscopy other than flexible nasolaryngoscopy ○ No use of smartphone adapters
Comparator	○ NA
Outcome	○ No reported outcomes
Study Design	○ Single case reports ○ Case series with $N < 10$ ○ Non-English language

baseline variables as well as primary outcomes measures (Tables 2, 3). All disagreements between reviewers were discussed and resolved by a consensus meeting including all four authors.

Data items

The baseline variables that were extracted from each article included: type of exams performed (scope adapter +/– endoscopy video tower recording), scope operator trainee level, model of scope adapter and (when applicable) endoscopy tower used, model of smartphone used, and safety/ privacy measures. Primary outcomes of interest were: 1) patient care impacts of scope adapter video recordings, 2) resident educational impacts of scope adapter video recordings, 3) diagnostic accuracy of flexible nasolaryngoscopy videos recorded with smartphone adapters, and 4) costs of smartphone adapters for flexible nasolaryngoscopy. Secondary outcomes of interest were: 1) Quality of videos recorded using smartphone adapters compared to endoscopy tower video recordings, and 2) patient satisfaction with the use of smartphone adapters for flexible nasolaryngoscopy.

Table 2 Included study characteristics

Study name	Year	Type of Study	Patients (N)	Exams recorded with endoscope adapter (N)	Exams recorded with endoscopy video tower (N)	Scope operator trainee level	Model of scope adapter	Model of endoscopy video tower	Model of smartphone	Safety/Privacy measures
Liu H et al..	2016	Prospective cohort	30	30	30	Staff, residents (all levels)	ClearScope (Clearwater Clinical Limited, Ottawa, Canada)	KayPentax (HOYA Corporation, Pentax Lifecare Division, Tokyo, Japan)	iPhone (Apple, Cupertino, CA)	Modica (Clearwater Clinical Limited, Ottawa, Canada)
Liu YF et al	2016	Prospective cohort	43	43	0	Residents (PGY-1, −2)	ClearScope	NA	NA	NA
Lozada et al	2017	Prospective cohort	79	79	0	Residents (PGY-1)	Mobile Optyx (MobileOptyx, Philadelphia, PA)	NA	iPhone	Dedicated team iPhone

Risk of Bias in individual studies

Internal validity of study design and conduct was assessed independently by two reviewers (A.Q., L.C.). For non-randomized studies, the Newcastle-Ottawa Quality Assessment Tool was used [3]. Discrepancies were resolved by a consensus meeting including all four authors.

Results

A total of 91 studies were screened (Fig. 1). Studies were excluded for: duplicates, different topic/ intervention, non-English language, and insufficient data (abstract only, single case reports, no outcomes data). Three cohort studies were deemed eligible for inclusion [4–6].

Study characteristics

The total of 152 examinations of patients using smartphone endoscope adapters were reported in the literature. Thirty of these patients also had endoscopy video tower recording of their flexible nasolaryngosocpy exams for direct comparison. The pertinent characteristics of the studies included for review are illustrated in Table 2.

Study outcomes

Two of the three studies assessed the diagnostic accuracy and quality of videos recorded using smartphone endoscope adapters (Table 3) [4, 6]. In one of these studies (Liu H et al), videos recorded using smartphone endoscope adapters were compared to those recorded using endoscopy video towers, and mean differences in percent correct diagnoses made by blinded observers

Table 3 Included study outcomes

Study name	Year	Primary Outcomes of Interest	Secondary Outcomes	Outcome Measures	Findings
Liu H et al	2016	Diagnostic accuracy	NA	Controlled blinded comparison of scope adapters and endoscope tower recorded videos	No significant difference between scope adapter and endoscopy tower videos (mean difference = 1.54%, p = 0.69).
		Video recording quality		5-point Likert scale across 7quality variables	No significant difference across 7 categories ($p = 0.11$–0.92)
Liu YF et al	2016	Resident Education	NA	Resident and attending self-ratings of educational value of scope adapter examinations (non-validated 5-point scale)	Residents felt that reviewing examinations recorded with scope adapters enhanced learning in 79% of cases, and that ability to discuss recorded exams with attendings enhanced learning in 88% of cases. Attendings felt discussing recordings enhanced learning in 81% of cases.
Lozada et al	2017	Diagnostic accuracy	NA	Event rates of discordant diagnoses between staff/ resident based on smartphone adapter recordings; χ^2 to compare frequency of discordant diagnoses across diagnostic categories	11% frequency of discordant exams; No statistically significant difference in number of discordant diagnoses among diagnostic categories
		Video recording quailty		Event rate of repeated examinations	1.3% of exams needed to be repeated due to poor recording quailty

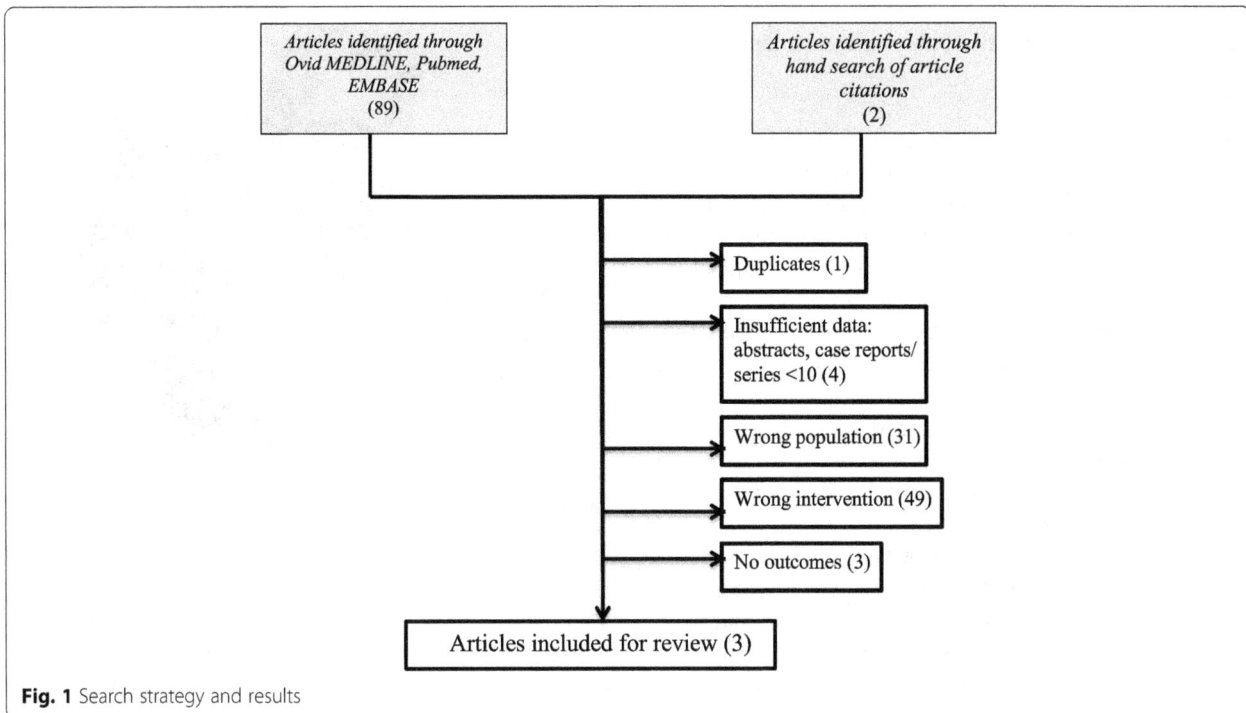

Fig. 1 Search strategy and results

(senior residents and staff attending physicians) was calculated. The authors found that there was no significant difference in correct diagnoses made between endoscopy video tower recordings and smartphone endoscope adapter recordings (mean difference = 1.54%, p = 0.69). This study assessed video quality subjectively using a 5-point Likert scale, with a linear mixed effects model to determine differences in mobile and tower video quality. No significant difference in video quality ratings was found across 7 quality categories (illumination and brightness; ability to identify camera orientation; ability to identify important landmarks/ structures; picture clarify and texture; artefact and background noise; contrast, border, and sharpness; overall satisfaction with video quality) [4]. In the other study (Lozara et al.), videos recorded by postgraduate year-1 residents using smartphone adapters were divided into diagnostic categories (airway evaluation, voice evaluation, dysphagia, aerodigestive tract mass) and were interpreted both by these same residents and staff attending physicians. Chi-squared statistics were used to compare the frequency of discordant exams. The authors found that there was an 11% frequency of discordant exams, with no statistical difference between diagnostic categories. They found that only 1 of 79 (1.3%) of exams had to be repeated due to poor quality [6]. One study (Liu YF et al.) assessed the ability of flexible nasolaryngoscopy videos recorded with smartphone adapters to enhance resident learning. Postgraduate year-1 and -2 residents recorded flexible nasolaryngoscopy exams using smartphone endoscope adapters and then reviewed recorded videos with staff attending physicians, and subsequently were surveyed using a 5-point Likert scale on whether they believed the discussions afforded by the use of smartphone adapters enhanced their learning. The authors found that residents reported that reviewing videos they had recording using adapters enhanced their learning in 79% of cases, and that the ability to discuss video findings with attending physicians enhanced their learning in 88% of cases as reported by attendings, and 81% of cases as reported by residents [5].

Two studies discussed methods employed to protect patient confidentiality. Liu H et al... used a Health Insurance Portability and Accountability Act (HIPAA)- compliant mobile application to record and store images and videos. Lozada et al. used a dedicated team iPhone, with encrypted email and password-secured files and computers. The third study (Liu YF et al) did not comment on the method used to ensure patient privacy and confidentiality.

Risk of Bias

The Newcastle-Ottawa Quality Assessment tool was used to appraise the selected studies (Additional file 1: Table S1) [3]. The strength of evidence was overall low to moderate quality, with a Newcastle-Ottawa score from 5 to 9 (range 0–9; a lower score indicates methodological weakness). The analysis of the methodologic quality indicated that the principal risks of bias were a lack of objective data comparing outcomes of smartphone endoscope adapter recordings to recordings made with endoscopy video towers, and lack of objective outcome assessment.

Discussion

Flexible nasolaryngoscopy is an essential tool to the practicing Otolaryngologist. Smartphone endoscope adapters which allow video recording of flexible nasolaryngoscopy examinations are relatively new devices with a number of potential benefits, including enhanced patient care and satisfaction by means of fewer repeat examinations; enhanced resident education by virtue of the ability to store, analyze, and discuss findings of videos recorded in remote locations such as emergency departments and inpatient wards; and decreased costs compared to fixed endoscopy towers. There have been very few studies objectively evaluating the effects of these devices in Otolaryngology practice.

In the present study, we have systematically reviewed the literature and found three studies which assessed the diagnostic accuracy, video quality, and educational benefits of smartphone endoscope adapters. These studies reported heterogeneous outcome data, but overall suggested a benefit of smartphone adapters on resident education, and demonstrated high diagnostic accuracy and video quality with the use of these devices. Lieu et al. [4] objectively compared diagnostic accuracy and quality between videos recorded with endoscopy towers and smartphone adapters and found no difference in either metric. A study of diagnostic accuracy and video quality of smartphone adapters, by way of demonstrating staff physician ability to come to diagnostic and management decisions based on videos recorded with smartphone adapters, identified a low rate of repeat examinations as a result of poor quality (Liu et al., 2016) [6]. Lozada et al. (2017) used self-reported surveys to show a resident educational benefit of smartphone adapters [5]. Outcome data was unable to be combined due to its heterogeneous nature. No study in the literature objectively examined resident educational benefits of smartphone adapters, patient care outcomes with the use of smartphone adapters, patient satisfaction with the use of adapters, or cost-effectiveness smartphone adapters.

At our own centre (The Ottawa Hospital, Department of Otolaryngology- Head & Neck Surgery), a tertiary care academic centre serving a catchment area of 1.2 million people, residents have been provided with and utilized smartphone endoscope adapters over a five-year period (ClearScope; Clearwater Clinical Limited, Ottawa, Canada) (Fig. 2). Since their introduction, smartphone endoscope adapters have improved cross-departmental communications, being used in grand rounds, interdisciplinary meetings, and teaching rounds. The recordings made using these devices are securely shared with healthcare professionals including members of the

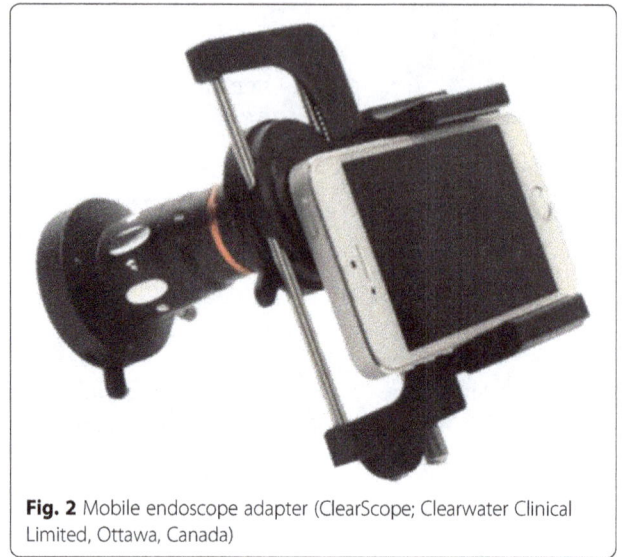

Fig. 2 Mobile endoscope adapter (ClearScope; Clearwater Clinical Limited, Ottawa, Canada)

OTOHNS team, anesthesiologists, and respiratory therapists, and have improved shared-decision making amongst airway consultants. Furthermore, a database of interesting cases has been curated, proving useful for medical education and research purposes. Endoscopic recordings are included in electronic medical records (EMRs) to ensure improved continuity of care in team handovers. Resident and staff physicians have reported that the frequency of repeat endoscopy by attending physicians to confirm resident diagnoses has decreased, as has the cleaning and maintenance costs associated with using a greater number of flexible scopes.

A variety of models of smartphone endoscope adapter are available on the market. We critically appraised the literature for commercially available smartphone endoscope adapters. There were no head-to-head comparisons of these products available in the published literature. Additional file 2: Table S2 summarizes commercially available devices.

Patient privacy and confidentiality is one concern which has increased in the era of omnipresent smartphone cameras and video recordings [7–9]. Smartphones can be misplaced or hacked, resulting in the breach of private medical information. Furthermore, images captured on smartphones are often stored in insecure mobile applications, many of which automatically sync the image to non-HIPAA-compliant cloud servers such as iCloud, Google+, and Dropbox. Conversely, encrypted mobile applications allow physicians to securely capture and save images and videos; some also provide HIPAA-compliant cloud sync services, allowing physicians to securely backup and share their photos and videos with the rest of the patient's healthcare team. Additional file 3: Table S3 summarizes available HIPAA-compliant mobile applications for storage of captured images and videos. In our own department, MODICA (Clearwater Clinical Limited; Ottawa, Canada) was formerly used.

There are several important limitations of the present study. There were only a small number of studies published in the literature examining the effects of smartphone endoscope adapters for FNL. Among existing studies, there was a lack of objective data examining our outcomes of interest, including lack of validated surveys; cost-effectiveness analyses; small patient populations; standardization between device operator level of training; and non-uniform use of a variety of different available adapters, endoscope video towers, and smartphones. Two of our three included studies were of poor quality based on Newcastle-Ottawa Scale ratings, due to lack of comparability data within the studies, and lack of objective outcome assessment (Additional file 1: Table S1). As well, among the three included studies, only two types of smartphone adapters were used (ClearScope, Clearwater Clinical Limited, Ottawa, Canada; and Mobile Optyx, MobileOptyx, Philadelphia, PA), and our own departmental experience is also with the ClearScope. The generalizability of our findings – especially scope video quality and diagnostic accuracy – is therefore limited by a lack of data derived from the use of other commercially available scope adapter products (Additional file 2: Table S2). Despite these limitations, we are able to conclude that the present study provides a sufficient overview of the current literature examining the use of smartphone adapters for flexible nasolaryngoscopy. In implementing our search strategy and study design as per the Cochrane handbook and PRISMA guidelines, we were able to effectively appraise the studies meeting our inclusion criteria.

Conclusion

The market for smartphone endoscope adapters has slowly evolved over the last decade such that new and innovative technology is now available for healthcare professionals to utilize. Accompanying these are a variety of HIPAA-compliant mobile applications to ensure the secure storage and sharing of captured images and videos. Few studies exist examining the utility of smartphone endoscope adapters in OTOHNS practice. This study has systematically reviewed the literature on the use of smartphone endoscope adapters. It has served to identify a significant lack of objective evidence exploring the use, benefits, and cost-effectiveness of these devices. However, we have shown that existing data supports the diagnostic accuracy, video quality, and educational benefits of smartphone endoscope adapters for flexible nasolaryngoscopy. Our study highlights the need for further research into the effects of incorporating these devices into practice.

Additional files

Additional file 1: Table S1. Summary of critical appraisal of included studies using the Newcastle-Ottawa Quality Assessment tool for cohort studies.

Additional file 2: Table S2. Commercially available smartphone endoscope adapters.

Additional file 3: Table S3. Commercially available Health Insurance Portability and Accountability Act (HIPAA)-compliant secure mobile applications.

Abbreviations
EMR: Electronic medical record; FNL: Flexible nasolaryngoscopy; HIPAA: Health Insurance Portability and Accountability Act; OTOHNS: Otolaryngology- Head & Neck Surgery; PRISMA: Preferred Reporting Items for Systematic reviews and Meta-analyses

Authors' contributions
AEQ participated in the design of the study, acquired data, and edited the manuscript. SK conceived the study and drafted the manuscript. LC participated in the design of the study, acquired data, and edited the manuscript. MB participated in the design of the study and edited the manuscript. All authors read and approved the final manuscript.

Competing interests
M.B. is the inventor of ClearScope and a shareholder in Clearwater Clinical, a company that manufactures a smartphone adapter for the purposes of endoscopy. No corporate funding was used for this project. The other authors have no conflicts of interest to declare.

Author details
[1]Department of Otolaryngology - Head and Neck Surgery, University of Ottawa, 501 Smyth Rd, Module S, Room M2566, Box 216, Ottawa, ON K1H 8L6, Canada. [2]Bringham and Women's Hospital, Department of Neuroendocrinology, 75 Francis St, Boston, MA 02115, USA. [3]Division of Otolaryngology – Head and Neck Surgery, Children's Hospital of Eastern Ontario, 401 Smyth Rd, Ottawa, ON K1H 8L1, Canada.

References
1. Cochrane Handbook for Systematic Reviews of Interventions. Online Kensaku 2014, 35(3):154–155.
2. Moher D, Liberati A, Tetzlaff J, Altman DG, Group P. Preferred reporting items for systematic reviews and meta-analyses: the PRISMA statement. BMJ. 2009;339:b2535.
3. Wells GA, Shea B, O'Connell D, et al. The Newcastle-Ottawa Scale (NOS) for assessing the quality of nonrandomized studies in meta-analyses. Ottawa Hospital Research Institute. 2011. Available at: http://www.ohri.ca/programs/clinical_epidemiology/oxford.asp.
4. Liu H, Akiki S, Barrowman NJ, Bromwich M. Mobile endoscopy vs video tower: a prospective comparison of video quality and diagnostic accuracy. Otolaryngol Head Neck Surg. 2016;155(4):575–80.
5. Liu YF, Kim CH, Bailey TW, Hondorp BM, Nguyen K, Krishnan M, et al. A prospective assessment of Nasopharyngolaryngoscope recording adaptor use in residency training. Otolaryngol Head Neck Surg. 2016;155(4):710–3.

6. Lozada K, Morton KM, Stepan K, Capo J, Chai R. Clinical impact of smartphone recording for flexible laryngoscopy. Otolaryngol Head Neck Surg. 2016;155:179.

7. Wang CJ, Huang DJ. The HIPAA conundrum in the era of mobile health and communications. JAMA. 2013;310:1121–2.

8. Rodriguez-Feliz JR, Roth MZ. The mobile technology era: potential benefits and the challenging quest to ensure patient privacy and confidentiality. Plast Reconstr Surg. 2012;130:1395–7.

9. Bromwich M, Bromwich R. Privacy risks when using mobile devices in health care. CMAJ. 2016;188:855–6.

20

A retrospective comparative study of endoscopic and microscopic Tympanoplasty

Ying-Chieh Hsu[1], Chin-Lung Kuo[2] and Tzu-Chin Huang[1,3]*

Abstract

Background: This study compares endoscopic and microscopic tympanoplasty for the treatment of chronic otitis media (COM) without cholesteatoma.

Methods: This retrospective study included 153 ears (139 patients) treated surgically (endoscopic or microscopic tympanoplasty) for COM in the absence of cholesteatoma at our hospital between January 2008 and October 2015. The adoption of transcanal endoscopic ear surgery (TEES) or microscopic ear surgery (MES) was divided temporally (before and since 2014). Comparisons between these groups focused on the following: (I) surgical outcomes, including successful tympanic membrane healing and post-operative complications; (II) restoration of hearing; and (III) consumption of medical resources, including the duration of surgery and anesthesia. All patients had a follow-up period of at least 3 months after surgery.

Results: No statistically significant differences were observed between the two groups regarding surgical outcome or hearing restoration. TEES resulted in the successful healing of 96.2% of ear drums, whereas MES led to successful healing in 92% ($p = 0.2826$) of cases. The average hearing gains following surgery were 10.27 ± 6.4 and 12.43 ± 7.46 dB in TEES and MES, respectively. The consumption of medical resources in the TEES group was lower than that of the MES group (TEES versus MES) regarding the average operating time (87.8 ± 19.01 min (mins) versus 110.2 ± 17.0 (mins) ($p < 0.0001$)) and the mean duration of anesthesia ((for general anesthesia patients) (122.1 ± 21.25 mins versus 145.8 ± 16.88 mins) ($p \leq 0.0001$)).

Conclusions: The results indicate that TEES can achieve surgical outcomes and hearing restoration comparable to those of MES. In addition, TEES appears to be associated with shorter surgical and anesthesia time, which makes it an ideal alternative for the management of COM without cholesteatoma.

Keywords: Endoscopic ear surgery, Microscopic, Tympanoplasty, Cost-efficacy

Background

A tympanoplasty is commonly performed to repair a perforated tympanic membrane and recover hearing loss in cases of chronic otitis media (COM) without cholesteatoma [1]. Conventional microscopic ear surgery (MES) using a post-auricular approach remains the most common tympanoplasty technique. However, it may require a large surgical incision, resulting in a visible scar and increased discomfort after surgery. Furthermore, the straight-line vision of microscopes greatly limits the surgeon's ability to visualize the middle ear through the ear canal.

Endoscopic ear surgery (EES) was introduced in 1960, although it did not attract much attention initially [1]. However, the evolution of endoscopes and other instruments has made EES far more powerful, particularly in the management of ear disease [2]. Transcanal endoscopic ear surgery (TEES) permits wide-angle vision at a high resolution while enabling magnification of the structures of the middle ear as well as the direct visualization of

* Correspondence: ab7801026@gmail.com
[1]Department of Otorhinolaryngology, Cathay General Hospital, 280 Ren-Ai Rd. Sec. 4, Taipei, Taiwan
[3]Department of Otorhinolaryngology, Hsinchu Cathay General Hospital, Hsinchu, Taiwan
Full list of author information is available at the end of the article

hidden areas, such as the hypotympanum, sinus tympani, epitympanum, and posterior part of the mesotympanum [3–5].

The feasibility of using EES to manage diseases of the ear has been widely discussed. However, most prior studies have focused on the outcomes of EES in the management of cholesteatomas. Few studies have compared the efficacy of endoscopic versus microscopic tympanoplasty [2, 6, 7]. This paper reports our experience using tympanoplasties to treat COM without cholesteatoma and compares the surgical outcomes, hearing restoration rates, and medical resource consumption of MES and TEES.

Methods

Patients

This retrospective study included 153 ears of 139 patients who had COM without cholesteatoma and underwent tympanoplasty at Hsinchu Cathay General Hospital, Taiwan between January 2008 and October 2015. Patients who had perforated tympanic membranes, with or without concomitant tympanic cavity pathology such as granulation, fibrotic bands, shallow retraction pocket or ossicular chain defects, and underwent tympanoplasty were included in this study. Those who had cholesteatoma, cholesterol granuloma, or had tympanic membrane retraction pocket that underwent atticotomy or mastoidectomy were excluded. The patients were divided into two groups: conventional microscopic tympanoplasty group (MES group: 100 ears; 92 patients) and endoscopic tympanoplasty group (TEES group: 53 ears, 47 patients). The adoption of TEES or MES had a clear temporal division (before versus since 2014). In our hospital, all patients treated before 2014 received MES. As of January 2014, TEES was adopted as the primary procedure, and MES was used as a salvage technique for patients who were not suitable for TEES. The surgeon was prepared to switch to MES (through a post-auricular approach) in cases where the situation warranted, such as in the case of ear canal stenosis or uncontrollable hemorrhage during surgery that might interfere with transcanal endoscopic manipulation. The data were collected and analyzed from the hospital database.

All surgical procedures, post-operative follow-up evaluations and management were performed by the senior author (corresponding author) alone, which may avoid the bias related to surgeries and treatment performed by different surgeons. Furthermore, the review of medical records and data collection and analyses were performed by the first author and a research assistant who were blinded to the patients and their clinical management to reduce observer bias. This study was approved by the institutional board of the hospital.

Exclusion criteria

Patients with a pre-operative or intra-operative diagnosis of cholesteatoma, cholesterol granuloma, and had tympanic membrane retraction pocket that underwent atticotomy or mastoidectomy were excluded. Moreover, patients who presented with facial paralysis or had a history of prior ear surgery were also excluded.

Audiological assessment

All patients underwent pure tone audiometry (PTA) analysis to evaluate their pre- and post-operative hearing status. The mean hearing level and air-bone gap (ABG) of each patient were measured by averaging their hearing thresholds at 0.5, 1, 2, and 4 kHz.

Anesthesia

Most of the tympanoplasties in our department were performed under general anesthesia (GA). Surgery was sometimes performed under local anesthesia (LA) for patients who were not suitable for GA for reasons such as old age, poor cardiopulmonary function or a difficult intubation. In some situations, LA was also performed in accordance with an individual patient's preference or willingness.

Surgical technique

All patients prior to 2014 underwent a conventional microscopic tympanoplasty for the treatment of COM without cholesteatoma, whereas all patients after January 2014 were managed with TEES. All surgical procedures, pre-operative assessments, and post-operative follow-up evaluations were performed by the senior author. In our department, TEES is indicated for almost all adult cases of COM without ear canal stenosis or congenital anomalies. These indications have been expanded to include the pediatric population, where TEES is initiated but the surgeon is prepared to switch to MES (post-auricular approach) if the situation warrants, such as in cases of ear canal stenosis or uncontrollable hemorrhage during surgery that might interfere with transcanal endoscopic manipulation.

In our hospital, all of the conventional microscopic tympanoplasties were performed via the post-auricular approach in order to obtain a wider surgical view. The procedure involves harvesting graft tissue from the areolar tissue layer above the temporalis fascia (loose areolar fascia) via a post-auricular incision. This is followed by the creation of a vascular strip in the ear canal, freshening the edges of the perforation, and the elevation of the tympanomeatal flap (TM flap) to gain access to the tympanic cavity. Following a thorough elimination of inflamed and infected tissue in the tympanic cavity, graft tissue is placed on the undersurface of the TM flap to reconstruct the tympanic membrane. Ossicular chains are assessed intra-operatively during all cases. If ossicular chain defects are noted during surgery, then a concomitant ossiculoplasty using an artificial total or partial ossicular replacement prosthesis (TORP or PORP) and cartilage may also be performed at the same time. Finally, the middle ear and external ear canals are packed with Gelfoam (absorbable gelatin sponge, USP, Pfizer, USA).

In contrast, TEES follows a transcanal approach using a rigid endoscope with an outer diameter of 3 mm and a length of 14 cm (HOPKINS II telescopes Karl Storz, Germany) at an angle of 0 or 30 degrees, in conjunction with a high definition (HD) video system. TEES at our facility involves the collection of graft tissue from three sources: areolar tissue above the temporalis fascia (through a post-auricular incision), cartilage from the perichondrium of the concha (through a retro-auricular wound), or the perichondrium of Tragus (from a wound within the ear canal). We then freshen the edges of the perforation, elevate the TM flap, and eliminate the inflamed and infected tissue in the tympanic cavity using an endoscope and various curved instruments, including needles, dissectors, and suction devices. Graft tissue is then placed on the undersurface of the TM flap to reconstruct the tympanic membrane. A concomitant ossiculoplasty with an artificial prosthesis (TORP or PORP) and cartilage may also be performed if an ossicular chain defect is noted during the surgery. The middle ear and external ear canals are also packed with Gelfoam at the end of the procedure.

Post-operative follow-up

All patients returned for follow-up 1, 2, 4, and 8 weeks after surgery. External ear canal packing was removed within 2 weeks, and patients were followed-up every 2 weeks until the end of their recovery period. The integrity of the tympanic membrane was assessed and an audiogram with PTA was performed 3 months after surgery.

Evaluation of outcomes

Retrospective medical record review and all subsequent data collection were conducted by an independent reviewer (the first author) who was not involved in the surgeries or post-operative follow-up, thereby diminishing possible observer bias. Analysis was performed by a research assistant who was blinded to the patients and interventions. The two groups were analyzed and compared from three perspectives: (I) surgical outcomes, including successful tympanic membrane healing and post-operative complications; (II) restoration of hearing function, including the average pre- and post-operative ABG, average hearing gain (dB), and percentage of patients with improved hearing (%, percentage of patients with post-operative hearing gain > 5 dB); and (III) consumption of medical resources, including the average

time spent in surgery (mins) and the average time spent under anesthesia (mins).

Statistical analysis

Statistical analysis was performed using SPSS for Windows (version 16.0; SPSS Inc., Chicago, IL, USA). Categorical variables were analyzed using a chi-squared or Fisher's exact test. Differences between groups were analyzed using a Mann-Whitney U test. A p-value < 0.05 was considered statistically significant.

Results

Our series included 139 patients (153 ears) (51 male (36.6%) and 88 females (63.3%)) between the ages of 6 and 78 years with a mean age ± standard deviation (SD) of 46.8 ± 14.5 years. Each subgroup presented with similar clinical and demographic characteristics (Table 1).

Comparison of surgical outcomes

Surgical procedures were adopted in accordance with the severity and extent of the pathology. The type of tympanoplasty was recorded and analyzed in accordance with a Wullstein classification of type I to V (Table 2) [8]. Since January 2014, TEES was adopted as the primary procedure for treating COM, and MES was used as the salvage technique for patients who were not suitable for TEES. The surgeons may need to switch to MES in cases where the situation warranted. However, none of the patients need to change

Table 1 Baseline clinical and demographic parameters

	TEES Group (n = 53 ears)	MES Group (n = 100 ears)	p-value
Sex			0.221
Male	22 (41.5%)	34 (34.0%)	
Female	31 (58.5%)	66 (66.0%)	
Lesion side			0.314
Left ear	30 (56.6%)	49 (49.0%)	
Right ear	23 (43.4%)	51 (51.0%)	
Average age ± SD (years)	48.9 ± 14.7	45.7 ± 14.2	0.1946
Average perforation size of tympanic membrane ± SD (%)[a]	51.6 ± 23.5	49.4 ± 21.1	0.5665
Comorbidity	7 (13.2%)	7 (7.0%)	0.2051
DM	4 (7.5%)	2 (2.0%)	
Hypertension	5 (9.4%)	4 (4.0%)	
Asthma	0	1 (1.0%)	
Hepatitis B	0	1 (1.0%)	
Average follow-up period ± SD (months)	3.5 ± 2.6	7.0 ± 10.4	0.016

[a]Perforation size was estimated through visual inspection of the percentage of perforation relative to the tympanic membrane area by the senior otologist (corresponding author)

Table 2 Surgical procedure

	Group		p
	TEES (n = 53)	MES (n = 100)	
Graft material			< 0.0001
Areolar temporalis fascia	12 (22.6%)	100 (100%)	
Concha perichondrium	23 (43.4%)		
Tragus perichondrium	18 (34.0%)		
Tympanoplasty type			0.1094
Type I	46 (88.5%)	94 (94.0%)	
Type III	3 (5.8%)	5 (5.0%)	
Type IV	2 (3.8%)	1 (1.0%)	
Type V	1 (1.9%)	0	
Ossiculoplasty	6 (11.3%)	6 (6.0%)	0.127
PORP	3 (5.8%)	5 (5.0%)	
TORP	2 (3.8%)	1 (1.0%)	
Piston wire	1 (1.9%)	0	

to MES during the study period. It is also worth mentioning that 13 of MES patients required bony canalplasty because of insufficient surgical views whereas none of the patients in the TEES group required the procedure.

The surgical outcomes of the two groups were compared in many categories. The rates of complete tympanic membrane healing in the TEES and MES groups were 96.2 and 92%, respectively ($p = 0.282$). We also compared the incidence of post-operative complications. The MES group included one patient with severe sensory neural hearing loss (SNHL) (SNHL > 70 dB), one patient with mastoiditis, and another patient with persistent otorrhea for 2 months after surgery (Table 3). We hypothesized that these three complications occurred due to a severe middle ear infection but were not relevant to the procedure itself. Overall, we were unable to detect any statistically significant differences ($p < 0.05$) between the two groups with respect to the rates of complete tympanic membrane healing or the incidence of post-operative complications.

Table 3 Surgical outcome

	Group		p
	TEES (n = 53)	MES (n = 100)	
Successful tympanic membrane healing	51 (96.2%)	92 (92.0%)	0.2826
Post-operative complications			0.2028
Severe SNHL	0	1 (1.0%)	
Mastoiditis	0	1 (1.0%)	
Persistent otorrhea (wet ear)	0	1 (1.0%)	

Comparison of hearing outcomes

We also assessed the restoration of hearing in the two groups. The average hearing gain was 10.3 ± 6.4 dB in the TEES group and 12.4 ± 7.5 dB in the MES group ($p = 0.1663$). We did not detect any statistically significant differences ($p < 0.05$) between the two groups with respect to the average pre- and post-operative ABG, average hearing gain, or percentage of patients with improved hearing (Table 4).

Comparison of medical resource consumption

Statistically significant differences were observed between the two groups regarding the consumption of medical resources. Compared to the MES group, a higher percentage of patients in the TEES group was treated under LA (TEES versus MES: 17.0% versus 2.0%, $p < 0.001$), and a higher percentage of TEES was performed as outpatient surgery (TEES versus MES: 22.6% versus 1.0%, $p < 0.0001$). The mean duration of surgery was significantly shorter in the TEES group (87.8 ± 19.01 mins) than in the MES group (110.2 ± 17.0 mins, $p < 0.0001$), as was the mean duration of anesthesia (for GA patients) (mins) (122.1 ± 21.3 versus 145.8 ± 16.9, $p \le 0.0001$) (Table 5). Overall, patients in the TEES group seemed to use fewer medical resources than those in the MES group with respect to shorter time spent in surgery and under anesthesia.

Discussion

The main goals of a tympanoplasty for COM are to eradicate infection, repair the perforated tympanic membrane, and improve hearing [9]. For decades, MES was the main modality for ear surgery, enabling two-handed manipulation as well as binocular vision along with an excellent stereoscopic surgical view. However, the vision of a microscope may be limited when using a transcanal approach, particularly in hidden areas such as the anterior margin of the tympanic membrane and the sinus tympani or facial recesses, which forces the surgeons to use the post-auricular approach in order to obtain a wider surgical view. In some cases,

Table 4 Restoration of hearing function

	Group		p
	TEES (n = 53)	MES (n = 100)	
Average pre-operative ABG ± SD (dB)	24.7 ± 8.1	25.0 ± 8.2	0.8217
Average post-operative ABG ± SD (dB)	14.4 ± 9.2	12.3 ± 6.2	0.2256
Average hearing gain ± SD (dB)	10.3 ± 6.4	12.4 ± 7.5	0.1663
Percentage of patients with improved hearing	51 / 53 (96.2%)	94 / 100 (94.0%)	0.4848

Table 5 Consumption of medical resources

	Group		p
	TEES (n = 53)	MES (n = 100)	
Outpatient/Admission			< 0.0001
Outpatient procedure	12 (22.6%)	1 (1.0%)	
Admission procedure	41 (77.4%)	99 (99.0%)	
Anesthesia method			0.0007
General (GA)	44 (83.0%)	98 (98.0%)	
Local (LA)	9 (17.0%)	2 (2.0%)	
Average surgical time ± SD (mins)	87.8 ± 19.0	110.2 ± 17.0	< 0.0001
Average time under anesthesia ±SD (mins) (GA patients)	122.1 ± 21.3	145.8 ± 16.9	< 0.0001

creating sufficient space necessitates a canalplasty and soft-tissue retraction [5].

TEES provides an excellent surgical view, uses a smaller surgical incision, and preserves more tissue. Kozin et al. reported that a clear benefit existed for observational EES [2]. Some studies have suggested that when treating COM with cholesteatoma, TEES enables surgeons to avoid unnecessary mastoidectomies and prevent external ear canal widening and soft-tissue injuries during ear surgery [5–7, 10, 11]. Nonetheless, TEES still has a number of disadvantages, such as the need for one-handed manipulation, reduced endoscopic vision in the setting of uncontrollable hemorrhage, and the potential for thermal injury to the middle or inner ear caused by the endoscopic light source [12, 13]. However, operative EES is still in its infancy. Previous studies on EES have focused mainly on the management of cholesteatomas. Few researchers have conducted a systematic comparison of microscopic and endoscopic tympanoplasties in the absence of cholesteatoma [14–17].

Surgical outcomes
In this study, the rate of successful tympanic membrane healing and the incidence of post-operative complications were similar in the TEES and MES groups. In the MES group, one patient presented with post-operative complication of severe SNHL, one had mastoiditis and another had persistent otorrhea for months after surgery. Overall, we observed no statistically significant differences in the surgical outcomes following MES and TEES. Choi et al. [14] concluded that the outcomes of microscopic and endoscopic tympanoplasties are similar, with graft success rates of 100 and 95.8% in the endoscopic and microscopic groups, respectively ($p = 0.304$). Dundar et al. [15] also reported that no significant differences in the condition of the graft were observed 12 months after surgery in pediatric patients who underwent a type 1 tympanoplasty through an endoscopic or

microscopic approach (graft success rate: 87.5% (endoscopic) versus 94.3% (microscopic), $p > 0.05$). These outcomes are also consistent with those obtained in our study (graft success rate: TEES: 96.2% versus MES: 92.0%, $p = 0.2826$).

Restoration of hearing function
Post-operative hearing restoration is another important indicator by which the outcomes of tympanoplasties can be evaluated. Dundar et al. [15] reported that there was no statistically significant difference in the pre-operative (20.40 versus 21.34 dB, $p \geq 0.05$) and post-operative ABG (8.12 versus 8.13 dB, $p \geq 0.05$) regardless of which procedure was performed. Similar to our results, we also observed no statistically significant differences between the TEES and MES groups in hearing restoration, including pre- and post-operative ABG, average hearing gain (dB) (10.3 ± 6.4 for TEES and 12.4 ± 7.5 for MES, $p = 0.1663$) and the percentage of patients with improved hearing after surgery (TEES versus MES: 96.2% versus 94.0%, $p = 0.4848$) (Table 3). This implies that TEES shows similar results to MES for the restoration of hearing after surgery.

Consumption of medical resources
A medical record review found that most of the patients in the MES group were treated under GA. In contrast, a much higher percentage of cases in the TEES group utilized LA. In addition, a higher percentage of outpatient surgery was performed in the TEES group when comparing with the MES group. Our findings show that TEES can reduce the consumption of medical resources by shortening the surgical time, and the anesthesia time. The mean operative time in the TEES group (87.8 ± 19.01 mins) was significantly lower than that of the MES group (110.2 ± 17.0 mins). This result is consistent with previous studies that have reported that the operative time of an endoscopic tympanoplasty is significant shorter than that of a microscopic tympanoplasty [14, 16]. These differences may be attributed to differences in the surgical approach for TEES and MES. Prior to 2014, we employed a post-auricular approach in MES that produced a wide surgical wound during the surgery and required considerable time to manage the soft tissues and close the wound. In contrast, TEES is based on a transcanal approach, which leaves only a tiny wound associated with graft harvesting. The minimally invasive transcanal approach of TEES saves time in the assessment of the middle ear and results in far less soft-tissue damage, thereby reducing the time required to complete the surgery and the time spent under anesthesia. In addition, when performing microscopic tympanoplasty, a bony canalplasty may be required in narrow or crooked ear canal patients in order to obtain a sufficient surgical view. While in TEES, the endoscope can

bypass the narrow part of the ear canal, provide greater visual access and wide-angle view of the middle ear, as well as sufficient manipulation space without the necessity of canalplasty, which can also help to save the surgical and anesthesia time significantly [5, 18].

TEES has also been shown to preserve the integrity of the outer ear and cause a less extensive injury to the cartilaginous ear canal, thereby reducing the incidence of post-operative complications such as tissue swelling, wound pain, bleeding, scaring, and ear canal stenosis [5, 18]. Choi also reported that patients who underwent an endoscopic tympanoplasty experienced far less pain the first day after the procedure than patients who underwent the microscopic procedure [14]. We infer that the minimally invasive nature of TEES can help to reduce the physical and psychological burden placed on patients, which may somewhat influence the patient's reliance on hospitalization and explain why physicians opt to perform TEES under LA or as an outpatient procedure. Although some confounding factors exist, we believe that the results of our study reflect clinical reality to some extent.

According to previous studies, the success rate of microscopic tympanoplasties ranges from 90 to 98% [19, 20]. However, the outcomes of TEES still lack sufficient acceptance. In our series, we achieved a graft success rate of 96% following an endoscopic tympanoplasty, with satisfying improvements in hearing and no post-operative complications. Shoeb et al. [17] reported graft success rates of 93% using TEES and MES. Dundar et al. [15] also reported that in pediatric patients undergoing a type 1 tympanoplasty, the endoscopic and microscopic approaches appear to be equal in terms of hearing gain and graft success rate, whereas the operative duration was shorter in the endoscopic group than in the microscopic group. These findings are also consistent with those observed in this study. We therefore believe that TEES not only achieves surgical outcomes that are at least as good as those of MES but also reduces the consumption of medical resources due to a shorter procedure time. TEES is likely a good alternative to MES in the management of COM without cholesteatoma.

Limitations

The selection bias in this study was minimized by adopting TEES and MES in a consecutive series, with a clear temporal division (before and since 2014) rather than one based on disease severity. When TEES was first adopted in our department in 2014, it was inevitable that part of the patients in the TEES group were within the learning curve of the operator which might cause bias in the results.

Furthermore, all surgical procedures, pre-operative assessments, and post-operative follow-up evaluations were performed by the senior author (corresponding author)

alone, which avoids a discrepancy between different surgeons. However, this might increase the risk of bias in the review process.

In addition, this study was limited by a number of factors. This is a retrospective study conducted at a single hospital with relatively small group of patients. The sample size might be too small to come up with a widely accepted conclusion. A more extensive survey of cases or a multi-hospital study would be beneficial. The relatively short follow-up period in both groups likely led to an underestimation of actual long-term results. Although close office-based examination was performed after surgery, regular follow-up over a longer time scale should still be considered if necessary. Furthermore, several limitations remain regarding the use of TEES in the management of COM including that (1) stenosis, narrowing or exostosis of the external ear canal and (2) coagulopathies are relative contraindications of TEES due to the increased complexity of the endoscopic transcanal approach.

Two additional issues need to be addressed. First, we did not report the location of tympanic membrane perforation because the data were either incomplete or non-objective. Second, MES via endaural approach was not mentioned throughout the study because all of the microscopic tympanoplasties in our hospital were performed via the post-auricular approach.

Conclusions

The results show that TEES can achieve satisfactory outcomes that are at least as good as those following traditional MES in the management of COM without cholesteatoma. Additionally, TEES appears to be associated with less consumption of medical resources in terms of shorter surgical and anesthesia time. However, further prospective studies should be conducted in the future to reinforce these conclusions.

Abbreviations
ABG: Air-bone gap; COM: Chronic otitis media; MES: Microscopic ear surgery; PORP: Partial ossicular replacement prosthesis; PTA: Pure tone audiometry; TEES: Transcanal endoscopic ear surgery; TORP: Total ossicular replacement prosthesis

Authors' contributions
GMS participated in the conceptualization of the experimental design, data analysis and manuscript preparation. CAEB participated in the data collection and manuscript preparation. DCM participated in the data analysis and manuscript preparation. All authors read and approved the final manuscript.

Competing interests
The authors declare that they have no competing interests.

Author details
[1]Department of Otorhinolaryngology, Cathay General Hospital, 280 Ren-Ai Rd. Sec. 4, Taipei, Taiwan. [2]Department of Otolaryngology, Taoyuan Armed Forces General Hospital, Taoyuan, Taiwan, Republic of China. [3]Department of Otorhinolaryngology, Hsinchu Cathay General Hospital, Hsinchu, Taiwan.

References
1. Zöllner F. The principles of plastic surgery of the sound-conducting apparatus. J Laryngol Otol. 1955;69:637–52.
2. Kozin ED, Gulati S, Kaplan AB, Lehmann AE, Remenschneider AK, Landegger LD, et al. Systematic review of outcomes following observational and operative endoscopic middle ear surgery. Laryngoscope. 2015;125:1205–14.
3. Thomassin JM, Duchon-Doris JM, Emram B, Rud C, Conciatori J, Vilcoq P. Endoscopic ear surgery. Initial evaluation. Ann Otolaryngol Chir Cervicofac. 1990;107:564–70.
4. Marchioni D, Alicandri-Ciufelli M, Piccinini A, Genovese E, Presutti L. Inferior retrotympanum revisited: an endoscopic anatomic study. Laryngoscope. 2010;120:1880–6.
5. Tarabichi M. Endoscopic middle ear surgery. Ann Otol Rhinol Laryngol. 1999;108:39–46.
6. Presutti L, Gioacchini FM, Alicandri-Ciufelli M, Villari D, Marchioni D. Results of endoscopic middle ear surgery for cholesteatoma treatment: a systematic review. Acta Otorhinolaryngol Ital. 2014;34:153–7.
7. Marchioni D, Mattioli F, Alicandri-Ciufelli M, Presutti L. Endoscopic approach to tensor fold in patients with attic cholesteatoma. Acta Otolaryngol. 2009; 129:946–54.
8. Wullstein H. The restoration of the function of the middle ear, in chronic otitis media. Ann Otol Rhinol Laryngol. 1956;65:1020–41.
9. Sheehy JL, Anderson RG. Myringoplasty. A review of 472 cases. Ann Otol Rhinol Laryngol. 1980;89:331–4.
10. Marchioni D, Villari D, Alicandri-Ciufelli M, Piccinini A, Presutti L. Endoscopic open technique in patients with middle ear cholesteatoma. Eur Arch Otorhinolaryngol. 2011;268:1557–63.
11. Ayache S, Tramier B, Strunski V. Otoendoscopy in cholesteatoma surgery of the middle ear. Otol Neurotol. 2008;29:1085–90.
12. Bottrill I, Perrault DF, Poe D. In vitro and in vivo determination of the thermal effect of middle ear endoscopy. Laryngoscope. 1996;106:213–6.
13. Kozin ED, Lehmann A, Carter M, Hight E, Cohen M, Nakajima HH, et al. Thermal effects of endoscopy in a human temporal bone model: implications for endoscopic ear surgery. Laryngoscope. 2014;124:E332–9.
14. Choi N, Noh Y, Park W, Lee JJ, Yook S, Choi JE, et al. Comparison of endoscopic tympanoplasty to microscopic tympanoplasty. Clin Exp Otorhinolaryngol. 2016;10:44–9.
15. Dündar R, Kulduk E, Soy FK, Aslan M, Hanci D, Muluk NB, et al. Endoscopic versus microscopic approach to type 1 tympanoplasty in children. Int J Pediatr Otorhinolaryngol. 2014;78:1084–9.
16. Lakpathi G, Reddy LS, Anand. Comparative study of endoscope assisted myringoplasty and microscopic myringoplasty. Indian J Otolaryngol Head Neck Surg. 2016;68:185–90.
17. Shoeb M, Gite V, Bhargava S, Mhashal S. Comparison of surgical outcomes of tympanoplasty assisted by conventional microscopic method and endoscopic method. Int J Otorhinolaryngology Head Neck Surg. 2016;2:184–8.
18. Tarabichi M. Principle of endoscopic ear surgery. In: Presutti L, Marchioni D, editors. Endoscopic ear surgery: principles, indications and techniques. Stuttgart: Thieme; 2015. p. 6–15.
19. Dornhoffer JL. Hearing results with cartilage tympanoplasty. Laryngoscope. 1997;107:1094–9.
20. Indorewala S, Adedeji TO, Indorewala A, Nemade G. Tympanoplasty outcomes: a review of 789 cases. Iran J Otorhinolaryngol. 2015;27:101–8.

21

Shared decision making and decisional conflict in the Management of Vestibular Schwannoma

M. Elise Graham[1*] ⓘ, Brian D. Westerberg[2], Jane Lea[2], Paul Hong[3], Simon Walling[4], David P. Morris[5], Andrea L. O. Hebb[4], Rochelle Galleto[2], Emily Papsin[5], Maeve Mulroy[5], Hannah Foggin[2] and Manohar Bance[5,6]

Abstract

Background: Patients with vestibular schwannomas (VS) are faced with complex management decisions. Watchful waiting, surgical resection, and radiation are all viable options with associated risks and benefits. We sought to determine if patients with VS experience decisional conflict when deciding between surgery or non-surgical management, and factors influencing the degree of decisional conflict.

Methods: A prospective cohort study in two tertiary ambulatory skull-base clinics was performed. Patients with newly diagnosed or newly growing vestibular schwannomas were recruited. Patients were given a demographic form and the decisional conflict scale (DCS), a validated measure to assess the degree of uncertainty when making medical decisions. The degree of shared decision making (SDM) experienced by the patient and physician were assessed via the SDM-Q-10 and SDM-Q-Doc questionnaires, respectively. Non-parametric statistics were used. Questionnaires and demographic information were correlated with DCS using Spearman correlation coefficient and Mann-Whitney U. Logistic regression was performed to determine factors independently associated with DCS scores.

Results: Seventy-seven patients participated (55% female, aged 37–81 years); VS ranged in size from 2 mm–50 mm. Significant decisional conflict (DCS score 25 or greater) was experienced by 17 (22%) patients. Patients reported an average SDM-Q-10 score of 86, indicating highly perceived level of SDM. Physician and patient SDM scores were weakly correlated ($p = 0.045$, Spearman correlation coefficient 0.234). DCS scores were significantly negatively correlated with a decision to pursue surgery, presence of a trainee, and higher SDM-Q-10 score. DCS was higher with female gender. Using logistic regression, the SDM-Q-10 score was the only variable associated with significantly reduced DCS.

Conclusions: About one fifth of patients deciding how to manage their vestibular schwannoma experienced a significant degree of decisional conflict. Involving the patients in the process through shared decision-making significantly reduced the degree of uncertainty patients experienced.

Keywords: Decisional conflict, Acoustic neuroma, Shared decision making, Vestibular schwannoma

Background

Vestibular schwannomas (VS) have an estimated incidence of 0.6–1.9 per 100,000 annually [1]. In tertiary neurotology practices, however, they can be a substantial part of the patient flow. Symptoms are variable, and it is therefore difficult to create a standardized management algorithm. Options include watchful waiting, stereotactic radiation

surgery (SRS) and conventional surgical approaches. The risks and benefits of each option may make management decisions challenging for both surgeons and patients.

Watchful waiting is a commonly employed treatment approach in the modern management of vestibular schwannomas. There are no identified factors to predict an individual's VS growth pattern at initial presentation or when the tumor first shows evidence of growth [2, 3]. Various series have shown that the majority (> 60%) of VSs do not grow if followed. If the tumor does grow, most grow slowly though some grow rapidly, with an overall estimated

---

* Correspondence: Elisegraham.md@gmail.com
[1]Division of Otolaryngology – Head and Neck Surgery, Western University and London Health Sciences Centre, 5010, 800 Commissioners Road E, London, Ontario, Canada
Full list of author information is available at the end of the article

annual growth between 0.4 and 2.9 mm per year [4–6]. When growth does occur, it can affect patient function and influence both the options and outcomes for future management.

Microsurgical resection is another management option for patients, via the translabyrinthine, retrosigmoid or middle cranial fossa approach, with each possessing its own set of advantages and disadvantages. Surgery places surrounding nerves and arteries at potential risk. Standard neurosurgical risks also apply, such as cerebrospinal fluid leak and meningitis [7]. Stereotactic radiation surgery (SRS) as an option has its own risks. SRS can cause acute hydrocephalus from tumor swelling, albeit rarely [8], or contribute to hearing loss [9, 10]. If SRS fails, salvage surgery may be more challenging [11]. There is also the low but real risk of malignant transformation in the radiation field [12, 13].

With multiple treatment options, all with their own inherent risks and benefits, and variable natural history, any treatment decision is complex and likely to involve significant anxiety and stress. The decision between treatment options must consider the patient's experiences, values and risk tolerance, in addition to tumor characteristics and local physician expertise. Shared decision-making (SDM) may play an important role in facilitating the management of VS. SDM is a collaborative approach that describes the process of patients working with healthcare providers to come to a consensus regarding their care. SDM has previously been shown to decrease uncertainty around management decisions and improve health-related quality of life [14, 15].

A related topic is "decisional conflict", which defines difficulties experienced by patients in coming to a decision regarding their care. Previous data has suggested that the degree of decisional conflict experienced by patients may be influenced by the degree of shared decision-making in patient consultation [16–18], with those patients perceiving more SDM experiencing less decisional conflict. Studies in other surgical decision-making contexts have showed that patients experience significant decisional conflict when deciding between surgical and non-surgical treatment for various conditions [17, 19, 20].

The objective of this study was to determine if patients experience decisional conflict when making management decisions for their VS, and to explore which factors, if any, influence the degree of conflict experienced. Given the benign nature of the tumors and the sometimes conflicting and confusing evidence surrounding management of patients with VS, we hypothesized that these patients may experience significant levels of decisional conflict.

Methods
Ethical considerations
Institutional ethics board approval was obtained at both participating centers. Written informed consent was obtained

from each patient and de-identified data was securely stored.

Aim
To assess the degree of shared decision making experienced by patients when deciding how best to manage their VS.

Participants
This study was carried out in two tertiary/quaternary academic centres. One centre (Halifax, Nova Scotia) involved a multi-disciplinary skull base clinic with fellowship trained neurotologists and neurosurgeons, whereas the second site (Vancouver, British Columbia) involved a neurotology clinic with fellowship trained neurotologists with referrals to other services being directed after the initial consultation.

All new patients with a clinical diagnosis of VS presenting to the two centers were approached. Follow-up patients with demonstrated recent VS growth on serial MRI scans were also approached, as they were faced with the need to make a new treatment decision. Patients were excluded if they declined to participate or were not fluent in English. Patients were not approached if they had previously undergone treatment of their VS.

All patients underwent a standardized clinic visit, which involved a neurotological history and examination, review of imaging, discussion of the diagnosis, and a review of possible treatment options, highlighting those felt to be most appropriate for the individual patient. Risks and benefits of each option were discussed by the attending surgeons. Following the consultation, patients who agreed to participate were referred to the research assistant who provided details of the study, obtained consent and administered the questionnaires to the patients.

Measures
Demographic form
Baseline demographic information was collected, including previous surgeries, education, and income. A separate demographic form was completed by the attending surgeons responsible for the consultation including maximum diameter of VS measured on MRI, presenting symptoms, presence of a trainee, and management options presented.

Decisional Conflict Scale (DCS)
This 16-item Likert-like measure is a validated scale that determines patient uncertainty about a medical decision. Sample items include the following: "I am clear about what benefits matter most to me," "I feel sure about what to choose," and "My decision shows what is important to me." It includes five subcategories, is context non-specific, and has been used in a variety of surgical settings [17–20]. Previous research has suggested that a score of 25 or greater is representative for significant decisional conflict [12].

Shared Decision Making Questionnaire-Patient Version (SDM-Q-9)

This is a validated measure with nine items on a Likert scale to assess the perception of patients regarding their involvement in clinical decision-making. Total score range from 0 (no shared decision-making) to 100 (a high degree of shared decision-making). Sample items include: "My doctor and I selected a treatment option together" and "My doctor made it clear that a decision had to be made." The SDM-Q-9 has been shown to have high reliability [19].

Shared Decision Making Questionnaire-Physician Version (SDM-Q-Doc)

This is a validated scale that was developed from SDM-Q-9 to make it applicable for healthcare providers. Its format is similar to the SDM-Q-9 with overall score also ranging from 0 to 100. This scale has demonstrated high reliability [20]. Sample items include: "I wanted to know exactly from my patient how he/she wants to be involved in making the decision" and "I told my patient that there are different options for treating his/her medical condition."

Data analysis

Power calculation indicated that 52 patients would be required to detect a correlation coefficient of 0.38 between shared decision-making and decisional conflict. This correlation coefficient has been established in previous research examining DCS and SDM [15]. To ensure adequate sample size, accounting for attrition and incomplete data, we set the recruitment goal at 75 patients.

Data entry was completed in Microsoft Excel ™ and analysis conducted in RStudio, Version 1.0.136 (Boston, MA).

DCS was not normally distributed; therefore, non-parametric statistics were used. Descriptive statistics such as median, interquartile range and standard error (SE) are reported. Scores greater than 25 on the DCS indicate significant decisional conflict. Mann-Whitney U test and Spearman's correlation coefficient were utilized to correlate DCS with demographic variables. Spearman's correlation coefficient was used to compare SDM-Q-9 and SDM-Q-Doc. Logistic regression was performed to determine which factors are independently associated with decisional conflict. Statistical significance was set at $p < 0.05$.

Results

Patient demographics

Seventy-seven patients participated, 62 of whom (79%) were presenting to the clinics for the first time, while 15 (19%) were follow-up patients with demonstrated VS growth. One patient did not have new/follow-up patient status recorded. Fifty-eight percent of patients were recruited from Halifax, with the remainder were from Vancouver. Seventy-one percent of patients (55/78) had undergone surgery previously,

with the most common surgery being a hysterectomy. Average patient age was 57.8 years old (range 37 to 81 years); 55% of patients were female and the majority (73%) were married. Patients had an average of 14 years of education (range 8 to 20 years).

Vestibular schwannoma characteristics

The participants' mean maximal diameter of vestibular schwannoma was 18.3 mm, with diameters ranging from 2 mm to 50 mm. The most common presenting complaint was hearing loss, noted in 92% of patients (72/78). Other presentations included vestibular dysfunction in 44%, tinnitus in 19%, and facial numbness in 17%.

Decisional conflict

Median decisional conflict across all patients was 4.69. Seventeen participants (22%) had significant decisional conflict, as defined by a score of 25 or more (Fig. 1). Thirty-two patients (41%) reported that they experienced zero decisional conflict. The DCS score did not significantly differ based on previous surgery, marital status, study site, or type of visit (first time vs. follow-up). Significant differences were noted in DCS scores between participants who decided upon surgery as a treatment and those who did not ($p = 0.034$), with the surgery group experiencing lower decisional conflict. There was also a significant difference noted between the degree of decisional conflict reported by female patients and male patients (male lower), and lower DCS scores were noted in those encounters where a trainee was present ($p = 0.035$).

DCS scores were not related to whether the patient felt they wanted surgery prior to the consultation, patient age, number of previous surgeries, years of education, size of VS, or number of symptoms. DCS was also not correlated with any individual presenting symptom, including hearing loss, vestibular dysfunction, tinnitus and facial numbness ($p > 0.05$).

Shared decision-making

Median SDM-Q-9 scores for patients was 88.89. Median SDMQ score for physicians was 75.56 (Fig. 2). There was a significant difference between patient and physician SDMQ scores ($p < 0.001$). The mean difference in score between physician and patients was 11.29 (95% CI, 7.98–14.61). Spearman's correlation between participant and physician shared decision-making scores was 0.234, $p < 0.05$, indicating they were weakly correlated (Fig. 3).

A significantly negative correlation between SDM-Q-9 scores and DCS scores was noted (Fig. 4). SDM-Q-Doc scores and DCS scores were not correlated.

Management decisions and decisional conflict

More than half of patients (40/78, 51%) decided on a watchful waiting approach. Twenty-one patients (27%) decided to

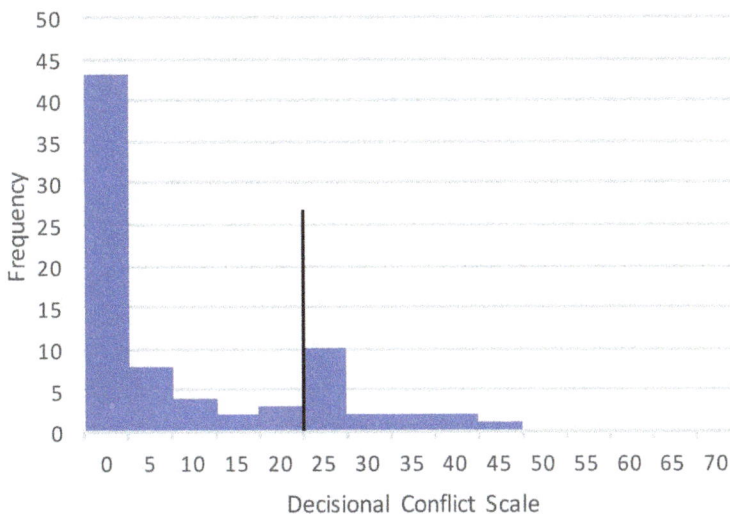

Fig. 1 Distribution of decisional conflict amongst patients. The black line represents significant decisional conflict (25), and 22% of patients exceeded this

proceed with surgery, and 8 patients (10%) decided on radiation. More than one option was usually discussed with each patient. Options discussed with patients were radiation with 88.3% of patients, surgery with 93.5%, and watchful waiting (W & W) with 85.7%. Seventy-one of 75 patients (95%) who responded to this question indicated that they knew surgery was an option prior to the consultation. Figure 5 shows the distribution of DCS by treatment decision.

Logistic regression

Logistic regression was performed to predict the presence of significant decisional conflict (DCS > 25). The best model

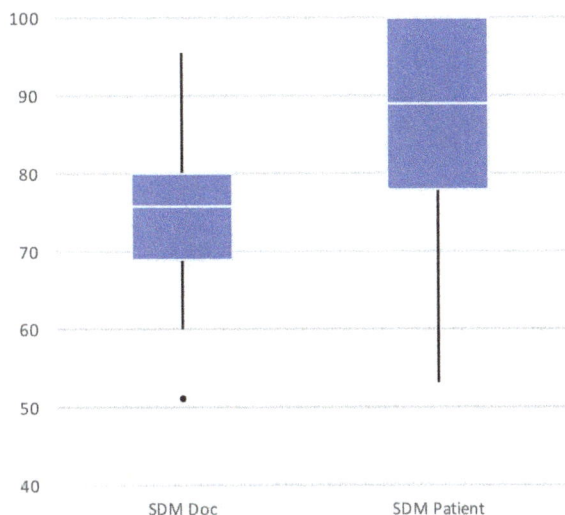

Fig. 2 Comparison of the self-reported shared decisional conflict between patients (SDM-Q-9 (right) and physicians SDM-Q-Doc (left). The upper and lower bars represent 25th and 75th centiles, with the black dot representing an outlier

generated, by lowest Akaike information criterion (51.77), incorporated patient sex, age, number of previous surgeries, years of education, SDM-Q-10 score and number of options discussed with the patients to predict the presence or absence of significant decisional conflict. Of the individual variables, only the patient's SDM-Q-10 score contributed significantly to prediction, with higher SDM-Q-10 scores predicting lower probability of significant decisional conflict.

Discussion
Synopsis of key findings
Given the benign nature of VS and the sometimes conflicting and confusing evidence surrounding management of VS, we hypothesized that these patients may experience significant levels of decisional conflict. The overall median decisional conflict in our study at 4.69 was well below the cut-off for significant decisional conflict. However, one of every five patients (22%) experienced significant decisional conflict (DCS > 25). Previous studies suggest that decisional conflict affects emotional wellbeing and may influence subsequent regret surrounding their management choices [21, 22].

In deciding whether to proceed with an intervention or conservative management for their VS, patients must weigh significant risks to hearing, balance, and facial nerve function. Risks of watchful waiting are that that growth may limit the ability to use SRS or that the patient may experience a general decline in health that increases the risks of surgery later. Because facial nerve and hearing outcomes from surgery are related to size of the tumor there are risks that the outcome will not be as optimal if the tumor grows prior to surgery [23]. Rates of growth are variable and not predictable. Not surprisingly, because we can only provide patients with probabilistic outcomes rather than

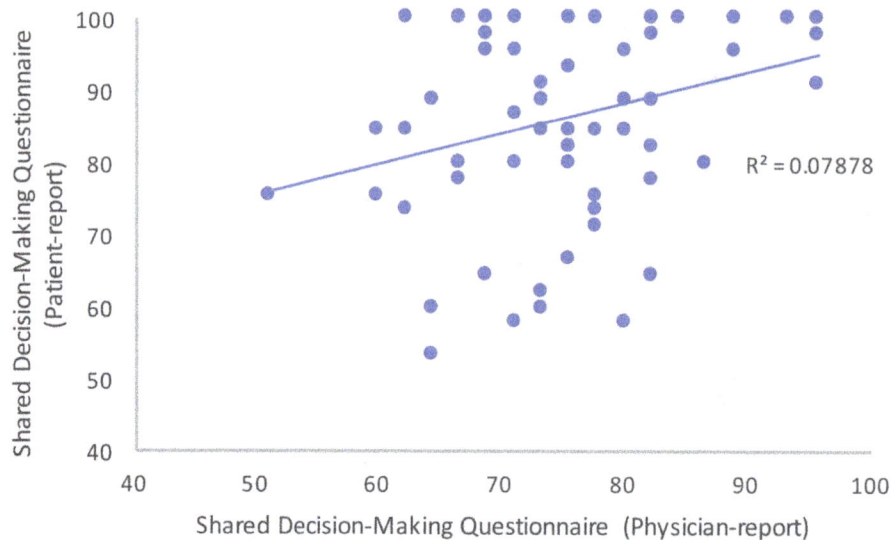

Fig. 3 Scatter plot of the correlation between patients' and physicians' perceptions of shared decision making (SDM-Q-9 and SDM-Q-Doc). The R^2 value is shown, correlation coefficient is 0.234

individualized precise trajectories, we often encounter significant anxiety associated with the watchful waiting choice. This has not been well explored in previous literature.

This study suggests, as in previous studies, that patient and physician estimates of SDM were not well correlated (correlation coefficient 0.234) [15, 18, 24]. Patients overall rated a higher level of SDM than physicians did. Physicians do not seem to have an accurate sense of how involved their patients felt, although in this case the physicians underestimated their success in sharing the clinical decision. After logistic regression, shared decision making was the only factor that was significantly correlated with reduced decisional conflict. This concept clearly must become a focus of clinical consultation to improve patient experience. Physicians should examine critically their technique for presenting management options, when equivocal, to involve the patients in deciding how to manage their care.

A novel finding in our study is that the presence of trainees in the consultation appeared to decrease the degree of decisional conflict experienced by patients. The presence of a trainee may remind the consultant to use non-medicalized language, or result in additional repetition of information if the trainee discusses management options prior to the consultant entering the room. Further

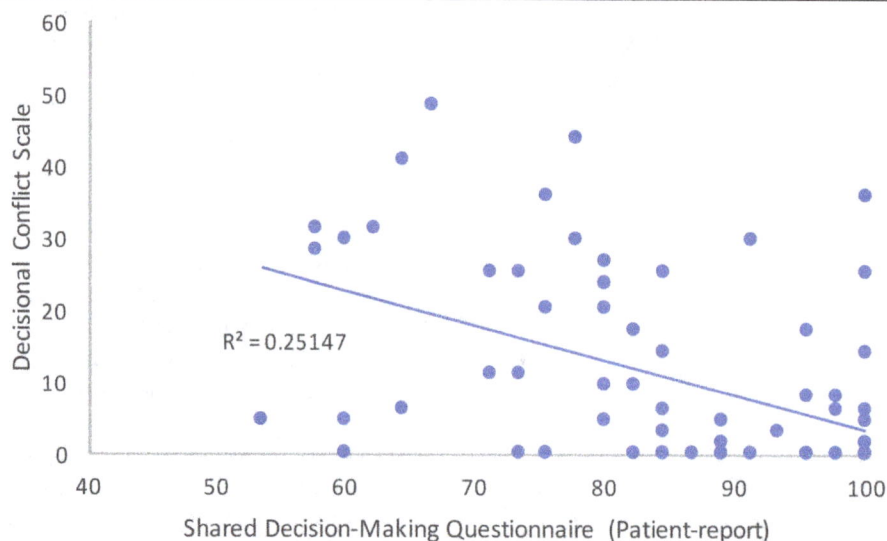

Fig. 4 Scatter plot of the correlation between SDM-Q-9 and DCS. The R^2 value is shown, correlation coefficient is − 0.539

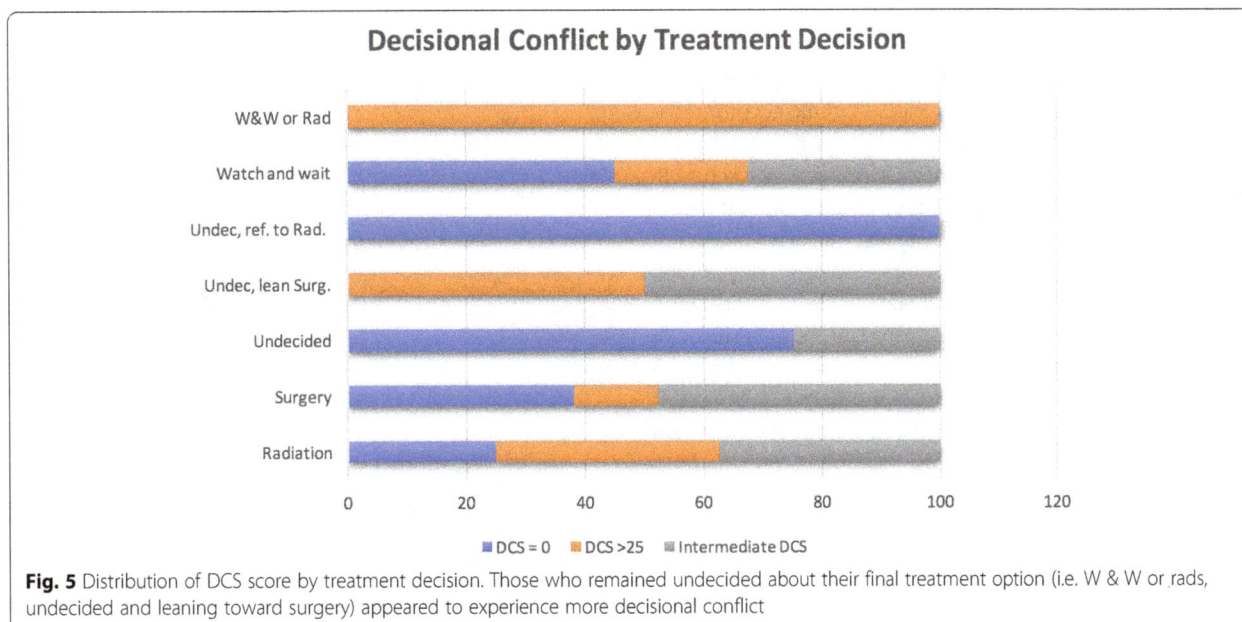

Fig. 5 Distribution of DCS score by treatment decision. Those who remained undecided about their final treatment option (i.e. W & W or rads, undecided and leaning toward surgery) appeared to experience more decisional conflict

study may be required to elucidate the mechanism of reduced DCS.

Comparison to other studies

Data on decisional conflict and shared decision making in patients with otolaryngology disorders is limited [15, 17, 18]. These, and studies in other surgical decision-making contexts have shown that patients experience significant decisional conflict when deciding between surgical and non-surgical treatment for various conditions [16]. For instance, almost one fifth of parents considering elective pediatric surgery for their child experienced a critical level of decisional conflict, with a DCS score greater than the predefined cutoff of 25 [15]. Decisional conflict was significantly correlated with parental perception of SDM, with patients feeling more involved in the surgical decision experiencing significantly less decisional conflict. In parents specifically considering bone anchored hearing devices for their child with aural atresia, over 40% reported experiencing significant decisional conflict [18]. This has also been shown in pediatric urology, with nearly a third of parents considering hypospadias repair for their child experiencing decisional conflict [16]. The proportion of patients with significant decisional conflict in the current study compares with data on pediatric patients undergoing elective procedures [15] but is less than adult patients considering thyroidectomy for indeterminate nodules, (34%) [17], or pediatric patients considering bone anchored hearing aids (43.5%) [18] or otoplasty (32.8%) [25]. The degree of conflict experienced by patients appears to vary considerably depending on the condition and ramifications of surgery.

Although research is increasingly showing that shared decision making is crucial in improving care, there are significant barriers to its implementation, both on the side of the healthcare provider and the patient. A systematic review by Legare et al. suggests that time constraints in a busy clinical practice remain the most frequent barrier to SDM cited by physicians [26]. Research does not presently exist showing that increasing SDM increases time of clinical encounters, however, so this may be a misconception. Physicians also may assume, at times based on socioeconomic status or other demographic factors, that patients may not desire involvement in the process of decision making [26]. Given we did not find that there was a difference in SDM or DCS based on these demographic factors, our study would strongly suggest providers not make such assumptions.

Patient identified barriers to shared decision making include inadequate provision of information to patients to allow them to make informed decisions [27]. Decision-aids are being developed in multiple areas to assist with this barrier, but improving information delivery in isolation is not enough. Other barriers identified include lack of patient knowledge that they may and should be involved in decisions regarding their care. This perception that the "doctor knows best", and the power imbalance perceived in the doctor-patient relationship may preclude patients from participating in decisions, thinking inclusion of their values is not needed or appropriate. In vestibular schwannoma management, the neurotologist must empower the patient to be a participant in the decision-making process, giving them "permission to participate", rather than just providing information.

Study strengths and limitations

There are limitations to this study. The inclusion of two sites may have resulted in differing patient experiences by geographic location given differences in clinic accommodation of patients with VS. Additionally, we did not have a standardized script delivered by each provider at each visit, meaning the information presented to each patient might vary. However, this is more in keeping with what occurs in clinical practice: each patient requires directed consultation based on their presentation, and standardizing information delivery would be likely to falsely estimate the prevalence of decisional conflict in these patients. Nonetheless, the DCS scores between these two sites were not found to be significantly different in our analysis. Alternatively, the inclusion of two sites would increase the likelihood our findings could be generalizable to other skull base clinics. Most patients decided on a watch and wait approach; this may bias the degree of decisional conflict present in patients as well.

In future studies, it would be useful to follow these patients longitudinally, to determine if decisional conflict is related to the degree of decisional regret associated with decisions patients make, as seen in some previous studies [16, 22, 25].

Conclusions

Approximately one in five patients with vestibular schwannoma experience significant decisional conflict. Increasing the degree to which the patient is involved in the decision-making process, through shared decision-making, may decrease the difficulty patients have and improve their experience in managing this potentially debilitating condition.

Abbreviations

DCS: Decisional conflict scale; SDM: Shared decision making; SDM-Q-10: Patient shared decision making questionnaire; SDM-Q-Doc: Physician version of the SDM-Q-10; SE: Standard error; SRS: Stereotactic radiation surgery; VS: Vestibular Schwannoma

Funding

A portion of the funding for this study was obtained through a grant from the Nova Scotia Health Authority Research Fund, and funding a research assistant for data collection and entry.

Authors' contributions

MEG conceptualized the study and the patient materials and drafted the manuscript. BDW, JL, and MB supervised the study, assisted in its conception, and provided editorial feedback. PH provided expertise on SDM/DCS surveys, performed manuscript revisions and assisted with study conception and grant approval. HF performed statistical analysis. EP and MM were responsible for Halifax site survey administration, data collection and entry, and revision of patient material. ALOH administered the survey at the Halifax site and assisted with manuscript editing. RG obtained ethical approval and administered the survey with data collection/entry at the Vancouver site. DPM and SW assisted with manuscript editing and survey administration. All authors read and approved the final manuscript.

Competing interests

The authors declare that they have no competing interests.

Author details

[1]Division of Otolaryngology – Head and Neck Surgery, Western University and London Health Sciences Centre, 5010, 800 Commissioners Road E, London, Ontario, Canada. [2]Division of Otolaryngology – Head and Neck Surgery, University of British Columbia, Vancouver, BC, Canada. [3]IWK Health Center and Division of Otolaryngology – Head and Neck Surgery, Dalhousie University, Halifax, NS, Canada. [4]Division of Neurosurgery, Dalhousie University, Halifax, NS, Canada. [5]Division of Otolaryngology, Head and Neck Surgery, Dalhousie University, Halifax, NS, Canada. [6]University of Cambridge, Cambridge, UK.

References

1. Babu R, Sharma R, Bagley JH, Hatef J, Friedman AH, Adamson C. Vestibular schwannomas in the modern era: epidemiology, treatment trends, and disparities in management. J Neurosurg. 2013;119:121–30.
2. Martin TP, Senthil L, Chavda SV, Walsh R, Irving RM. A protocol for the conservative management of vestibular schwannomas. Otol Neurotol. 2009;30:381–5.
3. Stangerup SE, Caye-Thomasen P, Tos M, Thomsen J. The natural history of vestibular schwannoma. Otol Neurotol. 2006;27:547–52.
4. Strasnick B, Glasscock ME 3rd, Haynes D, McMenomey SO, Minor LB. The natural history of untreated acoustic neuromas. Laryngoscope. 1994;104:1115–9.
5. Ansari SF, Terry C, Cohen-Gadol AA. Surgery for vestibular schwannomas: a systematic review of complications by approach. Neurosurg Focus. 2012;33:E14.
6. Vachhrajani S., Fawaz C., Mathieu D. et al. (2008) Complications of gamma knife surgery: an early report from 2 Canadian centers. J Neurosurg 109 Suppl, 2–7.
7. Carlson ML, Jacob JT, Pollock BE, et al. Long-term hearing outcomes following stereotactic radiosurgery for vestibular schwannoma: patterns of hearing loss and variables influencing audiometric decline. J Neurosurg. 2013;118:579–87.
8. Elliott A, Hebb AL, Walling S, Morris DP, Bance M. Hearing preservation in vestibular schwannoma management. Am J Otolaryngol. 2015;36:526–34.
9. Limb CJ, Long DM, Niparko JK. Acoustic neuromas after failed radiation therapy: challenges of surgical salvage. Laryngoscope. 2005;115:93–8.
10. Shamisa A., Bance M., Nag S. et al. (2013) Glioblastoma multiforme occurring in a patient treated with gamma knife surgery: case report and review of the literature. J Neurosurg 119 Suppl, 816–821.
11. Pollock BE, Link MJ, Stafford SL, Parney IF, Garces YI, Foote RL. The risk of radiation-induced tumors or malignant transformation after single-fraction intracranial radiosurgery: results based on a 25-year experience. Int J Radiat Oncol Biol Phys. 2017;97:919–23.
12. O'Connor A. (1993) User Manual - Decisional Conflict Scale.
13. Owings MF, Kozak LJ. Ambulatory and inpatient procedures in the United States, 1996. Vital Health Stat 13. 1998;139:1–119.
14. Joosten EA, DeFuentes-Merillas L, de Weert GH, Sensky T, van der Staak CP, de Jong CA. Systematic review of the effects of shared decision-making on patient satisfaction, treatment adherence and health status. Psychother Psychosom. 2008;77:219–26.
15. Chorney J, Haworth R, Graham ME, Ritchie K, Curran JA, Hong P. Understanding shared decision making in pediatric otolaryngology. Otolaryngol Head Neck Surg. 2015;152:941–7.
16. Lorenzo AJ, Braga LH, Zlateska B, et al. Analysis of decisional conflict among parents who consent to hypospadias repair: single institution prospective study of 100 couples. J Urol. 2012;188:571–5.
17. Taylor BA, Hart RD, Rigby MH, Trites J, Taylor SM, Hong P. Decisional conflict in patients considering diagnostic thyroidectomy with indeterminate fine needle aspirate cytopathology. J Otolaryngol Head Neck Surg. 2016;45:16.
18. Graham ME, Haworth R, Chorney J, Bance M, Hong P. Decisional conflict in parents considering bone-anchored hearing devices in children with unilateral aural atresia. Ann Otol Rhinol Laryngol. 2015;124:925–30.
19. Smith MY, Winkel G, Egert J, Diaz-Wionczek M, DuHamel KN. Patient-physician communication in the context of persistent pain: validation of a modified version of the patients' perceived involvement in care scale. J Pain Symptom Manag. 2006;32:71–81.
20. Scholl I, Kriston L, Dirmaier J, Buchholz A, Harter M. Development and

psychometric properties of the shared decision making questionnaire--physician version (SDM-Q-doc). Patient Educ Couns. 2012;88:284–90.

21. Carr MM, Derr JB, Karikari K. Decisional conflict and regret in parents whose children undergo tonsillectomy. Otolaryngol Head Neck Surg. 2016;155:863–8.

22. Ritchie KC, Chorney J, Hong P. Parents' decisional conflict, self-determination and emotional experiences in pediatric otolaryngology: a prospective descriptive-comparative study. Int J Pediatr Otorhinolaryngol. 2016;86:114–7.

23. Jacob A, Robinson LL Jr, Bortman JS, Yu L, Dodson EE, Welling DB. Nerve of origin, tumor size, hearing preservation, and facial nerve outcomes in 359 vestibular schwannoma resections at a tertiary care academic center. Laryngoscope. 2007;117:2087–92.

24. Hong P, Maguire E, Gorodzinsky AY, Curran JA, Ritchie K, Chorney J. Shared decision-making in pediatric otolaryngology: parent, physician and observational perspectives. Int J Pediatr Otorhinolaryngol. 2016;87:39–43.

25. Hong P, Gorodzinsky AY, Taylor BA, Chorney JM. Parental decision making in pediatric otoplasty: the role of shared decision making in parental decisional conflict and decisional regret. Laryngoscope. 2016;126(Suppl 5):S5–S13.

26. Legare F, Ratte S, Gravel K, Graham ID. Barriers and facilitators to implementing shared decision-making in clinical practice: update of a systematic review of health professionals' perceptions. Patient Educ Couns. 2008;73:526–35.

27. Joseph-Williams N, Elwyn G, Edwards A. Knowledge is not power for patients: a systematic review and thematic synthesis of patient-reported barriers and facilitators to shared decision making. Patient Educ Couns. 2014;94:291–309.

22

Mortality risk after clinical management of recurrent and metastatic adenoid cystic carcinoma

Melody J. Xu[1], Tara J. Wu[2], Annemieke van Zante[3], Ivan H. El-Sayed[4], Alain P. Algazi[5], William R. Ryan[4], Patrick K. Ha[4] and Sue S. Yom[1,4]*

Abstract

Background: Management of locoregional recurrence (LRR) and distant metastasis (DM) in adenoid cystic carcinoma (ACC) is guided by limited data. We investigated mortality risks in patients diagnosed and treated for recurrent ACC.

Methods: A retrospective review of ACC patients treated from 1989 to 2016 identified 36 patients with LRR or DM. High-risk disease was defined as skull base involvement (for LRR) or International Registry of Lung Metastases Group III/IV or extrapulmonary site of metastasis (for DM). Kaplan-Meier method, log-rank tests, and Cox proportional hazards were used for time-to-event analysis.

Results: Among 20 LRR and 16 DM patients, the median times to recurrence were 51 and 50 months, respectively. The median follow-up post-recurrence was 37.5 months (interquartile range (IQR)16.5–56.5). Post-recurrence 3-year overall survival (OS) was 78.5%, 73.3% for LRR and 85.1% for DM ($p = 0.62$). High-risk recurrences were associated with worse 3-year OS (68.8% for high-risk and 92.3% for low-risk, $\chi 2 = 10.4$, $p = 0.001$).
Among LRR patients, 90% had surgery as part of their treatment. Multimodality therapy, age, and histopathologic features (size, margins, solid histology, lymphovascular or perineural invasion) were not associated with PFS or OS. High-risk LRR was the only variable associated with OS ($\chi 2 = 5.9$, $p = 0.01$).
Among DM patients, six were initially managed with observation and ten received surgery, RT, or systemic therapy. Upfront therapy was not associated with improved PFS or OS. High-risk DM was the only variable associated with OS ($\chi 2 = 4.7$, $p = 0.03$).

Conclusions: High-risk LRR and DM were associated with decreased 3-year OS. More effective therapies are needed for high-risk ACC recurrences.

Keywords: Adenoid cystic carcinoma, Recurrence, Skull base, Lung metastases, Survival

Background

Adenoid cystic carcinoma (ACC) is an uncommon secretory gland malignancy arising from a variety of head and neck sites, including major and minor salivary glands, palate, maxilla, and trachea [1, 2]. Localized presentations of ACC are managed with surgery with or without postoperative radiation therapy (PORT) to improve local control [1–5].

The locoregional recurrence (LRR) rate is approximately 40% at 5 years, with T4 stage, nodal involvement, solid histology, perineural invasion (PNI) and positive surgical margins considered to be negative prognostic factors [6–10]. Lymph node metastases are uncommon [7, 11]. Distant metastases (DM) eventually occur in as many as 40% of patients, with the lung being the most common site of metastasis [1, 2, 8, 12]. While DM of ACC are traditionally thought to have indolent growth, reports suggest that solid histology, size greater than 3 cm, positive surgical margins, and presence of nodal

---

* Correspondence: Sue.Yom@ucsf.edu
[1]Department of Radiation Oncology, University of California San Francisco, San Francisco, CA, USA
[4]Division of Head and Neck Oncologic Surgery, Department of Otolaryngology-Head and Neck Surgery, University of California San Francisco, San Francisco, CA, USA
Full list of author information is available at the end of the article

involvement are associated with a more aggressive disease course [2, 13].

Limited data is available to guide management of LRR and DM. Metastasectomy of pulmonary metastases has been proposed, with promising results in patients with good performance status, young age, and long disease-free interval (DFI) prior to DM [14–18]. Systemic therapy outcomes have been reported in less than 500 patients over 20 years of publications but none have become a dominant standard of care; investigation of more effective therapeutics is needed [19].

To our knowledge, there are no reports focused on analyzing outcomes from local therapies such as surgery and/or radiation for recurrent and metastatic ACC patients. We therefore conducted a retrospective review to describe the LRR and DM management and outcomes of recurrent ACC treated at our institution.

Methods
Patient selection
We identified 85 patients with pathology-confirmed diagnosis of ACC treated at our center from 1989 to 2016 who had undergone surgical excision with or without PORT for initial treatment, and who had greater than six months of follow-up after initial treatment. Within this cohort of patients, we identified 36 patients (42.4%) who experienced LRR or DM.

Definition of variables
LRR was defined as recurrence at the initial site, immediately adjacent area, or regional draining nodal basin. DM was defined by radiographic findings consistent with metastatic disease and was confirmed with biopsy whenever possible. One patient had an orbital LRR and small lung DM diagnosed simultaneously and was treated aggressively at the orbit; this patient was categorized as having LRR as the primary first event after definitive treatment. Pathology reports were used to identify histologic subtype (e.g. tubular, cribriform, solid, etc.), margin status, PNI, and lymphovascular space invasion (LVSI).

High-risk LRR was defined as being at the skull base. High-risk DM was classified as International Registry of Lung Metastases (IRLM) Group III or IV (resectable but with DFI < 36 months and multiple metastases, or unresectable) or extrapulmonary site of metastasis. Older age was defined as age greater than the sample median of 63 years.

For the purposes of this report, follow-up time, progression-free survival (PFS), and overall survival (OS) were calculated from time of recurrence diagnosis. PFS was defined as progression of the initially recurrent tumor or development of new LRR or DM after treatment. PFS was censored at date of death or last follow-up and OS was censored at date of last follow-up in clinic or last known date of contact.

Statistical analysis
STATA (13th Edition, StataCorp, College Station, TX) was used for statistical analyses. Wilcoxon rank-sum tests were used for comparison of continuous variable distribution between LRR and DM recurrence types and Fisher's exact tests were used for comparison of categorical variable distribution between LRR and DM recurrence types. Kaplan-Meier method, log-rank tests, and Cox proportional hazards models were used for time-to-event analysis.

Results
Recurrence characteristics
Of the 36 identified patients with ACC recurrence, 20 (55.6%) had LRR and 16 (44.4%) had DM. Table 1 shows patient characteristics of this cohort, and Table 2 describes the treatment characteristics and outcome among patients who experienced LRR and DM. The median age at diagnosis for LRR or DM was 63.5 years (range, 30–85). Thirty-four patients (94%) had pathologic confirmation of LRR or DM. The other two patients had evident radiographic disease progression in the lung and cavernous sinus. On histopathologic review of recurrences, PNI was present in 11 recurrences (30.6%) and LVSI was present in four recurrences (11.1%). Histologic subtype was identified in 16 recurrences, with six of them (37.5%) having some solid component in the recurrent specimen.

Overall outcomes
After recurrence (LRR or DM) diagnosis, the median follow-up time was 37.5 months (interquartile range (IQR), 16.5–56.5). The overall 3-year PFS after diagnosis of recurrence was 71.7%; it was 82.1% for patients with LRR and 61.2% for patients with DM ($\chi2 = 2.36$, $p = 0.12$). Overall 3-year OS was 78.5%; it was 73.3% for patients with LRR and 85.1% for patients with DM ($\chi2 = 0.24$, $p = 0.62$).

High-risk recurrence (skull base LRR, IRLM Group III/IV lung DM, or extrapulmonary DM) was associated with worse OS, but not with worse PFS, although it should be noted that the absolute 3-year PFS difference between high- and low-risk groups was nearly 35%. The 3-year OS was 92.3% for low-risk and 68.8% for high-risk patients ($\chi2 = 10.4$, $p = 0.001$, Fig. 1a). The 3-year PFS was 90.0% for low-risk and 55.2% for high-risk patients ($\chi2 = 2.36$, $p = 0.12$).

Management strategies for Locoregional recurrence
After initial treatment for ACC, the median time to development of LRR was 51 months (IQR, 15–108). Six

Table 1 Characteristics of patients experiencing locoregional recurrence (LRR) or distant metastasis (DM) as first adenoid cystic carcinoma recurrence

	Overall	LRR	DM	p value
Characteristic	36	20	16	
Ethnicity				
White (incl. Hispanic)	25 (69.4%)	10 (50.0%)	15 (93.8%)	0.02
Asian/Pacific-Islander	8 (22.2%)	7 (35.0%)	1 (6.3%)	
African-American	1 (2.8%)	1 (5.0%)	0	
Other	2 (5.6%)	2 (10.0%)	0	
Female	24 (66.7%)	13 (65.0%)	11 (68.8%)	0.55
Male	12 (33.3%)	7 (35.0%)	5 (31.3%)	
Initial Stage				0.38
I-II	5 (22.7%)	1 (12.5%)	4 (28.6%)	
III-IV	15 (77.3%)	7 (87.5%)	10 (71.4%)	
Unknown	14	12	2	
Initial Treatment				
Surgery	7 (19.4%)	6 (30.0%)	1 (6.3%)	0.08
Surgery + PORT	29 (80.6%)	14 (70.0%)	15 (93.8%)	
Age at recurrence, Median (IQR)	64 (44–74)	66 (47–76)	60 (42–70)	0.48
Months to recurrence after initial treatment, Median (IQR)	50 (16–88)	51 (15–108)	50 (18–77)	0.58
Low-risk	14 (38.9%)	9 (45.0%)	5 (31.3%)	0.31
High-risk	22 (61.1%)	11 (55.0%)	11 (68.8%)	

IQR interquartile range, *RT* radiation therapy, *PORT* post-operative radiation therapy

Table 2 Treatment characteristics and outcomes of patients experiencing locoregional recurrence (LRR) or distant metastasis (DM) as first recurrence of adenoid cystic carcinoma

	LRR (n = 20)	p value	DM (n = 16)	p value
Treatment				
Surgery	10		5	
Surgery + PORT	8		0	
RT alone	1		4	
CF-RT	1		0	
SBRT	0		2	
Palliative RT	0		2	
Systemic therapy alone	1		1	
Observation	0		6	
3-year PFS	82.1%		61.2%	
3-year PFS				
Low-risk	100%	0.15	80.0%	0.48
High-risk	64.3%		44.4%	
3-year OS	73.3%		85.1%	
3-year OS				
Low-risk	87.5%	0.01	100%	0.03
High-risk	62.3%		76.2%	

CF-RT conventionally fractionated radiation therapy, *RT* radiation therapy, *PFS* progression-free survival, *PORT* post-operative radiation therapy, *OS* overall survival

of these 20 LRR patients were initially treated with surgery alone and 14 patients initially received surgery with PORT. Only eight patients had detailed pathologic information from their primary surgical resection, but all eight had positive margins and PNI, while six had pathologic T4 disease and one patient had > 30% solid histology.

Histopathologic evaluation of LRR after surgical resection of the recurrence was performed for 17 patients and found a median size of 3.0 cm (IQR, 1–3.5), 11 patients with positive margins, 11 with PNI, two with LVSI, and four with solid component. Eleven patients (55%) had high-risk LRR involving the skull base. Treatments for LRR consisted of surgery with PORT in 10 patients (50%), surgery only in eight patients (40%), high-dose radiation only in one patient (5%) and systemic therapy only in one patient (5%). Of the 10 patients receiving PORT, only five received standard-course fractionated external beam radiation; the remaining five received stereotactic radiosurgery (SRS), stereotactic body radiotherapy (SBRT), intra-operative radiation, or external beam radiation using altered fractionation. One patient who received surgery and PORT also received adjuvant chemotherapy. There was no clear association between high-risk LRR and delivery of multimodality therapy although a trend to improved outcome was likely limited by sample size ($\chi2 = 2.55$, $p = 0.11$).

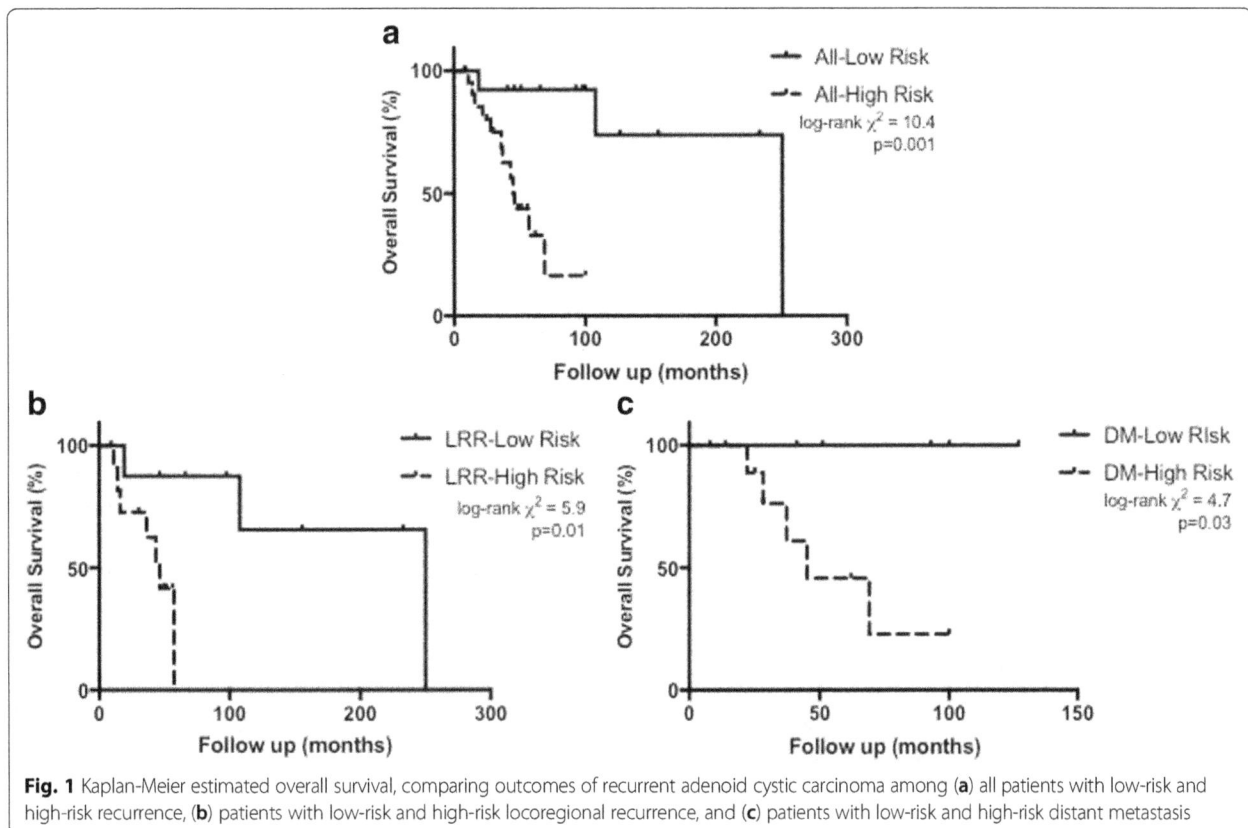

Fig. 1 Kaplan-Meier estimated overall survival, comparing outcomes of recurrent adenoid cystic carcinoma among (**a**) all patients with low-risk and high-risk recurrence, (**b**) patients with low-risk and high-risk locoregional recurrence, and (**c**) patients with low-risk and high-risk distant metastasis

The median follow-up time after LRR diagnosis was 38 months (IQR, 11.5–53.5), with three patients developing re-progression after their treatment for LRR. One patient had a parotid ACC that was re-excised at first recurrence, recurred seven years later, and was re-excised with PORT. Despite durable local control of over 13 years at the parotid, this patient eventually developed lung, spleen, kidney, and soft tissue metastases. One patient had a maxillary ACC initially treated with surgery and PORT, who recurred locally and underwent repeat surgical excision three times in two years before succumbing to recurrent skull base disease. The third patient had a hard palate ACC initially treated with surgery and PORT who developed a pterygopalatine fossa recurrence involving V1 and V2 nerves and was treated with surgery and SBRT, but eventually developed re-progression of local disease and was started on a systemic therapy clinical trial. Lung DM was found concurrently in one patient and was diagnosed eight months after treatment of LRR in a second patient.

Multimodality therapy was not found to be associated with PFS or OS outcomes. We therefore investigated whether older age, size of recurrence, positive margins at time of LRR resection, histopathologic factors of the primary or at the time of recurrence (solid histology, LVSI, PNI), or high-risk LRR were associated with PFS or OS. The only factor associated with PFS was size of recurrence < 3 cm (log rank $\chi2 = 5.0$, $p = 0.03$); Cox proportional hazards ratios could not be calculated due to too few progression events. High-risk LRR was the only variable with OS. The 3-year OS was 87.5% for low-risk and 62.3% for high-risk patients (log-rank $\chi2 = 5.9$, $p = 0.01$, Cox HR 10.1, 95%CI 1.1–90.0, $p = 0.038$, Fig. 1b). The 3-year PFS was 100% for low-risk and 64.3% for high-risk patients ($\chi2 = 2.1$, $p = 0.15$).

Management strategies for metastatic disease

After initial treatment for ACC, the median time to development of DM was 50 months (IQR, 18–77). The initial pathology of the 16 patients with DM was reviewed and two (12.5%) had positive nodes, eight (50.0%) were pT3 or pT4, six (37.5%) had ≥30% solid histological component, and 13 (81.3%) had close or positive margins. Of the 9 patients with core biopsies or surgical specimens of DM available for in-depth pathologic analysis, 2 had solid component subtypes, 0 had PNI, 2 had LVSI, and 1 had a positive margin.

Fourteen patients (87.5%) had recurrent lung metastases, nine of which were classified as IRLM Group III/IV. Other observed sites of metastases included bone, central nervous system, and subcutaneous tissue. In total, 11 patients (68.8%) were considered to have high-risk DM with IRLM Group III/IV or non-lung metastases.

Six patients with small-volume bilateral lung disease were initially managed with observation. Four eventually received treatment with surgery (1), radiation (1), chemotherapy (1), or were enrolled in a clinical trial (1). Of these patients initially deemed safe for initial management by observation, the median OS after recurrence diagnosis was 65.5 months (IQR, 28–100).

Among 10 DM patients receiving upfront treatment, five (50%) received surgery, two (20%) received SBRT, two received systemic therapy only (20%) and one received palliative radiation therapy (10%). The seven patients treated with upfront surgery or non-palliative radiation had a median survival of 45 months (IQR, 28–93) and four were disease-free for the remainder of their follow-up, which ranged from 25 to 51 months.

Upfront treatment with surgery or non-palliative radiation therapy was not found to be associated with PFS or OS. We therefore investigated whether older age, size of dominant DM, positive margins at time of DM resection, histopathologic factors of the primary or at the time of metastasis (solid histology, LVSI, PNI), or high-risk DM were associated with PFS or OS. We found no significant association between pre-treatment or treatment-related factors with PFS. High-risk DM was the only variable significantly associated with OS. The 3-year OS was 100% for low-risk patients compared to 76.2% for high-risk patients (log-rank $\chi2 = 4.7$, $p = 0.03$, Fig. 1c). Cox proportional hazard ratios could not be calculated as no patients with low-risk DM died during the follow-up period (median 37.5 months, IQR 22–64). The 3-year PFS was 80.0% for low-risk and 44.4% for high-risk patients ($\chi2 = 0.51$, $p = 0.48$).

Discussion

Limited data is available to guide the clinical management of locally recurrent or metastatic ACC. We therefore analyzed 36 consecutive cases of recurrent ACC at a single tertiary care institution to describe treatment outcomes and prognostic variables. In LRR, the most common treatments were surgery with or without PORT; high-risk disease at the skull base was often aggressively treated in an attempt to maintain local control. In DM, lung metastases were the most common sites of disease managed with observation, surgery, or SBRT, depending on resectability, bilaterality, and whether the metastases were singular or multiple in number. While no treatment paradigms or histopathologic factors were identified as prognostic for PFS or OS after recurrence, stratifying patients by high- and low-risk classifications found that a high-risk pattern of disease recurrence was associated with significantly decreased survival. Based on our institutional practices, we propose risk-stratified treatment considerations in Fig. 2.

In our study population, the median time to first recurrence (whether LRR or DM) was approximately 50 months from initial treatment. After a recurrence diagnosis, we observed a 3-year OS of 79% overall, with LRR patients having lower Kaplan-Meier estimates of OS (73%) compared to DM patients (85%). Although not significantly different, these findings indicate that the time to LRR is comparable to that of DM with an equally decreased or potentially worse subsequent survival outcome. Our findings are in keeping with observations from large retrospective reviews indicating that local recurrence is a critical issue associated with cause-

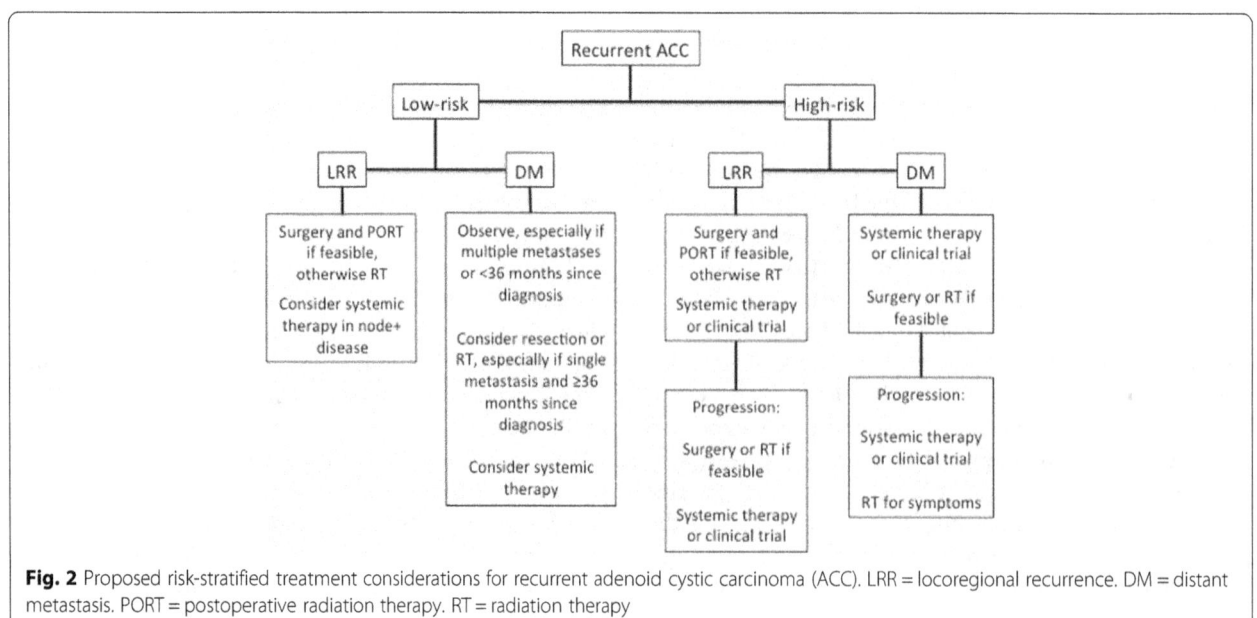

Fig. 2 Proposed risk-stratified treatment considerations for recurrent adenoid cystic carcinoma (ACC). LRR = locoregional recurrence. DM = distant metastasis. PORT = postoperative radiation therapy. RT = radiation therapy

specific survival. [10, 20]. Yet, whereas many studies have sought to define survival prognostics related to DM [2, 13, 21–23], very little literature exists to describe survival prognostics or management strategies for LRR.

At our institution, LRR was often treated in an aggressive and multimodal fashion (Fig. 2) with 90% of patients receiving resection and 50% of patients receiving PORT. Due to the use of prior full-course radiation, only five patients were able to receive fully fractionated PORT. The other five were re-irradiated using extremely conformal techniques such as SRS, SBRT, or intraoperative radiotherapy. We found that traditional prognostic variables such as age, histology, margin status, LVSI, and PNI were not associated with PFS or OS (size < 3 cm was associated with worse PFS on log-rank testing, but there were too few progression events to determine whether this was a real effect in Cox proportional hazards modeling). However, due to our small sample size and unavailable pathologic information on six specimens, we could not entirely rule out the prognostic value of traditional pathologic characteristics. The only prognostic factor we were able to detect was based on worse survival in LRR from high-risk recurrent disease involving the skull base. While this finding may support an approach of treating skull base LRR early and aggressively, it should be noted that progressive local and metastatic disease continued despite our efforts to maximize local control in these patients. There is an urgent need for more effective combinatorial and systemic therapies to enhance the principal strategy of surgical resection.

Although the patients with DM in this cohort had heterogeneous treatments ranging from observation to metastasectomies to chemotherapy, the observed outcomes remained consistent with those reported in literature. The majority of patients with DM (80%) had lung metastases [1, 2, 8, 12]. Many with low-volume lung disease were initially managed with observation and these carefully selected patients did not have significantly poorer outcomes compared to upfront surgery or non-palliative radiation [15, 24]. Of patients who received metastasectomies or non-palliative radiation, 4 of 7 (57%) enjoyed disease-free intervals of 2–4 years.

We confirmed that patients with extrapulmonary [12, 21] or IRLM Group III/IV lung metastases [18] constitute a high-risk group with significantly worse OS outcomes. The inverse was also true, as we found that the low-risk group was associated with a good prognosis with no deaths observed in the follow-up period.

When managing lung metastases, our institution considers resectability, number of metastases, bilaterality, and pace of disease (Fig. 2). In patients with Group III or IV lung metastases (high-risk DM), we favor starting with systemic therapy with limited resection or radiation if safe and feasible, or for palliation. In patients with Group I low-risk DM (resectable, DFI ≥36 months, and single metastasis), we consider this to represent oligometastatic disease and favor early metastasis-directed therapy with resection or radiation. In Group II low-risk DM (resectable, DFI < 36 months or multiple metastases), we favor observation with ascertainment of disease stability before deciding upon a course of further observation, resection/radiation, or initiation of systemic therapy. This is supported by our findings that initial observation for low-volume bilateral lung disease did not have significantly poorer outcomes compared to upfront treatment.

Overall, in the two cohorts of patients experiencing LRR and DM, an initial recurrence with high-risk disease was highly associated with OS ($p = 0.001$). Therefore, for patients with skull base recurrences, extrapulmonary metastases, or multiple lung metastases that develop within 36 months of initial treatment, better prognostic markers and effective treatments are urgently needed.

Our study is limited by small sample size, heterogeneous treatment paradigms, and selection bias as a tertiary care institution. To maximize completeness of the analysis, we restricted our population to a cohort of patients whose recurrences were treated and followed at our institution, but this may have introduced biases related to the patient population and/or our treatment policies. Some patients did not have full pathologic characteristics available at time of recurrence. Slides from the initial surgical specimen may not always be available, as recurrences at our institution are often diagnosed by fine needle aspiration (thereby limiting pathologic analysis of PNI and LVSI) and/or are treated with non-surgical approaches (thereby limiting available tissue for pathologic analysis). Where possible, we maximized the pathologic information available to us, but further studies incorporating full pathologic review and confirmation of these findings would be useful.

Conclusion

Recurrences, both local and distant, can be life-limiting in patients with ACC. At our institution, LRR is commonly managed with surgical excision and PORT. Metastases are managed heterogeneously with observation, metastasectomy, radiation, or systemic therapy depending on number, bilaterality, and resectability. We developed a set of criteria designating high-risk disease (skull base recurrence, extrapulmonary metastases, and IRLM Group III/IV lung metastases), which were significantly prognostic of OS; enhanced treatments are needed for these patients. Additional studies are needed to validate these findings and identify better prognostic markers and therapeutics.

Abbreviations

ACC: Adenoid Cystic Carcinoma; DFI: Disease-free interval; DM: Distant metastases; IQR: Interquartile range; IRLM: International Registry of Lung Metastases; LRR: Locoregional recurrence; LVSI: Lymphovascular space invasion; OS: Overall survival; PFS: Progression-free survival; PNI: Perineural invasion; PORT: Postoperative radiation therapy; SBRT: Stereotactic body radiotherapy; SRS: Stereotactic radiosurgery

Funding

This study was supported by the National Institute of Dental & Craniofacial Research, National Institutes of Health (NIH), through Grant Number R01DE023227–02 (P.K.H.). Administrative support from the Lu Family Salivary Gland Cancer Research Fund and the Etter Family Radiation Oncology Database and Analysis Fund (S.S.Y.).

Authors' contributions

MJX, TJW, PKH, and SSY: conception and design, data interpretation. MJX, TJW, AvZ, PKH: data acquisition. MJX, TJW, AvZ, IHE, APA, WRR, PKH, SSY: manuscript drafting and revision. MJX, TJW, AvZ, IHE, APA, WRR, PKH, SSY: manuscript approval.

Competing interests

IHE is a consultant for Stryker Corporation. WRR is a consultant for Ziteo and on the Head and Neck Advisory Board for Medtronic. PKH is a consultant for Bristol-Myers Squibb. SSY receives research support from Genentech, Merck and Bristol-Myers Squibb. All other authors report no conflicts of interest.

Author details

[1]Department of Radiation Oncology, University of California San Francisco, San Francisco, CA, USA. [2]Department of Head and Neck Surgery, University of California Los Angeles, Los Angeles, CA, USA. [3]Department of Pathology, University of California San Francisco, San Francisco, CA, USA. [4]Division of Head and Neck Oncologic Surgery, Department of Otolaryngology-Head and Neck Surgery, University of California San Francisco, San Francisco, CA, USA. [5]Department of Medicine, University of California San Francisco, San Francisco, CA, USA.

References

1. Coca-Pelaz A, Rodrigo JP, Bradley PJ, Vander Poorten V, Triantafyllou A, Hunt JL, et al. Adenoid cystic carcinoma of the head and neck–An update. Oral Oncol. 2015;51(7):652–61.
2. Dillon PM, Chakraborty S, Moskaluk CA, Joshi PJ, Thomas CY. Adenoid cystic carcinoma: a review of recent advances, molecular targets, and clinical trials. Head Neck. 2016;38(4):620–7.
3. Mendenhall WM, Morris CG, Amdur RJ, Werning JW, Hinerman RW, Villaret DB. Radiotherapy alone or combined with surgery for adenoid cystic carcinoma of the head and neck. Head Neck. 2004;26(2):154–62.
4. Silverman DA, Carlson TP, Khuntia D, Bergstrom RT, Saxton J, Esclamado RM. Role for postoperative radiation therapy in adenoid cystic carcinoma of the head and neck. Laryngoscope. 2004;114(7):1194–9.
5. Balamucki CJ, Amdur RJ, Werning JW, Vaysberg M, Morris CG, Kirwan JM, Mendenhall WM. Adenoid cystic carcinoma of the head and neck. Am J Otolaryngol. 2012;33(5):510–8.
6. Chen AM, Bucci MK, Weinberg V, Garcia J, Quivey JM, Schechter NR, et al. Adenoid cystic carcinoma of the head and neck treated by surgery with or without postoperative radiation therapy: prognostic features of recurrence. Int J Radiat Oncol Biol Phys. 2006;66(1):152–9.
7. He S, Li P, Zhong Q, Hou L, Yu Z, Huang Z, et al. Clinicopathologic and prognostic factors in adenoid cystic carcinoma of head and neck minor salivary glands: a clinical analysis of 130 cases. Am J Otolaryngol. 2016;38(2): 157–62.
8. Kokemueller H, Eckardt A, Brachvogel P, Hausamen JE. Adenoid cystic carcinoma of the head and neck–a 20 years experience. Int J Oral Maxillofac Surg. 2004;33(1):25–31.
9. Ju J, Li Y, Chai J, Ma C, Ni Q, Shen Z, et al. The role of perineural invasion on head and neck adenoid cystic carcinoma prognosis: a systematic review and meta-analysis. Oral Surg Oral Med Oral Pathol Oral Radiol. 2016;122(6): 691–701.
10. van Weert S, Bloemena E, van der Waal I, de Bree R, Rietveld DH, Kuik JD, Leemans CR. Adenoid cystic carcinoma of the head and neck: a single-center analysis of 105 consecutive cases over a 30-year period. Oral Oncol. 2013;49(8):824–9.
11. International head and neck scientific group. Cervical lymph node metastasis in adenoid cystic carcinoma of the sinonasal tract, nasopharynx, lacrimal glands and external auditory canal: a collective international review. J Laryngol Otol. 2016;130(12):1093–7.
12. van der Wal JE, Becking AG, Snow GB, van der Waal I. Distant metastases of adenoid cystic carcinoma of the salivary glands and the value of diagnostic examinations during follow-up. Head Neck. 2002;24(8):779–83.
13. van Weert S, Reinhard R, Bloemena E, Buter J, Witte BI, Vergeer MR, Leemans CR. Differences in patterns of survival in metastatic adenoid cystic carcinoma of the head and neck. Head Neck. 2017;39(3):456–63.
14. Locati LD, Guzzo M, Bossi P, Massone PP, Conti B, Fumagalli E, et al. Lung metastasectomy in adenoid cystic carcinoma (ACC) of salivary gland. Oral Oncol. 2005;41(9):890–4.
15. Spiro RH. Distant metastasis in adenoid cystic carcinoma of salivary origin. Am J Surg. 1997;174(5):495–8.
16. Syed IM, Howard DJ. Should we treat lung metastases from adenoid cystic carcinoma of the head and neck in asymptomatic patients? Ear Nose Throat J. 2009;88(6):969–73.
17. Yotsukura M, Kinoshita T, Kohno M, Asakura K, Kamiyama I, Emoto K, et al. Survival predictors after resection of lung metastases of head or neck cancers. Thorac Cancer. 2015;6(5):579–83.
18. Girelli L, Locati L, Galeone C, Scanagatta P, Duranti L, Licitra L, Pastorino U. Lung metastasectomy in adenoid cystic cancer: is it worth it? Oral Oncol. 2016;65:114–8.
19. Laurie SA, Ho AL, Fury MG, Sherman E, Pfister DG. Systemic therapy in the management of metastatic or locally recurrent adenoid cystic carcinoma of the salivary glands: a systematic review. Lancet Oncol. 2011;12(8):815–24.
20. Zhang CY, Xia RH, Han J, Wang BS, Tian WD, Zhong LP, et al. Adenoid cystic carcinoma of the head and neck: clinicopathologic analysis of 218 cases in a Chinese population. Oral Surg Oral Med Oral Pathol Oral Radiol. 2013; 115(3):368–75.
21. Sung MW, Kim KH, Kim JW, Min YG, Seong WJ, Roh JL, et al. Clinicopathologic predictors and impact of distant metastasis from adenoid cystic carcinoma of the head and neck. Arch Otolaryngol Head Neck Surg. 2003;129(11):1193–7.
22. Sur RK, Donde B, Levin V, Pacella J, Kotzen J, Cooper K, Hale M. Adenoid cystic carcinoma of the salivary glands: a review of 10 years. Laryngoscope. 1997;107(9):1276–80.
23. Gao MW, Hao Y, Huang MX, Ma DQ, Luo HY, Gao Y, et al. Clinicopathological study of distant metastases of salivary adenoid cystic carcinoma. Int J Oral Maxillofac Surg. 2013;42(8):923–8.
24. Bobbio A, Copelli C, Ampollini L, Bianchi B, Carbognani P, Bettati S, et al. Lung metastasis resection of adenoid cystic carcinoma of salivary glands. Eur J Cardiothorac Surg. 2008;33(5):790–3.

23

A systematic approach to the recurrent laryngeal nerve dissection at the cricothyroid junction

Oleksandr Butskiy[1,2]* (iD), Brent A. Chang[1], Kimberly Luu[1], Robert M. McKenzie[1] and Donald W. Anderson[1]

Abstract

Background: To describe and evaluate a four step systematic approach to dissecting the recurrent laryngeal nerve (RLN) starting at the cricothyroid junction during thyroid surgery (subsequently referred to as the retrograde medial approach).

Methods: All thyroidectomies completed by the senior author between August 2014 and January 2016 were retrospectively reviewed. Patients were excluded if concurrent lateral or central neck dissection was performed. A follow up period of 1 year was included.

Results: Surgical photographs and illustrations demonstrate the four steps in the retrograde medial approach to dissection of the RLN in thyroid surgery.

Three hundred forty-two consecutive thyroid surgeries were performed in 17 months, including 213 hemithyroidectomies, 91 total thyroidectomies, and 38 completion thyroidectomies. The rate of temporary and permanent hypocalcemia was 13% (95% confidence interval [CI]: 8–20%) and 3% (95% CI: 1–8%) respectively. The rate of temporary and permanent vocal cord palsy was 9% (95% CI: 6–12%) and 0.3% (95%CI: 0.01–2%) respectively. The median surgical times for hemithyroidectomy, total thyroidectomy, and completion thyroidectomy were 39 min (Interquartile range [IQR]: 33–47 min), 48 min (IQR: 40–60 min), and 40 min (IQR: 35–51 min) respectively. 1% of cases required conversion to an alternative surgical approach.

Conclusion: In a tertiary endocrine head and neck practice, the routine use of the retrograde medial approach to RLN dissection is safe and results in a short operative time, and a low conversion rate to other RLN dissection approaches.

Keywords: Surgical technique, Thyroidectomy, Recurrent laryngeal nerve, Retrograde dissection, Surgical anatomy

Background

Thyroid surgeries are the most frequent operations performed by head and neck surgeons in the United States [1]. 2015 American Thyroid Association Guidelines recommend "Visual identification of the recurrent laryngeal [RLN] during dissection in all cases" on moderate-quality evidence [2]. Three approaches to RLN identification have been described: lateral approach, inferior approach, and the superior approach [3].

The lateral approach is routinely used by most surgeons for uncomplicated thyroid surgery and was

advocated since the time of Theodor Kocher (Fig. 1) [4]. In this approach the thyroid lobe is retracted medially, middle thyroid vein is divided, and the RLN is identified at the mid-polar level.

For revision cases and for goiter surgery, the inferior approach is often used. In this approach the RLN is found in the soft areolar tissue in the tracheoesophageal groove proximal to the inferior thyroid artery crossing point. One advantage of this technique is that the RLN is found proximally prior to extra-laryngeal branching and away from thyroid bed scarring that might have been caused by prior surgery [3].

The superior Superior approach is the least used approach. In this approach, the RLN is identified as it enters under the inferior constrictor muscle proximal to

* Correspondence: butskiy.alex@gmail.com
[1]Division of Otolaryngology – Head & Neck Surgery, University of British Columbia, Vancouver, BC, Canada
[2]Gordon & Leslie Diamond Health Care Centre, 4th. Fl. 4299B-2775 Laurel Street, Vancouver, BC V5Z 1M9, Canada

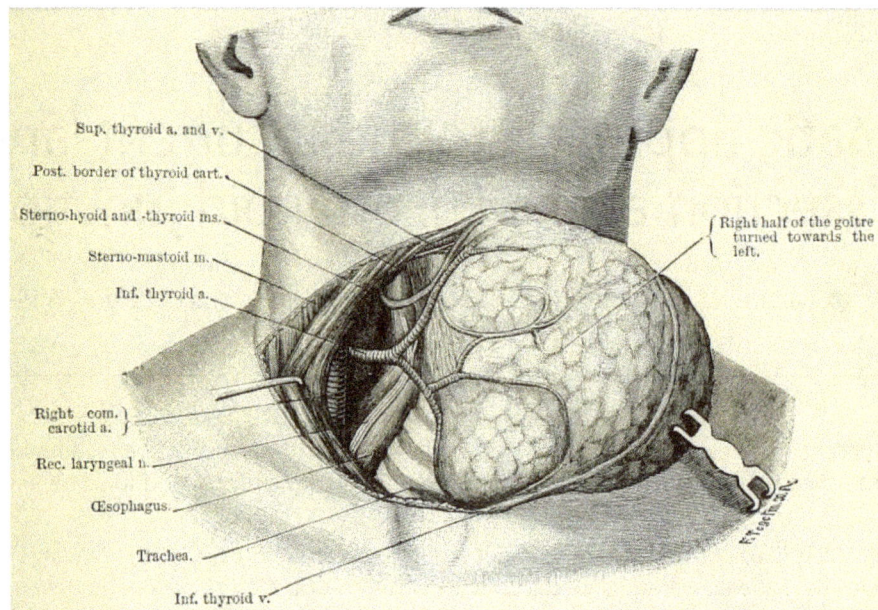

Fig. 1 Illustration to Theodor Kocher's 1895 surgical textbook demonstrating the dissection in the tracheo-esophageal groove after the thyroid is swept medially [4]

the cricothyroid junction [3]. This approach is advantageous as the RLN position relative to the cricothyroid junction is consistent regardless of thyroid pathology and congenital variations [5–8].

The surgical technique for the superior approach has not been described in sufficient detail and its outcomes have not been documented well in literature. Only three studies report on the routine use of the superior approach: one study used a single sentence to describe the surgical technique [9], and the authors of the other two studies followed a technique that appears to be a modification of the lateral approach [6, 10]. In this technique the thyroid is retracted medially, and the RLN is found by searching between Zukerkandl's tubercle and the cricopharyngeus muscle [6]. Thus, the RLN is not found right at the cricothyroid junction. While a method of identifying the RLN at the cricothyroid junction is likely known to experienced thyroid surgeons, this method has not been described in detail nor evaluated previously in literature.

The main objective of this study was to describe a four step standardized surgical technique to identifying the RLN at the cricothyroid junction (subsequently referred to as the retrograde medial approach). The primary outcome of interest was the rate of surgical complications (temporary and permanent hypocalcemia and vocal cord palsy). The secondary outcomes were surgical time and conversion rate to other techniques.

Methods

The University of British Columbia (UBC) Research Ethics Board granted approval (H15–01667) for the study.

STROBE Statement for cohort studies was followed in reporting the study [11]. Study was designed as a retrospective review of a cohort of consecutive thyroidectomy patients. All eligible patients were referred to a tertiary head and neck surgical practice affiliated with the University of British Columbia (UBC) for consideration of a thyroidectomy.

All thyroidectomies were performed at teaching hospitals where residents assumed increasing responsibility to complete the procedure as their experience developed. The operations were performed between August 2014 and January 2016.

Participants

All patients who underwent a hemi-, total, or completion thyroidectomy between August 2014 and January 2016 were selected. To obtain an estimate of the surgical time attributed solely to thyroid dissection, patients were excluded if concurrent lateral or central neck dissection was performed. Pre-operatively all patient underwent visual examination of the larynx, but PTH, Calcium and Vitamin D levels were not routinely measured.

Post-operative care

After hemithyroidectomy, all patients were observed for 4 hours and were discharged home barring complications. Completion thyroidectomy and total thyroidectomy patients were admitted overnight and their ionized calcium level was checked in the morning. Patients were discharged if the ionized calcium level was above

1.00 mmol/L. Routine calcium/vitamin D supplementation and surgical drains were not used.

Follow-up

Post-operative follow-up consisted of an office visit 2 weeks after the operation or earlier on patient request. Post-operative larynx visualization was performed only if patients described voice or swallowing abnormalities on specific questioning. If any abnormality was detected on the first post-operative visit, such as hypocalcemia or vocal cord palsy, the patients were followed monthly for up to a year or until the abnormality resolved.

Data collection, variables and data sources

Four co-investigators (OB, BAC, RMM, and KL) collected data retrospectively from August 2016 to May 2017. Patient demographic and surgical indications data was obtained from clinic notes. Procedures performed, surgical times, and admission duration data were obtained from hospital records. Surgical time was defined as the time from first incision to wound closure completion as documented by the nursing staff.Operative dictations were used to establish if conversion to an alternative RLN dissection technique occurred. Pathological diagnoses and thyroid weights were determined reviewing the final pathology reports.

Data on the following complications were extracted from hospital and clinic records: temporary and permanent hypocalcemia and vocal cord palsy, hematoma, seroma, wound infection, and subcutaneous emphysema. Superior laryngeal neve palsy was not looked for during the follow up visit unless deemed necessary. Temporary hypocalcemia was defined as any hypocalcemia requiring calcium or vitamin D supplementation within 6 months of surgery. Permanent hypocalcemia was defined as any hypocalcemia requiring supplementation for greater than

6 months after surgery. Temporary vocal cord palsy was defined as the loss of true vocal cord adduction lasting less than 6 months of surgery, after which the palsy was deemed permanent. Hematoma was defined as any bleeding requiring reoperation or drain placement. In addition, the provincial health care database was screened for post-operative complications related hospital visits that might not have been captured in clinic charts. Patients with missing data were included in the study.

Surgical technique

Skin incision, elevation of subplatysmal flaps, separation of strap muscles, and release of the sternothyroid muscles to expose the thyroid gland were performed in the usual manner. Unless invaded by the tumor, sternothyroid muscles were not cut. All vessel ligation was performed with Adson insulated bipolar forceps (Kirwan Surgical Products, Marshfield, MA) without routine use of suture ties or surgical clips. RLN monitor was not used. The next four steps are critical to the described technique.

1. Isolation and division of the isthmus:

The thyroid isthmus is isolated and divided over the trachea using bipolar cautery.

2. Subtotal division of Berry's suspensory ligaments and exposure of the cricothyroid region (Fig. 2):

The divided edge of the isthmus is grasped with Babcock clamps and retracted laterally (Fig. 2a). Inferior to the first tracheal ring, Berry's suspensory ligaments are divided to separate the thyroid away from the trachea (Fig. 2b). Retraction of the trachea toward the contralateral side

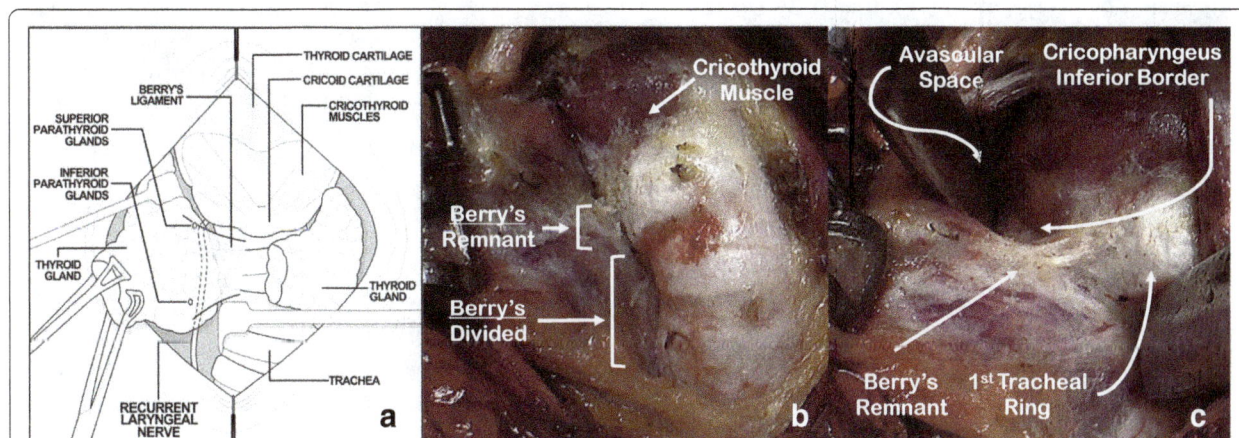

Fig. 2 Subtotal division of Berry's suspensory ligaments and exposure of the cricothyroid region. **a** Schematic demonstrating anatomy and instrument orientation; **b** Subtotal division of Berry's ligaments; **c** Placing Berry's ligament remnant on the stretch with avascular space open

facilitates performance of this step. Care is taken to dissect directly on the trachea, as the RLN will be protected by a layer of fascia and ligamentous tissue. Lateral to the first tracheal ring the full thickness of Berry's suspensory ligament is left intact (Fig. 2c).

The avascular space between the superior pole and the cricothyroid muscle is developed avoiding damage to the superior laryngeal nerve and the cricothyroid muscle (Fig. 2c). Differential traction between the superior pole and the trachea (demonstrated by the Langenbeck retractors in Fig. 2a & c) is critical for exposure and identification of the anatomical structures. Bowstring tension promotes isolation and identification of the Berry's ligament remnant. Subsequent to injury-free identification of the cricothyroid muscle, care is then taken to expose the inferior border of the cricopharyngeus muscle, a critical landmark for RLN identification (Fig. 2c).

3. Identification and dissection of the recurrent laryngeal nerve (Fig. 3):

At this point, the remnant of the Berry's ligament tethers the thyroid to the superior portion of the first tracheal ring and protects the RLN from the stretch of the retractors (Fig. 3a). Deep to the remnant are the RLN and the inferior thyroid artery terminal branches. The RLN runs in a plane posterior to Berry's ligaments and then turns medially to enter the larynx at the superior aspect of the ligamentous tissue, forming an anatomical 'genu' [8]. Careful dissection through the superior portion of this ligamentous tissue using a fine mosquito forceps and bipolar cautery allows identification of the RLN insertion under the inferior constrictor (Fig. 2b). Inferior border of the cricopharyngeus muscle is visualized at all times and serves as a landmark for the depth at which the RLN is found. Dissection is facilitated by

judicious and careful control of the inferior thyroid artery terminal branches to avoid bleeding that can make RLN visualization difficult. We use bipolar cautery to control the terminal branches, with tips cooled with a wet gauze between applications. As the remnant of the Berry's ligament is transected, the retraction is reduced to avoid stretch injury to the RLN. Once the RLN branches are identified, they are traced inferiorly by dividing the remainder of the Berry's suspensory ligament and releasing the RLN from the thyroid gland. The maximum extent of RLN dissection is 1 to 2 cm (Fig. 3c).

4. Capsular dissection with preservation of parathyroid tissue and ligation of superior pole vessels (Fig. 4):

The thyroid gland is then swept medially, delivered through the wound, and retracted in an anterosuperior direction (Fig 4a). With the RLN in direct view, a capsular dissection is undertaken from inferior to superior direction. Elevation of the gland assists in exposure and isolation of the blood vessels feeding the parathyroid glands, helping their preservation under direct visualization (Fig. 4a).

The thyroid lobe remains pedicled on the superior pole vessels (Fig. 4b). Gentle retraction of the lobe inferiorly allows for their ligation and division, releasing the thyroid from the wound (Fig. 4c). Hemostasis is achieved and multi-layered closure is performed in the usual fashion.

Results

Three hundred sixty-seven operations were eligible for inclusion. Twenty-five operations were excluded as either a central or a lateral neck dissection was performed concurrently. Out of 342 surgeries included in the analysis, 213 (62%) were hemi-, 91 (27%) were total, and 38

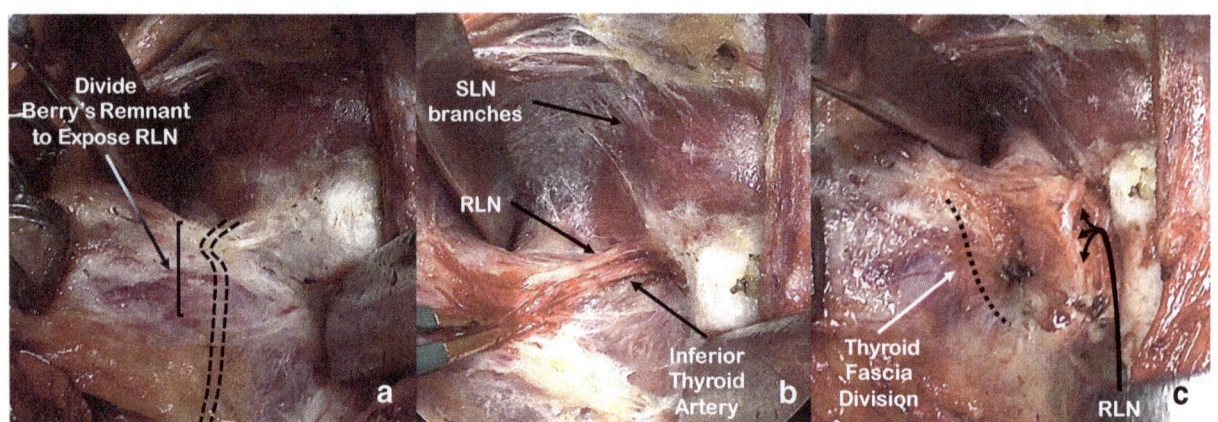

Fig. 3 Identification and dissection of the recurrent laryngeal nerve (RLN). **a** RLN path deep to the Berry's ligament remnant; **b** Berry's ligament remnant dissected to reveal the RLN and the terminal branch of the inferior thyroid artery (nerve is placed on retraction to demonstrate anatomy to the photographer); **c** Thyroid fascia divided. Superior Laryngeal Nerve (SLN)

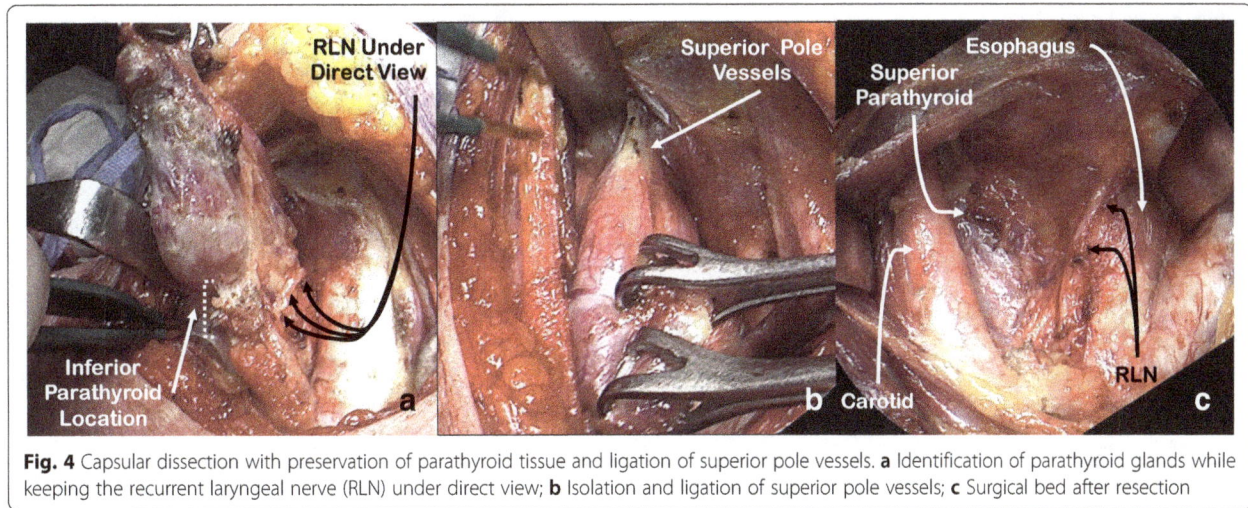

Fig. 4 Capsular dissection with preservation of parathyroid tissue and ligation of superior pole vessels. **a** Identification of parathyroid glands while keeping the recurrent laryngeal nerve (RLN) under direct view; **b** Isolation and ligation of superior pole vessels; **c** Surgical bed after resection

(11%) were completion thyroidectomies. The mean age of the patients was 50 years (range: 13–89 years), and 84% of patients were female.

The most common indications for a total thyroidectomy were papillary thyroid carcinoma (40%) and thyromegaly (27%) (Table 1). The most common indications for a hemithyroidectomy were nodules of intermediate suspicion for malignancy (54%) and thyromegaly (38%) (Table 1).

The final pathology results showed a variety of benign and malignant conditions (Table 2). The median surgical times for a total, hemi-, and completion thyroidectomy were 48 min (Interquartile range [IQR]: 40–60 min),

39 min (IQR: 33–47 min) and 40 min (IQR: 35–51 min) respectively (Table 3).

Complications experienced by the patients are summarized in Table 4. Out of 129 patients who underwent total or completion thyroidectomy, 17 (13%; 95% confidence interval [CI]: 8–20%) experienced transient and 4 (3%; 95% CI:1–8%) experienced permanent hypocalcemia. Out of 342 patients, 30 (9%; 95% CI: 6–12%) experienced temporary (i.e. 7% of nerves at risk), and 1 experienced permanent vocal cord palsy (0.3%; 95%CI: 0.01–2%). There were no instances of bilateral vocal cord palsy. It was unclear what caused the majority of temporary vocal cord palsies. In a minority of cases of

Table 1 Indications for surgery

	Total thyroidectomy n = 91	Hemi-thyroidectomy n = 213	Completion thyroidectomy n = 38	Total n = 342
Nodules requiring diagnosis				
Intermediate suspicion for malignancy	–	114 (54%)	2 (5%)	116 (34%)
High suspicion for malignancy	15 (16%)	2 (1%)	1 (3%)	18 (5%)
Thyromegaly				
Obstructive/Symptomatic	20 (22%)	73 (34%)	6 (16%)	99 (29%)
Substernal goiter	5 (5%)	8 (4%)	–	14 (4%)
Malignancy				
Papillary carcinoma	36 (40%)	2 (1%)	17 (45%)	55 (16%)
Follicular carcinoma	–	–	8 (21%)	8 (2%)
Poorly differentiated carcinoma	–	–	1 (3%)	1 (0.3%)
Lymphoma	–	–	1 (3%)	1 (0.3%)
Endocrinological diseases				
Graves' disease	13 (14%)	1 (0.5%)	1 (3%)	15 (4%)
Hashimoto thyroiditis	1 (1%)	2 (1%)	–	3 (1%)
Other				
Symptomatic cyst	–	9 (4%)	–	9 (3%)
PET incidentaloma	1 (1%)	2 (1%)	–	3 (1%)

Table 2 Pathological diagnoses

	Total thyroidectomy (n = 91)	Hemi-thyroidectomy (n = 213)	Completion thyroidectomy (n = 38)	Total (n = 342)
Malignancies				
Papillary	50 (54%)	22 (10%)	12 (32%)	84 (25%)
Follicular	1 (1%)	11 (5%)	2 (5%)	14 (4%)
Poorly differentiated	1 (1%)	1 (0.5%)	–	2 (1%)
B-Cell lymphoma	–	1 (0.5%)	–	1 (0.3%)
Renal cell carcinoma	1 (1%)	–	–	1 (0.3%)
Goiters				
Multinodular goiter	16 (18%)	73 (34%)	9 (24%)	98 (29%)
Diffuse goiter	1 (1%)	5 (2%)	1 (3%)	7 (2%)
Endocrine diseases				
Graves' disease	8 (9%)	1 (0.5%)	–	9 (3%)
Hashimoto's thyroiditis	7 (8%)	10 (5%)	1 (3%)	18 (5%)
Other benign pathology				
Follicular adenoma	4 (4%)	65 (31%)	1 (3%)	70 (20%)
Thyroid cyst	–	5 (2%)	–	5 (2%)
Not otherwise specified	2 (2%)	19 (9%)	12 (32%)	33 (10%)

temporary vocal cord palsy, the dictating surgeon commented on the difficulty due to inflammation and bleeding. In the single instance of permanent vocal cord paralysis, a RLN nerve branch was cut.

In 3 patients (1%) a conversion to an alternative method of RLN dissection was needed, this was due to difficulty in controlling bleeding (2 cases) and dense scarring superior to Berry's ligament (1 case).

Discussion

In this study we introduce a systematic approach to dissecting the RLN at the cricothyroid junction, referred to here as the retrograde medial approach. The outcomes of this approach were investigated through a retrospective review of a single surgeon's cohort of patients. The rates of transient and permanent vocal cord palsy were 9% (95% CI: 6–12%) and 0.3% (95%CI: 0.01–2%) respectively, while the rates of transient and permanent hypocalcemia were

13% (95% CI: 8–20%) and 3% (95% CI: 1–8%) respectively. The retrograde medial approach appears to be fast, with a median surgical time of 41 min.

Three previous studies have described using the superior approach to finding the RLN. While the authors of one study do not describe the specific technique [9], the authors of the other two studies followed the technique first described by Shindo et al [6, 10]. This technique involves releasing the superior pole, finding and releasing the tubercle of Zuckerkandl, retracting the gland medially, and then searching for the RLN as it courses towards the cricothyroid junction. Shindo et al. acknowledged the variability in the angle that the RLN takes as it approaches the cricothyroid junction and classified it into four categories. The authors also acknowledged that their technique is difficult in cases of nonrecurrent RLN, presence of large tubercle of Zuckerkandl, and extrathyroidal extension of cancer along the distal RLN segment.

Table 3 Surgical times

	Total thyroidectomy Median (IQR)	Hemi-thyroidectomy Median (IQR)	Completion thyroidectomy Median (IQR)	Total Median (IQR)
All indications	48 min (40–60 min)	39 min (33–47 min)	40 min (25–93 min)	41 min (35–51 min)
Nodules requiring diagnosis	42 min (39–50 min)	38 min (32–44 min)	29 min (27–56 min)	39 min (32–45 min)
Thyromegaly				
Obstructive/Symptomatic	57 min (47–66 min)	41 min (35–50 min)	41 min (33–54 min)	44 min (37–53 min)
Substernal goiter	84 min (50–98 min)	60 min (52–65 min)	93 min	64 min (51–81 min)
Malignancy	47 min (40–53 min)	51 min (45–55 min)	39 min (36–46 min)	43 min (38–51 min)
Graves' disease	55 min (43–63 min)	60 min	67 min	56 min (43–65 min)

Abbreviations: IQR interquartile range, min minutes

Table 4 Course in hospital and complications

	Total thyroidectomy n = 91	Hemi–thyroidectomy n = 213	Completion thyroidectomy n = 38	Total n = 342
Nights in hospital – median (Range)	1 (0–30)	0 (0–3)	1 (1–7)	1 (0 – 30)
Conversion to alternative approach – n (%)	2 (2%)	–	1 (3%)	3 (1%)
Complications – n (%)				
Transient hypocalcemia	16 (18%)	–	1 (3%)	17 (5%)
Permanent hypocalcemia	1 (1%)	–	2 (5%)	3 (1%)
Temporary vocal cord paresis/Paralysis	13 (14%)	14 (7%)	3 (8%)	30 (9%)
Permanent vocal cord paresis/Paralysis	1 (1%)	–	–	1 (0.3%)
Hematoma	1 (1%)	4 (2%)	1 (3%)	6 (2%)
Seroma	–	1 (0.5%)	–	
Wound infection	5 (6%)	3 (1%)	1 (2.6%)	9 (3%)
Subcutaneous emphysema	1 (1%)	2 (1%)	–	3 (1%)

In the presented retrograde medial approach, the RLN nerve is found early prior to the release of the superior pole and exploration of the thyroid's lateral side. Given that the RLN is found superior to the Berry's ligament, the variability in the angle that RLN takes in its approach has no impact on the dissection. Furthermore, the retrograde medial approach is preferential in cases with nonrecurrent RLN, large Zuckerkandl's tubercle, and in the majority of cases with extrathyroidal extension of cancer along the distal RLN segment (with exception of cricothyroid junction involvement). We find the retrograde medial approach especially useful in cases of large goiters. Finally, an additional advantage of the retrograde medial approach is that no thyroid tissues is left unresected at the cricothyroid junction.

Some surgical situations make the use of retrograde medial approach difficult. The method relies on splitting the thyroid isthmus and identifying the inferior border of the cricopharyngeal muscle. If a surgeon is unable to complete these steps, either due to fear of tumor spillage with the isthmus division or extensive scarring, bleeding, or presence of tumor at the cricopharyngeus muscle or the cricothyroid junction, it is advisable that the lateral or inferior approach to the thyroidectomy is used.

With the use of the retrograde medial approach, the rates of permanent vocal cord palsy and hypocalcemia are similar to the rates reported with other superior approaches to finding the RLN; however, the rates of temporary vocal cord palsy and hypocalcemia appear higher. With regard to the permanent complications, in a study of 181 patients, Sykes et al. reported permanent vocal cord palsy and hypocalcemia rates of 0.4% and 2.2% respectively [10]. In a study of 67 patients, Veyseller et al. reported the corresponding rates to be 0 [9].

With regard to the transient complications, Sykes et al. reported a 2.2% rate of temporary vocal cord palsy [10]; whereas Veyseller et al. reported temporary vocal cord palsy and hypocalcemia rates of 0% and 8.3% respectively [9].

There are a number of possible reasons to why the rates of temporary complications were higher in the presented study than in the studies discussed above. First, given different sizes and compositions of populations studied, the difference could be secondary to sampling variability. Second, the difference might be due to different definitions of temporary complications. Specifically, compared to the mentioned studies we used a more liberal definition of hypocalcemia – requirement for calcium or vitamin D supplementation regardless of the reason. Finally, the technique described in this paper could be the reason for higher temporary complication rates. For example, the exclusive use of bipolar cautery could be responsible for transient RLN and parathyroid gland heat damage. Some surgeons might also suggest that traction at the Berry's ligament transferred to the RLN might be responsible for higher transient vocal cord palsy rate. However, there is no tension on the nerve until the suspensory ligament is divided. Recognizing this is a point of importance and teaching. After division of the suspensory ligament the nerve is dissected out from top to bottom while on the slack at the fixation point at entrance to larynx.

Comparing the outcomes of the retrograde medial technique to the outcomes of the two other approaches (lateral and inferior) is difficult given that one approach is rarely used exclusively. Perhaps the best estimate of thyroidectomy complication rates comes from national studies. For example, the 2008 study of Scandinavian Quality Register for Thyroid and Parathyroid Surgery reported complication rates based on 3660 thyroidecto-mies [12]. In this report, the authors presented data on hypocalcemia defined identically to our study – the use of supplemental calcium and/or vitamin D at the first post-operative visit and 6 months after surgery. Using this definition, the rates of transient and permanent hypocalcemia in the Scandinavian study (17% and 6% respectively) appear similar to our study (13% and 3% respectively). With regard to vocal cord palsy, the authors of the Scandinavian study report temporary palsy rates lower than in our study (3.9% versus 9% respectively), but the permanent palsy rates appear similar to our study (0.9% versus 1% respectively).

With regard to surgical time, the authors of the studies described above do not report on the surgical speed. The speed of the described technique appears similar to the techniques described in recent meta-analyses and reviews of ultrasonic and electrothermal devices in thyroid surgery [13, 14]. For example, the authors of a recent meta-analysis concluded that a total thyroidectomy is performed faster with the use of Harmonic Focus® (Ethicon Inc., Cincinnati OH) than with the use of clips and ties [13]. The pooled average time for a total thyroidectomy using the Harmonic Focus® was 66 min and the average time for the conventional technique was 95 min [13]. In comparison, the average time for a total thyroidectomy in our series was 48 min.

Short operative time with the retrograde medial approach is possibly due to early RLN identification in a consistent location. The remaining dissection can then proceed quickly without concern of RLN injury. This is in contrast to the lateral approach in which complete RLN dissection is one of the last operating steps. We acknowledge that aside from the RLN dissection technique there might be other reasons for shorter operative time. These include the use of bipolar cautery in place of clips and ties and the surgical experience of the author.

The presented study has strengths. First, the described approach, while likely known to experienced thyroid surgeons, has not been previously reported in surgical literature. Second, while the presented technique is not meant to be prescriptive, prior to this study there has been no attempt to standardize identification of RLN at the cricothyroid junction. Finally, this study reports on the largest cohort of patients in literature for whom the superior approach to identifying RLN was used.

This series has limitations. First, a retrospective review might have resulted in missing data for complications. . Second, the study represents a single surgeon's experience, possibly limiting the generalizability of the findings. Finally, our study excluded patients requiring lateral and central neck dissection; therefore, further investigation is required to determine the utility of the retrograde medial approach in such cases.

Conclusion

A retrograde medial approach to identifying the RLN at the cricothyroid junction is described. This technique is useful in dissecting large goiters and when lateral RLN identification is difficult. In a tertiary endocrine head and neck practice, the routine use of the retrograde medial approach is safe and results in short operative time and a low conversion rate to other RLN dissection approaches.

Acknowledgment

We would like to thank Mr. Callum Faris for encouragement to publish the retograde medial approach and his assistance with study design.

Authors' contributions

All authors contributed to study design. All authors with exception of DWA participated in data collection. OB analyzed the data and prepared the manuscript. All other authors edited the manuscript for publication. All authors read and approved the final manuscript.

Competing interests

The authors declare that they have no competing interests.

References

1. Bhattacharyya N. The increasing workload in head and neck surgery: an epidemiologic analysis. Laryngoscope. 2011;121(1):111–5. https://doi.org/10.1002/lary.21193.
2. Haugen BR, Alexander EK, Bible KC, et al. 2015 American thyroid association management guidelines for adult patients with thyroid nodules and differentiated thyroid cancer: the American thyroid association guidelines task force on thyroid nodules and differentiated thyroid cancer. Thyroid. 2015;26(1):1–133. https://doi.org/10.1089/thy.2015.0020.
3. Richer SL, Randolph GW. Management of the recurrent laryngeal nerve in thyroid surgery. Oper Tech Otolaryngol-Head Neck Surg. 2009;20(1):29–34. https://doi.org/10.1016/j.otot.2009.02.006.
4. Kocher T, Stiles HJ. Text-book of operative surgery. London: Adam and Charles Black; 1895. http://archive.org/details/textbookofoperat00koch
5. Çakir BÖ, Ercan I, Şam B, Turgut S. Reliable surgical landmarks for the identification of the recurrent laryngeal nerve. Otolaryngol Head Neck Surg. 2006;135(2):299–302. https://doi.org/10.1016/j.otohns.2006.03.026.
6. Shindo ML, Wu JC, Park EE. Surgical anatomy of the recurrent laryngeal nerve revisited. Otolaryngol Head Neck Surg. 2005;133(4):514–9. https://doi.org/10.1016/j.otohns.2005.07.010.
7. Ardito G, Revelli L, D'Alatri L, Lerro V, Guidi ML, Ardito F. Revisited anatomy of the recurrent laryngeal nerves. Am J Surg. 2004;187(2):249–53. https://doi.org/10.1016/j.amjsurg.2003.11.001.
8. Sasou S, Nakamura S, Kurihara H. Suspensory ligament of berry: its relationship to recurrent laryngeal nerve and anatomic examination of 24 autopsies. Head Neck. 1998;20(8):695–8. https://doi.org/10.1002/(SICI)1097-0347(199812)20:8<695::AID-HED6>3.0.CO;2-3.
9. Veyseller B, Aksoy F, Y Y KA, Özturan O. EFfect of recurrent laryngeal nerve identification technique in thyroidectomy on recurrent laryngeal nerve paralysis and hypoparathyroidism. Arch Otolaryngol Neck Surg. 2011;137(9):897–900. https://doi.org/10.1001/archoto.2011.134.
10. Sykes RF, Moorthy R, Olaleye O, Black IM. Identification of the recurrent laryngeal nerve at the cricothyroid joint: our experience of 181 thyroid procedures. Clin Otolaryngol. 2014;39(3):174–7. https://doi.org/10.1111/coa.12254.
11. von Elm E, Altman DG, Egger M, et al. The Strengthening the Reporting of Observational Studies in Epidemiology (STROBE) statement: guidelines for

reporting observational studies. Ann Intern Med. 2007;147(8):573. https://doi.org/10.7326/0003-4819-147-8-200710160-00010.

12. Bergenfelz A, Jansson S, Kristoffersson A, et al. Complications to thyroid surgery: results as reported in a database from a multicenter audit comprising 3,660 patients. Langenbeck's Arch Surg. 2008;393(5):667–73. https://doi.org/10.1007/s00423-008-0366-7.

13. Cheng H, Soleas I, Ferko NC, Clymer JW, Amaral JF. A systematic review and meta-analysis of harmonic focus in thyroidectomy compared to conventional techniques. Thyroid Res. 2015;8:15. https://doi.org/10.1186/s13044-015-0027-1.

14. Butskiy O, Wiseman SM. Electrothermal bipolar vessel sealing system (LigaSure) for hemostasis during thyroid surgery: a comprehensive review. Expert Rev Med Devices. 2013;10(3):389–410. https://doi.org/10.1586/erd.13.6.

24

Management of epistaxis in patients with ventricular assist device

Clifford Scott Brown* ⓘ, Ralph Abi-Hachem and David Woojin Jang

Abstract

Background: Patients with a ventricular assist device (VAD) are at risk for epistaxis due to the need for anticoagulation. Additionally, these patients develop acquired von Willebrand syndrome (AvWS) due to these devices. Management is complicated by the risk of thrombosis if anticoagulation is reversed. This study sought to characterize the clinical features and management of epistaxis in this high-risk population.

Methods: Retrospective review of adults with VAD and epistaxis necessitating inpatient consultation with the otolaryngology service were included.

Results: 49 patients met inclusion criteria. All patients had a presumed diagnosis of AvWS. An elevated INR (> 2.0) was present in 18 patients (36.7%). Anticoagulation was held in 14 (28.6%) patients, though active correction was not necessary. Multiple encounters were required in 16 (32.7%) patients. Spontaneous epistaxis was associated with multiple encounters ($p = 0.02$). The use of hemostatic material was associated with a lower likelihood of bleeding recurrence ($p = 0.05$), whereas cauterization with silver nitrate alone was associated with a higher likelihood of re-intervention ($p = 0.05$). Surgery or embolization was not required urgently for any patient. Endoscopy under general anesthesia was performed for one patient electively. Mean follow up time was 16.6 months ($\sigma = 6.3$). At six months, 18 (36.7%) patients were deceased.

Conclusion: While these patients are at risk for recurrent spontaneous epistaxis, nonsurgical treatment without active correction of INR or AvWS was largely successful. Placement of hemostatic material, as opposed to cautery with silver nitrate, should be considered as a first-line treatment in this group. Multidisciplinary collaboration is critical for successful management.

Keywords: Epistaxis, von Willebrand syndrome, Ventricular assist device, Anticoagulation

Background

Epistaxis remains the most frequent otolaryngologic emergency and the second most common reason for referral to an otolaryngologist [1]. Over the years, many studies have sought to develop algorithms for treatment and prevention. Despite this, management of epistaxis remains a controversial and evolving topic. For example, there are no standard guidelines on duration of nasal packing and whether prophylactic antibiotics are necessary [2]. More recently, the advent of endoscopic sphenopalatine artery ligation (ESPAL) and vascular interventional procedures raises the question of when such interventions should be pursued [3].

Epistaxis in the setting of coagulopathy is difficult to manage, as patients often require management of systemic coagulopathy in addition to intranasal interventions. Regardless of whether patients are medically anticoagulated or suffer from an acquired or hereditary coagulopathy, they have longer average inpatient hospital stays and require more invasive measures of local hemorrhage control when they develop epistaxis [4]. The incidence is high, with 10–17% of patients developing epistaxis during long-term vitamin K antagonist therapy [5]. Given that there are 2.83 million quarterly

---

* Correspondence: clifford.brown@duke.edu
Division of Head and Neck Surgery & Communication Sciences, Department of Surgery, Duke University Medical Center, DUMC 3805, Durham, NC 27710, USA

visits with anticoagulation use in the United States, the at-risk population is significant [5–7].

One patient population that is especially at risk for epistaxis are those with ventricular assist devices (VAD). Patients with heart failure may receive a VAD as either a bridge to transplantation or as destination therapy. They often require multiple anti-coagulant and anti-platelet medications, with a goal international normalized ratio (INR) of 2.5 [8]. While bleeding is a major risk in these patients, sub-therapeutic levels can lead to devastating thromboembolic consequences, with a reported incidence of 2–47% [9]. Therefore, a delicate balance must be maintained. To make matters more complex, virtually all of these patients develop acquired von Willebrand syndrome (AvWS) as a result of the device itself. Patients with VAD are also poor surgical candidates due to their cardiac co-morbidities. All of the above factors create a complex situation when such a patient develops epistaxis.

Patients may develop von Willebrand disease (VWD) from a variety of etiologies, including hereditary and acquired origins. Given that VWD the most common hereditary blood-clotting disorder, its incidence is only increased by the multiple medical conditions that contribute to its development. On the most basic level, a deficiency in either the quantity or quality of von Willebrand factor (vWF) results in impaired platelet adhesion, and even in the mildest subtypes, epistaxis is a frequent symptom.

To our knowledge, this study would be the first to describe patient characteristics and management of epistaxis in this unique and complex patient population. We aimed to determine the efficacy of current treatment modalities as well as to identify risk factors for recurrence of epistaxis. Based on the findings of Smith et. Al [4], we hypothesized that patients with VAD would be more likely to require aggressive measures such as operative intervention.

Methods

This is a retrospective review of adult patients (age greater than 18 years old) with an LVAD who required inpatient consultation with the otolaryngology service at Duke University Medical Center for epistaxis between July 1, 2006 and July 1, 2016. Institutional review board approval was obtained through Duke University. Patients were identified through the Duke Enterprise Data Unified Content Explorer (DEDUCE). All patients with LVAD were initially selected based on CPT code 0048 T or ICD codes V43.21 and Z95.811. From this group, those with a documented diagnosis of epistaxis (ICD codes 784.7 or R04.0) and associated otolaryngology inpatient consultation were selected.

Electronic medical records for these patients were then reviewed. Demographic information was recorded as well as information related to the LVAD (LVAD type, date of LVAD surgery). Furthermore, anticoagulant and antiplatelet medications, as well as vital signs and lab values at the time of consultation were extracted. Epistaxis was categorized as spontaneous versus traumatic. Additionally, the bleeding location, interventions performed, outpatient follow-up after discharge, and the outcomes of each intervention were extracted.

Statistical analysis

Data were grouped categorically and analyzed with Pearson's chi-squared test. Tests of independence assessed for correlations between data points. Statistical analyses were performed with SPSS 23.0 software (SPSS Inc., Chicago, IL), with $P < 0.05$ considered significant.

Results

A total of 49 patients met the inclusion criteria, with 37 male and 12 female patients. Median age was 58 years (range: 18–85 years). The types of LVAD included 39 (79%) HeartMate II (HMII), seven HeartWare (14%), two Centimag (4%), and one VentrAssist (2%). The median time between LVAD placement and consultation for epistaxis was 46 days (range 2–2886). There were 15 (30%) patients who required consultation within 10 days of placement. Primary reasons for admission included cardiac symptoms (79.6%), epistaxis (12.2%), and other (8.2%). Forty-six patients were seen in an inpatient unit and three patients were seen in the emergency room.

Spontaneous non-traumatic bleeds occurred in 37 (75.5%) patients. The presence of spontaneous epistaxis was associated with multiple interventions (Chi-square = 5.345, p-value = 0.02). The most common site of bleeding was the anterior septum, with 31 (63.2%) patients bleeding from the unilateral septum, and 10 (20.4%) from the bilateral anterior septum (Fig. 1). Sixteen (32.7%) patients required multiple interventions from the otolaryngology service. Age, gender, and VAD type did not correlate significantly with spontaneous bleeding or the need for multiple interventions. Bleed location and the time between LVAD surgery and consultation did not correlate with spontaneous bleeding or need for multiple interventions. Mean follow-up time after initial consultation was 16.6 ($\sigma = 6.3$) months. 18 (36.7%) patients died prior to six month follow-up due to various causes, none of which were directly attributed to epistaxis. These findings are summarized in Table 1.

Each subject had an average of 1.59 ($\sigma = 1.09$) encounters. Interventions included use of oxymetazoline spray with application of direct pressure as an initial measure in all patients. Cauterization with silver nitrate was performed in 35 (71.4%) patients. The use of cautery alone was associated with a need for repeat interventions (Chi-square = 3.998, p-value 0.05). Dissolvable hemostatic material was used in 23 (46.9%) patients, with Surgicel (Ethicon, NJ, USA) used

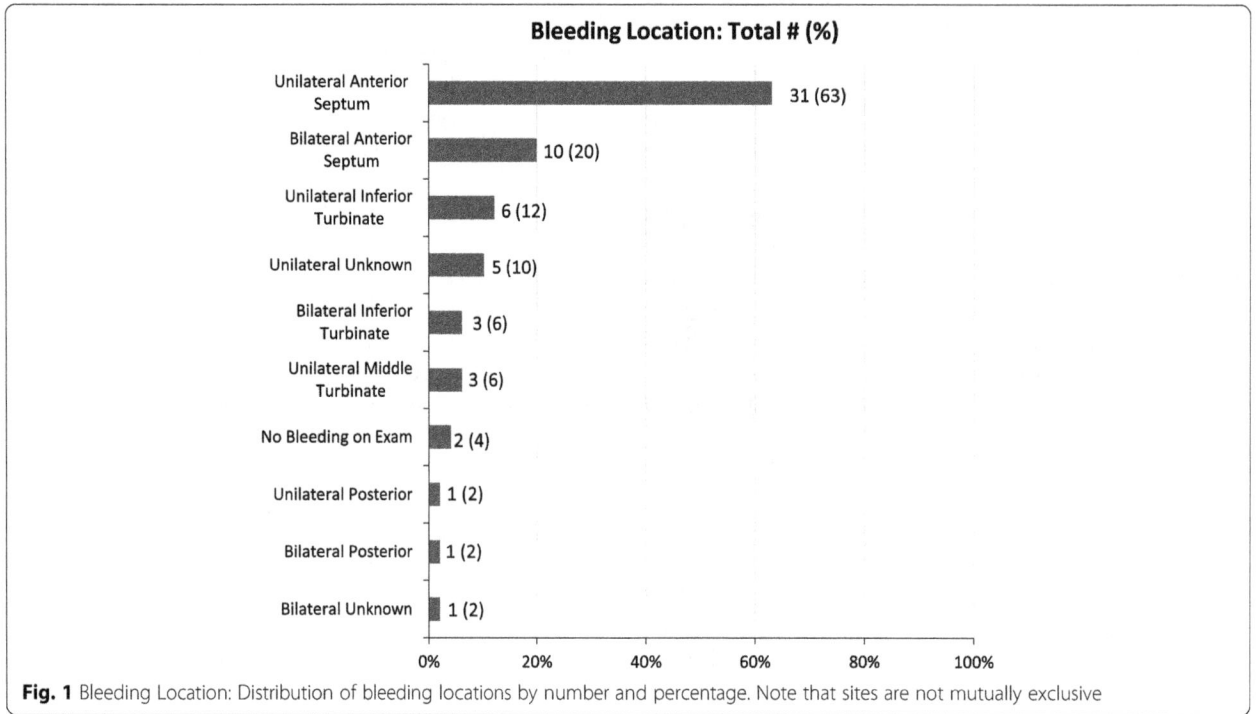

Fig. 1 Bleeding Location: Distribution of bleeding locations by number and percentage. Note that sites are not mutually exclusive

in 7 (14.3%) patients, and Nasopore (Stryker, MI, USA) used in 17 (34.7%) patients. Hemospore, which contains chitosan lactate, was not utilized. Non-dissolvable packing was used in 14 (28.6%) patients, with 8 (16.3%) patients receiving Merocel (Medtronic, MN, USA) and 7 (14.3%) receiving Rapid Rhino (ArthroCare, TX, USA). The use of dissolvable or non-dissolvable hemostatic material was associated with a lower likelihood of bleeding recurrence (Chi-square = 4.204, p-value = 0.04), however this effect was not significant when assessing either dissolvable and

non-dissolvable packing alone. Conservative, or non-surgical, therapy was successful in all patients. There was a single patient who was taken to the operating room for an elective lysis of synechiae that had resulted from prior interventions, requiring general anesthesia secondary to the amount of scarring and prior failure of bedside attempts. Dissolvable packing was placed in the nose at the conclusion of the procedure. No patient required urgent operative intervention or angiography with embolization (Fig. 2).

All patients had an a priori diagnosis of AvWS as a result of the LVAD. Thirty-four patients (69.4%) were concurrently on warfarin, but only 18 (36.7%) of these had a therapeutic INR (between 2.0 and 3.0) at the time of epistaxis and only 4 (8.2%) had a supratherapeutic INR (greater than 3.0). Twenty-one (42.9%) patients were concurrently on heparin with 12 (24.5%) of these having prolonged partial thromboplastin time (greater than 40 s). Thirty-three (67.3%) patients were taking aspirin. Anticoagulant and antiplatelet medications were held in 14 (28.6%) patients because of epistaxis. Twenty-seven (55.1%) patients had normal platelet numbers (greater than 150,000) and 7 (14.3%) patients had platelet counts less than 100,000. No patient required active correction of anticoagulation with fresh frozen plasma, vitamin K, or protamine sulfate. There was no association between spontaneous bleeding or need for multiple interventions and the PTT, INR, or platelet count.

Discussion

This study is the first to describe epistaxis management in patients with LVAD. Patients with LVAD represent a

Table 1 Patient and Epistaxis Characteristics

Sex:	VAD Type:
Male: 37 (75%)	HMII: 39 (79%)
Female: 12 (25%)	HeartWare: 7 (14%)
Total: 49	CentriMag: 2 (4%)
	VentrAssist: 1 (2%)
Reason For Admission:	Cause:
Cardiac: 39 (79%)	Spontaneous: 37 (75%)
Epistaxis: 6 (12%)	Traumatic: 12 (25%)
Other: 4 (8%)	
Location:	Recurrence:
Anterior Septum: 41 (84%)	< 7 Days: 6 (12%)
Inferior Turbinate: 9 (18%)	7–30 Days: 6 (12%)
Other: 2 (4%)	1–6 Months: 4 (8%)
	> 6 Months: 28 (57%)
	Death < 6 Months: 18 (37%)

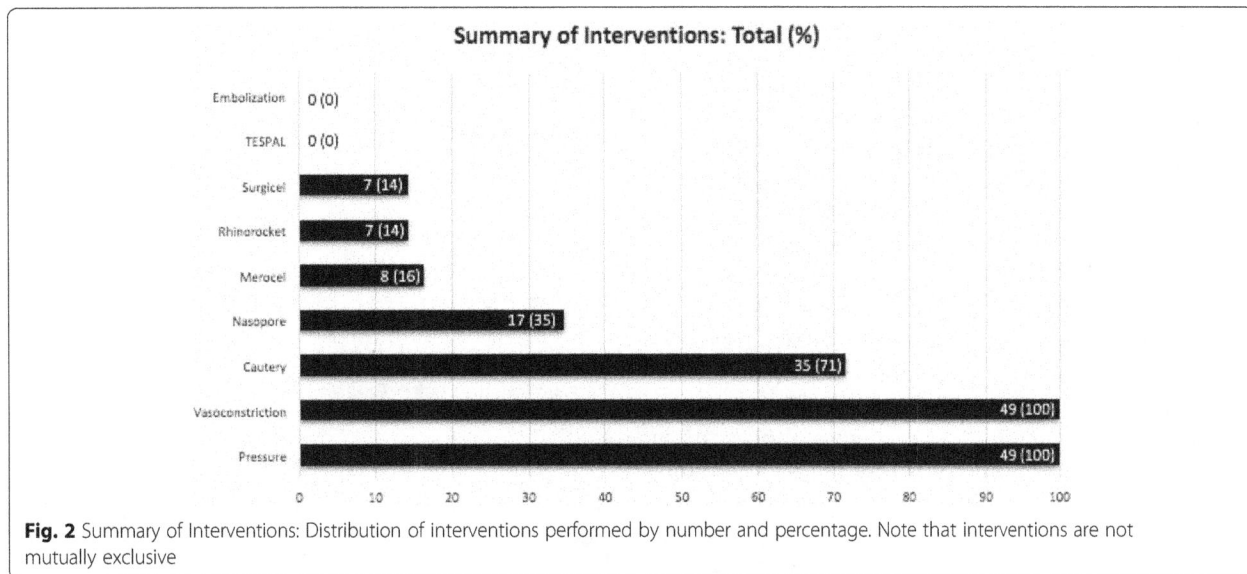

Fig. 2 Summary of Interventions: Distribution of interventions performed by number and percentage. Note that interventions are not mutually exclusive

complex patient population due to the need for continuous anticoagulation and the development of AvWS. Moreover, these patients have end-stage heart failure and are poor candidates for general anesthesia.

In several ways, our results are consistent with the existing literature. The majority (75.5%) of our patients had spontaneous, non-traumatic epistaxis. This is consistent with the findings by Parajuli [10], who noted that 80–90% of general epistaxis patients had no identifiable cause. Also, 83.6% of episodes reported in our study occurred at the anterior nasal septum. This is consistent with the distribution seen in the general population, with literature reports of 80–90% of bleeds occurring at this location [1, 11]. Moreover, the presence of spontaneous epistaxis in our patients was associated with multiple interventions ($P = 0.02$), with 32.7% requiring multiple interventions. Similarly, Anghel et. Al [1] noted that patients with an idiopathic cause had the highest rate of recurrence over two years (26%). As for interventions, local cauterization with silver nitrate was performed in the majority of LVAD patients (71.4%). However, those undergoing cauterization alone without placement of hemostatic material were likely to require additional interventions at a later date. In their systematic review, Spielmann et al. noted that cautery was typically ineffective in patients receiving antiplatelet therapy [3].

In our study, the use of hemostatic material, both absorbable and non-absorbable, was associated with a lower likelihood of bleeding recurrence. However, there was no difference in efficacy amongst the type of material placed. This is consistent with existing literature demonstrating no significant difference in efficacy of various types of nasal packing [12, 13]. Moreover, there were no adverse events related to nasal packing in our study. Based on these findings, hemostatic material should be considered

as initial management in patients with LVAD who present with epistaxis.

Recently, ESPAL has been shown to be associated with a reduction in cost and length of hospitalization in comparison to non-surgical treatment [14–17]. However, ESPAL should be considered carefully in patients with LVAD, given the high cardiac risks with general anesthesia and the bleeding risk from the surgery itself. For example, HeartMate II (HMII) devices have been associated with a significantly higher incidence of bleeding complications during surgical procedures [18]. In addition, the risk of postoperative infection is substantial in the LVAD population, as infection can seed the hardware [19]. Patients with LVAD who develop an infection have cumulative survival rates of 66.9% at 2 years compared to 81.3% for patients without an infection [20]. Although recent reviews suggest that patients with LVAD can safely undergo non-cardiac surgery [21], other studies showed that perioperative death occurred in a range of 6.4–16.7% [22]. Given these risks, surgery should be considered with caution in this patient population.

Because of the associated co-morbidities and need for anticoagulation with LVADs, a multi-disciplinary approach must be taken in management of epistaxis. In our study, holding anticoagulation was required in some patients, while it was continued in other instances. Interestingly, only 4 (8.2%) patients in this cohort had a supratherapeutic INR, and no association between spontaneous bleeding or multiple interventions with elevated INR was identified. This is consistent with the US-TRACE (STudy of Reduced Anti-Coagulation/Anti-platelEt therapy) study, which found that recurrent bleeding occurred in 52% of cases despite reduced antithrombotic therapy [23], suggesting alternative contributing factors to hemorrhagic complications.

Given the lack of association between INR and recurrent epistaxis, an important contributor may be AvWS, which results from the LVAD itself. LVADs produce continuous blood flow along an axial path using an internal rotor in the blood [24]. This results in the loss of large von Willebrand factor (vWF) multimers via a cleavage mechanism. In this situation, AvWS occurs immediately after implantation, and only resolves after device explantation [25, 26]. Serious bleeding, defined as episodes that result in death, reoperation, hospitalization, or transfusion, occurs in 19–40% of patients with the HMII, making it the most frequent complication [27], with the gastrointestinal tract and the nasal cavity being the most common sites [28]. The proteolytic mechanism that reduces VWF multimers also occurs in those with aortic valve stenosis, pancreatitis, liver cirrhosis, and leukemia [29]. According to the International Society on Thrombosis and Haemostasis, AvWS is most frequently associated with lymphoproliferative (48%), cardiovascular (21%), myeloproliferative (15%), other neoplastic (5%), and autoimmune disorders (2%) [30]. Importantly, AvWS must be distinguished from von Willebrand disease (VWD), an inherited disorder, due to different treatment approaches [31]. Diagnosis favors AvWS when patients have late onset of bleeding, typically after an uneventful surgery, along with an associated condition and a negative family history of bleeding. Desmopressin and VWF-containing concentrates are treatment options in VWD, but are ineffective in LVAD patients, with removal of the device being the only definitive treatment. Overall, AvWS is a condition that has implications beyond the LVAD population and should be recognized by otolaryngologists.

One limitation of this study is its retrospective nature. Another limitation is that we included only inpatient and emergency room consultations, which were mainly seen by residents of various training levels. Additionally, return visits to the emergency department that did not involve a consultation to otolaryngology were not included. However, we believe that our findings can be applied to care in the outpatient setting.

Conclusion

Patients with LVAD present a unique challenge in the management of their epistaxis. Based on our findings, this difficulty stems from a variety of factors, including the need for anticoagulant or antiplatelet medication, development of irreversible AvWS, and high anesthetic risk. From the otolaryngologic perspective, use of hemostatic packing should be considered as a first-line intervention. Overall, a non-surgical multidisciplinary approach was successful in managing this complex patient population.

Abbreviations

AvWS: Acquired von Willebrand syndrome; ESPAL: Endoscopic sphenopalatine artery ligation; HMII: HeartMate II; INR: International normalized ratio; PTT: Partial thromboplastin time; VAD: Ventricular assist device; VWD: Von Willebrand disease; VWF: Von Willebrand factor

Acknowledgements
not applicable.

Funding
There are no sources of funding for the research conducted in this study.

Author's contributions
CSB performed the study design, literature review, manuscript drafting and review, data analysis and interpretation, accountability for all aspects of the work.
RAH performed manuscript review, interpretation of data, accountability for all aspects of work.
DWJ oversaw the research project, was instrumental in study design, manuscript drafting and review, accountability for all aspects of the work. All authors read and approved the final manuscript.

Competing interests
The authors declare that they have no competing interests.

References

1. Anghel AG, Soreanu CC, Dumitru M, Anghel I. Treatment options for severe epistaxis, the experience of the Coltea ENT clinic. Maedica (Buchar). 2014 Jun;9(2):179–82.
2. Shrestha I, Pokharel M, Dhakal A, et al. Study of microorganism growth Patten in nasal pack of patients visiting the department of ENT, head and neck surgery. Kathmandu Univ Med J (KUMJ). 2015 Oct-Dec;13(52):303–7.
3. Spielmann PM, Barnes ML, White PS. Controversies in the specialist management of adult epistaxis: an evidence-based review. Clin Otolaryngol. 2012 Oct;37(5):382–9. Doi: 10.111/coa.12024.
4. Smith J, Kim D, Dyer C, Siddiq S. Epistaxis in patients taking oral anticoagulant and antiplatelet medication: prospective cohort study. J Laryngol Otol. 2011 Jan;125(1):38–42. https://doi.org/10.1017/S0022215110001921.
5. Rubboli A, Becattini C, Verheugt FWA. Incidence, clinical impact and risk of bleeding during oral anticoagulation therapy. World J Cardiol. 2011 Nov 26; 3(11):351–8. https://doi.org/10.4330/wjc.v3.i11.351.
6. Kirley K, Qato DM, Kornfield R, Stafford RS, Alexander GC. National trends in oral anticoagulant use in the United States, 2007 to 2011.
7. Barnes GD, Lucas E, Alexander GC, Goldberger ZD. National Trends in Ambulator Oral Anticoagulant Use. Am J Med. 2015 Dec;128(12):1300–5.e2. doi: https://doi.org/10.1016/j.amjmed.2015.05.044.
8. Rossi M, Serraina GF, Jiritano F, Renzuli A. What is the optimal anticoagulation in patients with a left ventricular assist device? Interact Cardiovasc Thorac Surg. 2012 Oct;15(4):733–40. https://doi.org/10.1093/icvts/ivs297.
9. Van den Bergh WM, Lanskin-Hartgring AO, Van Duijin AL, Engström AE, Lahpor JR, Slooter AJC. Thromboembolic stroke in patients with a HeartMate –II left ventricular assist device – the role of anticoagulation. J Cardiothorac Surg. 2015;10:128. https://doi.org/10.1186/s13019-015-0333-7.
10. Parajuli R. Evaluation of etiology and treatment methods for epistaxis: a review at a tertiary Care Hospital in Central Nepal. Int J Otolaryngol. 2015; https://doi.org/10.1155/2015/283854.
11. Rudmik L, Smith TL. Management of intractable spontaneous epistaxis. Am J Rhinol Allergy. 2012 Jan-Feb;26(1):55–60. https://doi.org/10.2500/ajra.2012.26.3696.
12. Badran K, Malik TH, Belloso A, Timms MS. Randomized controlled trial comparing Merocel and RapidRhino packing in the management of anterior epistaxis. Clin Otolaryngol. 2005 Aug;30(4):333–7.
13. Wang J, Cai C, Wang S. Merocel versus Nasopore for nasal packing: a meta-analysis of randomized controlled trials. PLoS One. 2014 Apr 7;9(4):e93959. https://doi.org/10.1371/journal.pone.0093959.
14. Moshaver A, Harris JR, Liu R, Diamond C, Seikaly H. Early operative

intervention vs. conventional treatment in epistaxis: randomized prospective trial. J Otolaryngol. 2004 Jun;33(3):185–8.

15. Zou Y, Deng YQ, Xia CW, Kong YG, Xu Y, Tao ZZ, Chen SM. Comparison of outcomes between endoscopic surgery and conventional nasal packing for epistaxis fornix of the inferior nasal meatus. Pak J Med Sci. 2015 Nov-Dec; 31(6):1361–5. Doi: https://doi.org/10.12669/pjms.316.8340.

16. Rudmik L, Leung R. Cost-effectiveness analysis of endoscopic sphenopalatine artery ligation vs arterial embolization for intractable epistaxis. JAMA Otolaryngol Head Neck Surg. 2014;140(9):802–8. https://doi. org/10.1001/jamaoto.2014.1450.

17. Liu J, Zhong G, Wang Y. A retrospective analysis of 163 cases with intractable epistaxis managed by nasal endoscopic surgery. Lin Chung Er Bi Yan Hou Tou Jing Wai Ke Za Zhi. 2013 Jun;27(11):590–2. Chinese.

18. Topkara VK, Kondareddy S, Malik F, Wang IW, Mann DL, Ewald GA, Moazami N. Infectious complications in patients with left ventricular assist device: etiology and outcomes in the continuous-flow era. Ann Thorac Surg. 2010;90:1270–7.

19. Kaplan JA. Ventricular Assist Devices, Cardiac Transplants, and Implanted Electrical Devices in Noncardiac Surgery. Chapter 45. Section 7. Kaplan's Cardiac Anesthesia: For Cardiac and Noncardiac Surgery. Seventh Edition. 2017.

20. Uriel N, et al. Acquired von Willebrand syndrome after continuous-flow mechanical device support contributes to a high prevalence of bleeding during long-term support and at the time of transplantation. J Am Coll Cardiol. 2010 Oct 5;56(15):1207–13. https://doi.org/10.1016/j.jacc.2010.05.016.

21. Nelson EW, et al. Management of LVAD patients for noncardiac surgery: a single-institution study. J Cardiothorac Vasc Anesth. 2015 Aug;29(4):898–900. https://doi.org/10.1053/j/jvca.2015.01.017.

22. Davis J, Sanford D, Schilling J, Hardi A, Colditz G. Systematic review of outcomes after noncardiac surgery in patients with implanted left ventricular assist devices. ASAIO J. 2015 Nov-Dec;61(6):648–51. https://doi. org/10.1097/MAT.0000000000000278.

23. Katz JN, Adamson RM, John R, et al. TRACE study. Safety of reduced anti-thrombotic strategies in HeartMate II patients: a one-year analysis of the US-TRACE study. J Heart Lung Transplant. 2015;34(12):1542–8.

24. Nascimbene A, Neelamegham S, Frazier OH, Moake JL, Dong JF. Acquired von Willebrand syndrome associated with left ventricular assist device. Blood. 2016 Jun 23;127(25):3133–41. https://doi.org/10.1182/blood-2015-10-636480.

25. Goda M, et al. Time course of acquire von Willebrand disease associated with two types of continuous-flow left ventricular assist devices: HeartMate II and CicuLite synergy pocket micro-pump. J Heart Lung Transplant. 2013 May;32(5):539–45. https://doi.org/10.1016/j.healun.2013.02.006.

26. Steinlechner B, et al. Platelet dysfunction in outpatients with left ventricular assist devices. Ann Thorac Surg. 2009 Jan;87(1):131–7. https://doi.org/10. 1016/j.athoracsur.2008.10.027.

27. Starling RC, Naka Y, Boyle AJ, et al. Results of the post-U.S. Food and Drug Administration-approval study with a continuous flow left ventricular assist device as a bridge to heart transplantation: a prospective study using the INTERMACS (interagency registry for mechanically assisted circulatory support). J Am Coll Cardiol. 2011;57(19):1890–8.

28. Suarez J, Patel CB, Felker GM, Becker R, Hernandez AF, Rogers JG. Mechanisms of bleeding and approach to patients with axial-flow left ventricular assist devices. Circ Heart Fail. 2011;4(6):779–84.

29. Federici AB, Berkowitz SD, Lattuada A, Mannucci PM. Degradation of von Willebrand factor in patients with acquired clinical conditions in which there is heightened proteolysis. Blood. 1993;81(3):720–5.

30. Federici AB, Rand JH, Bucciarelli P, et al. Acquired von Willebrand syndrome: data from an international registry. Thromb Haemost. 2000;84(2):345–9.

31. Tiede A, Rand JH, Federici AB, et al. How I treat the acquired von Willebrand syndrome. Blood 2011 117:6777–6785; doi: https://doi.org/10.1182/blood-2010-11-297580.

25

Improving vaccination uptake in pediatric Cochlear implant recipients

Lisa Jin[1], Paula Téllez[2], Ruth Chia[3], Daphne Lu[1], Neil K. Chadha[1,2], Julie Pauwels[2], Simon Dobson[4], Hazim Al Eid[5] and Frederick K. Kozak[1,2]* (iD)

Abstract

Background: An Infectious Disease vaccine specialist joined our institution's Cochlear Implant Team in 2010 in order to address the high percentage of non-compliance to immunization prior to surgery identified previously from an internal review. The purpose of this study was to (1) review the immunization status of cochlear implant recipients in 2010–2014, (2) assess if introducing a vaccine specialist made a significant change in vaccination compliance and (3) elucidate any barriers to vaccination compliance.

Methods: Retrospective chart review and a telephone survey. Medical records of 116 cochlear implant recipients between 2010 and 2014 were reviewed. A telephone survey was conducted to obtain the current vaccination status in children who required post-operative vaccinations with incomplete records on chart review and, if applicable, the reason for non-compliance.

Results: Between 2010 and 2014, 98% of children were up-to-date at the time of surgery, compared to 67% up-to-date at the time of surgery between 2002 and 2007. 27 children were included in our post-operative immunization analysis. 29.6% (8/27) failed to receive necessary vaccinations post-surgery. Pneumovax-23, a vaccine for high-risk patients (such as cochlear implant candidates) was missed in all cases.

Conclusion: Pre-operative vaccination for cochlear implant recipients improved dramatically with the addition of a vaccine specialist. However, a significant proportion of patients requiring vaccinations post-surgery did not receive them. The main reason for non-compliance was due to parents being unaware that their children required this vaccine postoperatively by being "high-risk".

Although improvement was demonstrated, a communication gap continued to impede the adequacy of vaccination uptake in pediatric cochlear implant recipients following surgery at age 2 when the high-risk vaccine was due.

Keywords: Cochlear implant, Meningitis, Otolaryngology, Preventative medicine, Paediatrics, Public health, Vaccination

Background

Advances in technology over the last few decades have greatly impacted patient care and quality of life; cochlear implants prove to be an excellent example. A cochlear implant (CI) is a 2-part electrode with an external microphone and an internal electrode implanted in the cochlea that provides direct electric stimulation to the auditory nerve fibers [1, 2]. CIs allow those with profound sensorineural hearing loss to appreciate hearing and to develop the ability to communicate through spoken language [1, 2]. However, as with any invasive intervention, there lies the risk of infection. Due to the close proximity of the cochlea to the brain, post-operative bacterial pneumococcal meningitis is and has been a significant concern for CI surgeons and recipients.

The incidence of *Streptococcus pneumoniae* meningitis in children with CIs has been reported to be 16 to 30 times higher than the general population due to multiple predisposing risk factors. Cochleovestibular malformation, a major risk factor for pneumococcal meningitis, is a common cause for children with sensorineural hearing loss. Electrode insertion, failure to seal the cochleostomy, and the lack of appropriate meningitis vaccines

* Correspondence: fkozak@cw.bc.ca
[1]Faculty of Medicine, University of British Columbia, 317-2194 Health Sciences Mall, Vancouver, BC V6T 1Z3, Canada
[2]Division of Pediatric Otolaryngology-Head and Neck Surgery, BC Children's Hospital, 4480 Oak St, Vancouver, BC V6H 3N1, Canada
Full list of author information is available at the end of the article

strictly for high-risk populations are additional identified risk factors [1, 3, 4]. Moreover, a much lower inoculation threshold of *S. pneumoniae* is required to induce meningitis through the cochlea compared to other means of entry [5]. Although many of these factors are beyond control, ensuring these children are properly immunized against the highly virulent *S. pneumoniae* subtypes before and after surgery is critical in harm-reduction for the CI population. Currently CI recipients in our province follow the provincial high-risk vaccination schedule for pneumococcal meningitis prevention. Under the high-risk schedule, CI patients receive 2 additional vaccines, an additional dose of 13-valent pneumococcal conjugate vaccine (PCV-13) at 6 months and the 23-valent pneumococcal polysaccharide vaccine (PPV-23) at 24 months of age, for greater protection against *S. pneumoniae*.

A previous internal review of vaccination rates in pediatric CI patients at our institution, implanted between 2002 and 2007 [unpublished], revealed that 33% of patients were not up-to-date with their meningitis vaccinations at the time of their surgery. Reported barriers to vaccination compliance included confusion from changes in provincial vaccination schedules, the language barrier associated with the province's high immigration rate, difference in vaccination requirements between provinces and lack of communication between patients' families and health providers. Recognizing that inadequate vaccination of CI patients largely stemmed from confusion and lack of communication over the high-risk schedule requirements, in 2008 the Cochlear Implant Team at our hospital partnered with a vaccine specialist to address this significant concern. As a result, a structured plan was put into place utilizing a preoperative template with both the routine and high risk vaccine

schedules clearly outlined to be confirmed by either the vaccine infectious disease specialist or the cochlear implant surgeon (Fig. 1). Any confusion surrounding the vaccine status of the patient was reviewed with the vaccine specialist. Situations where implant candidates either came from a different province or another country where in both instances vaccine schedules differ were closely reviewed and modifications made to comply with the province's standards. In order to improve the confusion and lack of adequate vaccination after the internal review, our institution created a policy that required patients to be up-to-date with their pneumococcal meningitis vaccinations prior to surgery. In some instances this may result in a delay in implantation. The option to vaccinate patients those vaccines that are missing on the day of surgery is not an optimal scenario as it takes between two to eight weeks depending on the vaccine to achieve adequate immune response to the vaccine and obtain maximal immunity. Although there is no firm data to support this stance that is taken by our program the above reasoning is why this position has been taken. The resultant delay is felt not to be significant enough to affect the long term outcome of the patient's cochlear implantation.

This study aimed to i) review the current immunization status of recently implanted patients at our institution since the aforementioned change was made, ii) assess if this change made a significant impact on the number of patients with inadequate vaccinations and iii) elucidate any barriers that continue to exist in vaccination compliance pre- and post-CI surgery. Of note, the high-risk immunizations and vaccinations referred in this review are specific to those for pneumococcal meningitis.

Vaccination	# Doses Required	Date of Dose 1	Date of Dose 2	Date of Dose 3	Date of Dose 4	Series Completed: Y/N
HiB Part of Pediacel ® (TdaP-IPV-HiB) or Infanrix hexa™ (TdaP-HB-IPV-HiB)	4 doses	2 months	4 months	6 months	18 months	
PCV-13[1] Pneumococcal conjugate Prevnar™	4 Doses (High Risk Schedule)	2 months	4 months	6 months[2]	12 months	
PPV-23 Pneumococcal polysaccharide Pneumovax-23®	1 Dose (High Risk Schedule)	>2 years				

Fig. 1 Vaccination schedule for children at high risk for meningitis (ie – Cochlear Implant Recipients). Additional high-risk vaccine doses are circled and outlined in red text. [1]Pneumococcal conjugate (PCV-13) is required for children under the age of 5. [2]The high-risk schedule for PCV-13 series only applies to patients < 1 years of age at the time of candidacy assessment. If a child is over the age of 1 at the time of cochlear implant candidacy assessment, only 3 doses are required

Methods

The objectives of this study were to review the vaccination status of CI patients implanted between 2010 and 2014, compare findings with the previous internal review (2002–2007) and identify barriers to vaccination compliance. Ethical approval was obtained by the Institutional Ethics Board and informed verbal or written consent was obtained from the parents and/or legal guardians of children who participated in the telephone interview.

The study consisted of two parts:

(1) *Chart Review:* A retrospective Chart Review was conducted to determine the vaccination status for all CI recipients operated on at our institution between 2010 and 2014 i) at the initial candidacy assessment, ii) during surgery and iii) postoperatively, if appropriate. Post-operative vaccination status was only collected if patients required additional meningitis immunizations after surgery. These include children that were operated on with missing vaccinations and children who were not old enough at the time of surgery to have completed the high-risk meningitis vaccination series (due at 24 months of age). For children who received two CIs during the study period at different times, the vaccination status (at candidacy assessment, during surgery and post-operatively) for their first CI was collected.

(2) *Telephone Survey:* All children identified with missing vaccination information on post-implant vaccinations that could not be found on the chart review were contacted for a telephone survey. Information was collected regarding current vaccination status and the reason for non-compliance, if applicable.

Chart review

The study population included all children (19 years or younger at time of their procedure) who had received a cochlear implant at our institution between January 1, 2010 and December 31, 2014, inclusive. Re-implanted recipients were excluded from the study. A total of 116 children met the study criteria. Hospital and clinic records were reviewed for basic demographics (gender, place of birth, date of immigration), clinical history of hearing loss, records of meningitis vaccination series (*Haemophilus influenzae* type 2, 13-valent pneumococcal conjugate vaccine, 23-valent pneumococcal polysaccharide vaccine), and focused pre-surgical, surgical and post-surgical details.

Once children are considered candidates for CI at our institution, they are required to follow the high-risk meningitis vaccination schedule thereafter. Children with a CI received prior to the study period are considered high-risk

for pneumococcal meningitis and thus are required to follow the high-risk schedule during the initial candidacy assessment for their second CI. The high-risk meningitis vaccination schedule includes four doses of *Haemophilus influenzae* type 2 vaccine (HiB), four doses of 13-valent pneumococcal conjugate vaccine (PCV-13) and a single dose of 23-valent pneumococcal polysaccharide vaccine (PPV-23) for children over the age of 2 who have completed the PCV-13 series. Figure 1 shows the additional doses required in the high-risk schedule. There are two exceptions to this schedule: i) a fourth PCV-13 dose is not required for children identified as a CI candidate after the age of 1 and ii) PCV-13 is recommended for children under the age of 5 only. Since the PCV-13 vaccine became part of the standard immunization series in 2000, PCV-13 records of children born prior to 2000 were not reviewed as they are over the age of 5 during the study period (2010–2014).

A child was deemed "up-to-date" with his or her vaccinations at the time of assessment with the cochlear implant team if all immunization series were completed or if the most recent age-appropriate dose of each immunization series was received at the time of this visit. This definition was also applied in the assessment of vaccination status at the time of surgery.

For children who were not "up-to-date" with their vaccinations, individualized immunization catch-up programs were implemented to ensure the most appropriate vaccines are received prior to surgery. A vaccine infectious disease specialist was consulted to determine whether or not these individuals were up-to-date with their vaccinations at the time of surgery on a case-by-case basis. The catch up vaccines prior to surgery were given by either the local public health unit, by the patient's family practitioner, or on rare occasions, by the vaccine infectious disease specialist.

Telephone survey

A telephone survey was administered to the parent and/or legal guardian of cochlear implant recipients with missing vaccination information after the chart review. These include children who were missing vaccines at the time of surgery or children who were not old enough to complete the immunization series prior to surgery and records were not updated in the chart during the review. A record of any additional vaccines (HiB, PCV-13 and PPV-23) received after surgery was recorded and if applicable, reasons for vaccine non-compliance were documented. Parents were made aware of any vaccine their child was missing. A letter outlining the vaccines each child was missing was also sent out to these families to be taken into Public Health or their family physician for appropriate vaccination catch-up. Public Health Records were also reviewed with permission.

Statistical analysis

Descriptive statistics including means, ranges and standard deviation were used to summarize continuous variables. Categorical variables were summarized with percentages. Absolute percentage change and odds ratio were used to compare results from this study and the 2008 internal review.

Results

One hundred sixteen children received cochlear implants at our institution between 2010 and 2014. The age range of the children was less than 1 year of age to 19 years (median 5.72 years; SD 4.77 years). The male to female ratio was 1.2:1 (63:53).

Of these 116 children, 37 had a cochlear implant prior to the study period and received a second CI between 2010 and 2014. These children were considered high-risk patients at the time of candidacy assessment for the second implant. From the remaining 79 patients, 48 received one CI and 31 received two CIs during the study period. Twelve children received both implants at the same surgery (bilateral simultaneous CI) and 19 children underwent two separate cochlear implant surgeries (bilateral sequential CI).

Vaccination status at time of candidacy assessment with the CI team

A total of 19/116 patients (16%) were not up-to-date at the time of candidacy assessment (Table 1). From the 79 patients who received their first CI during the study period, 9 were not up-to-date with their vaccinations at the time of their candidacy assessment. Ten out of the 37 children who were receiving a second implant were not up-to-date with their vaccinations. A greater proportion of children receiving a second implant during the study period were not up-to-date with vaccinations (OR 2.35). The vaccines most commonly missed at the initial visit for first time CI recipients were HiB and/or PCV-13, whereas for those children receiving their second implant, PPV-23 was the most commonly missed vaccine (Fig. 2).

Vaccination status at the time of surgery

The Cochlear Implant Team at our institution requires all children to be up-to-date with their vaccinations

prior to surgery. If the child is missing any vaccines at the time of candidacy assessment, the CI team will work closely with a vaccine specialist to develop an individualized vaccine catch-up schedule. Despite this policy, two children received a cochlear implant without being appropriately vaccinated. In both cases, the child was receiving their first CI and was missing PPV-23. All recipients who had a CI prior to the study period were up-to-date with their vaccinations at the time of the second CI surgery (Table 1).

Vaccination status after surgery

A total of 32 children required vaccinations post-operatively. These included the two children who were operated on with missing vaccines and 30 children who were not old enough at the time of surgery to have completed their meningitis vaccination series.

Completed immunization documentation was on file for 13 children, thus we attempted to contact the remaining 19 for the telephone survey. Five children did not complete the survey; 27/32 (84.4%) children were included in our post-operative immunization analysis (Fig. 3).

Out of the 27 children in our post-operative immunization analysis, 8 (29.6%) did not receive the necessary vaccination(s) after surgery. In all eight cases, the missing vaccine post-surgery was PPV-23. Four of the eight children missing PPV-23 also required additional HiB or PCV-13 vaccines, in which they received.

As previously mentioned, PPV-23 is only a requirement for high-risk children, whereas HiB and PCV-13 are part of the routine childhood immunization schedule. When asked the reason why the child missed this vaccine, the responses from the parents were similar: none of the parents were aware this vaccine was required for their child as they followed the vaccination schedule for a normal-risk child. This indicates that the main reason for non-compliance is that parents as well as Public Health were not following the high-risk schedule for cochlear implant recipients in our province.

Comparison with previous study internal review (2002–2007)

Between 2010 and 2014, 84% (97/116) of children receiving CI were up to date with their vaccines at time of candidacy assessment with the CI team. Through

Table 1 Patients missing vaccinations at time of candidacy assessment and at surgery

	Patients missing vaccines at the time of assessment	Patients missing vaccines at surgery
Assessment for 1st CI		
(Normal risk patients)	9/79 (11.4%)	2/79 (2.5%)
Assessment for 2nd CI		
(High risk patients)	10/37 (27.0%)	0/37 (0%)
Total	19/116 (16.4%)	2/116 (1.7%)
Odds Ratio	OR 2.35, 95% CI:0.96–5.75, $p = 0.06$	OR 0.42, 95% CI:0.02–9.05, $p = 0.58$

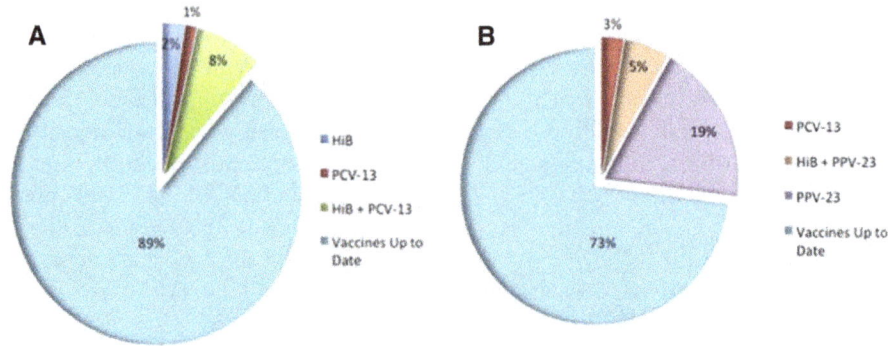

Fig. 2 Vaccines missing at time of candidacy assessment with the Cochlear Implant team. **a**–First time CI recipients. **b**–Patients receiving their second CI. Vaccines up to date – either the individual has completed all vaccinations or has received the most recent age-appropriate vaccination. HiB – Can be part of Pediacel ® or Infranrix Hexa depending on the age. PCV-13 – Pneumococcal Conjugate (Prevnar™). PPV-23 – Pneumococcal Polysaccharide (Pneumovax-23 ®)

individualized vaccination catch-up programs, 98% (114/116) of CI recipients were up-to-date at the time of their surgery. In comparison with the previous internal review, there was a 31% absolute increase in children being appropriately vaccinated at the time of CI surgery, from 67 to 98% (OR 28.5) (Table 2).

Discussion

Following a high-risk vaccination schedule is imperative to protect children with cochlear implants against the risk of serious, potentially life-threatening infection such as pneumococcal meningitis. Ensuring CI recipients are properly vaccinated before and after surgery is challenging due to multiple reasons. These factors, identified in our internal review, include the confusion over changes in the high-risk vaccination requirements over the years, the language barrier associated with our province's high

immigration rate, differences in the schedules among the provinces where a child might begin a schedule in one province and then move to BC. Adding to this complexity, immunizations are given in primary care settings, either by public health or family practitioners, however children are made high-risk status by the CI Team. Primary care providers need to be made aware that the patient is being considered for CI, otherwise the trigger of 'High Risk status' is not made.

A review of vaccination rates of CI patients at our institution in 2008 revealed that vaccination requirements were not being met and, as such, an Infectious Diseases vaccine specialist was enlisted to assist the CI Team in addressing this concern. This recent review of vaccination rates at our institution since the change was implemented indicates that pre-operative immunizations for meningitis, particularly pneumococcal meningitis, under

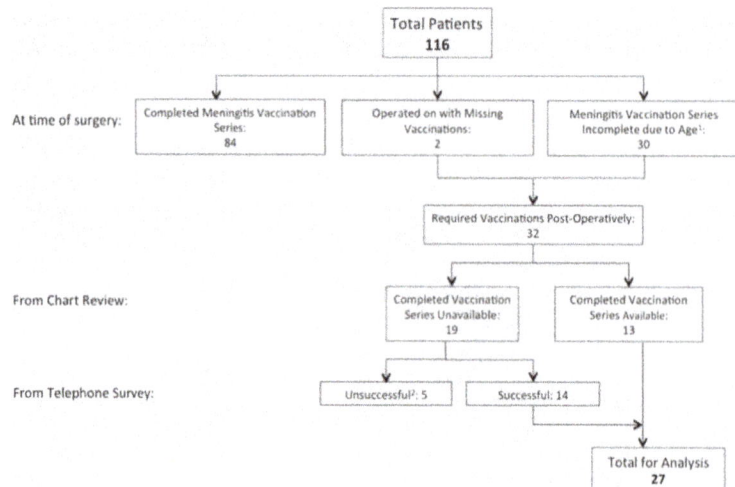

Fig. 3 Flowchart to establish patient for post-operative immunization analysis. [1]Children who are age-appropriately up-to-date with immunizations; however, still require additional vaccines post-operatively to complete meningitis immunization series. [2]No consent = 1, unable to reach = 4

Table 2 Patients up-to-date with vaccinations at candidacy assessment and at Cochlear Implant (CI) surgery

	CI surgeries 2002-2007[a]	CI surgeries 2010-2014[b]	Comparison
Time of candidacy assessment	N/A	97/116 (84%)	–
Time of Cochlear Implant Surgery	67%	114/116 (98%)	Absolute Increase: 31% Relative Odds: 28.5

Data outlined in Table 2 compares findings from the 2008 internal review of cochlear implant surgeries between 2002 and 2007[a] and from the current study, which reviews cochlear implant surgeries between 2010 and 2014[b]

the high-risk schedule improved significantly. There was a 31% absolute increase in the percentage of recipients who were up-to-date with vaccinations at the time of CI surgery; only 1.7% of children were operated on without having received the required vaccinations prior to surgery. Our finding highlights the success that can be achieved with the introduction of a designated specialist to monitor immunizations and provide individualized catch-up programs.

However, significant challenges remain in ensuring post-CI vaccination compliance. The 23-valent-pneumococcal-polysaccharide vaccine (PPV-23), a vaccine given specifically to patients at high risk of meningitis, is the only immunization that was reported missing in CI recipients who required immunizations post-operatively. Interestingly, children that missed PPV-23, but required other scheduled meningitis immunizations as part of the regular routine vaccines such as HiB and PCV-13 received the latter vaccinations in a timely manner. The odds of a child missing critical pneumococcal meningitis vaccinations at their visit for assessment double once the child is considered "high-risk". This also highlights the need to follow the high-risk vaccination schedule after surgery is not well communicated to the parent or to the immunizers in primary care.

In all eight cases of missed vaccinations post-surgery, the parents reported that they were unaware this vaccine was required for their child. These parents continue to follow the vaccination schedule for a normal-risk child provided by Public Health. The parents of the children who received PPV-23 after surgery indicated that the CI team informed them of this requirement during a follow-up appointment. Only one parent reported having followed the high-risk vaccination sheet given to them during the initial consult with the CI Team. The language barrier that was previously recognized as a barrier to vaccination compliance from our internal review was no longer an active problem, as it was not identified in this study. In the initial internal review between 2002 and 2007 Cantonese and Mandarin were the two main languages that posed difficulty. Repeat calls after working day hours improved acquisition of data as English speaking parents were at home at this time. In this study, perhaps improvement was a result of the fact that in instances where the initial contact of families was with a non English speaking person, we were fortunate enough to have two of the authors who spoke Mandarin to facilitate the interaction. There are an abundant number of resources in British Columbia and specifically the Vancouver area for interpreter services and one could speculate that this has assisted in compliance as well, however our study did not address this aspect directly.

Ensuring appropriate vaccination post-surgery still remains a current issue. The key reasons for non-compliance seems to be a communication gap between the CI team, parents, family physicians and Public Health. In our province, immunizations are generally obtained at a Public Health Clinic or at a primary care clinic. During the telephone survey, we clarified to the parents which vaccination schedule their child is recommended to follow and provided them with a letter to present to the Public Health Clinic or their family physician for appropriate vaccination catch-up. However, greater measures need to be taken to close the communication gap. Solutions to bridge this gap include providing families with updated high-risk vaccination schedules post-surgery, sending reminder notifications to family members, notifying Public Health or the patient's primary care physician regarding his/her high-risk status, or assigning a designated person or program to manage post-operative vaccinations in a similar manner to which is used in our pre-operative vaccination compliance management.

Our study revealed that immunization rates at time of surgery significantly improved after the introduction of an infectious disease vaccine specialist. Once a child was identified to be missing vaccinations during the initial candidacy assessment, individualized catch-up programs were created to ensure these children were appropriately vaccinated and would not prolong the wait time for surgery. An interesting future direction would be to assess whether this administrative change significantly impacted on the wait times for CI surgery. Our group acknowledges the difficulty of recruiting a specialist to assist in the implement of a vaccination program. Alternatively, the use of a Registered Nurse or Nurse Practitioner may exhibit similar benefits. Nonetheless, it is important to have a designated person to oversee and manage the vaccination status of a small group of high-risk individuals, such as Cochlear Implant recipients.

Conclusion

This study showed a significant improvement was made in pre-operative vaccination rates after the introduction of a specialist. However, it is evident that a communication gap regarding which vaccination schedule to follow post-operatively continues to exist. Post-operative vaccinations are not being appropriately managed and in turn, CI patients continue to occasionally miss vaccines critical to their health. Based on the significant success in increasing pre-operative vaccination rates, one may consider creating a designated program to improve post-operative vaccinations, specifically for PPV-23. At our institution, we have ensured that all patients implanted prior to the age of 2 are seen in follow-up at 2 years of age to ensure that they are up to date for their PPV-23 vaccine.

Abbreviations

CI: Cochlear Implant; HiB: *Haemophilus influenzae* type 2 vaccine; PCV: 13: 13-valent pneumococcal conjugate vaccine; PPV: 23: 23-valent pneumococcal polysaccharide vaccine

Acknowledgements

The authors acknowledge current and former members of the Cochlear Implant Team at BC Children's Hospital for their assistance over the years related to vaccination of the cochlear implant patient population.

Funding

This study was supported by the University of British Columbia under the Florence E Heighway Summer Research Award in the study and collection.

Authors' contribution

FKK, LJ and JP designed the study. LJ and PT performed the chart review with the guidance from RC, FKK and SD. LJ and DL collected consents and conducted the telephone survey. LJ, JP, PT and FKK wrote the manuscript and all authors read and approved the final manuscript.

Competing interests

The authors declare that they have no competing interests.

Author details

[1]Faculty of Medicine, University of British Columbia, 317-2194 Health Sciences Mall, Vancouver, BC V6T 1Z3, Canada. [2]Division of Pediatric Otolaryngology-Head and Neck Surgery, BC Children's Hospital, 4480 Oak St, Vancouver, BC V6H 3N1, Canada. [3]Department of Audiology, BC Children's Hospital, 4480 Oak St, Vancouver, BC V6H 3N1, Canada. [4]Sidra Medical and Research Centre, Doha, Qatar. [5]Department of Surgery, Division of Otolaryngology King Fahad Specialist Hospital, Dammam, Kingdom of Saudi Arabia.

References

1. Ou H, Cleary P, Sie K. Assessing the immunization status of pediatric cochlear implant recipients using a state-maintained immunization registry. Otolaryngol Head Neck Surg. 2010. https://doi.org/10.1016/j.otohns.2010.05.020.
2. Gluth MB, Driscoll CLW, Lalwani AK. Cochlear implants. In: Lalwani AK, editor. CURRENT Diagnosis & Treatment in Otolaryngology—Head & Neck Surgery. 3rd ed. New York: United States. McGraw-Hill Education; 2011.
3. Reefhuis J, Honein MA, Whitney CG, Chamany S, Mann EA, Biernath KR, et al.. Risk of bacterial meningitis in children with cochlear implants. N Engl J Med. 2003. https://doi.org/10.1056/NEJMoa031101.
4. Lalwani AK, Cohen NL. Does meningitis after cochlear implantation remain a concern in 2011? Otol Neurotol. 2011;33:93–5.
5. Wei BP, Shepherd RK, Robins-Browne RM, Clark GM, O'Leary SJ. Pneumococcal meningitis threshold model: A potential tool to assess infectious risk of new or existing inner ear surgical interventions. Otol Neurotol. 2006. https://doi.org/10.1097/01.mao.0000227898.80656.54.

26

Rates and causes of 30-day readmission and emergency room utilization following head and neck surgery

Vincent Wu[1] and Stephen F. Hall[2*]

Abstract

Background: Unplanned returns to hospital are common, costly, and potentially avoidable. We aimed to investigate and characterize reasons for all-cause readmissions to hospital as in-patients (IPs) and visits to the Emergency Department (ED) within 30-days following patient discharge post head and neck surgery (HNS).

Methods: Retrospective case series with chart review. All patients within the Department of Otolaryngology – Head and Neck Surgery who underwent HNS for benign and malignant disease from January 1, 2010 to May 31, 2015 were identified. The electronic medical records of readmitted patients were reviewed for reasons of readmission, demographic data, and comorbidities.

Results: Following 1281 surgical cases, there were 41 (3.20%) IP readmissions and 109 (8.43%) ED visits within 30-days after discharge for HNS. For IP readmissions, most common causes included infection (26.8%), respiratory symptoms (17.1%), and pain (17.1%). Most common reasons for ED visits were for pain (31.5%), bleeding (17.6%), and infection (14.8%). Readmitted IPs had significantly higher health burden at pre-operative baseline as compared to patients who visited the ED when assessed with the American Society of Anesthesiology scores ($p = 0.002$) and the Cumulative Illness Rating Scale ($p = 0.004$).

Conclusion: Rate of 30-day IP readmission and ED utilization was 3.20 and 8.43%, respectively. Pain and infection were common causes for returns to hospital. Discharge planning may be improved to target common causes for post-surgical hospital visits in order to decrease readmission rates.

Keywords: Rates, Causes, 30-day, Readmission, Emergency department, Otolaryngology, Head and neck surgery

Background

Unplanned returns to hospital, including readmissions as in-patients (IPs) and visits to the Emergency Department (ED) are identified as costly, common, and potentially avoidable with proper planning and patient education [1–6]. The Canadian Institute for Health Information (CIHI) identified 30-day readmission rates to be a measure of a hospital's quality and patient care [6]. From its 2012 report, surgical patients were identified as having the second highest overall rate of readmission as IP and return to the ED, contributing to the $1.8 billion dollar annual cost associated with 30-day readmissions in Canada [6]. While studies having indicated that between 9 to 59% of all unplanned readmissions are potentially avoidable, identifying these causes are necessary in order to reduce rates and the associated healthcare spending [5, 7–10].

In general, it is known that readmitted patients are older and have more medical comorbidities [11–13]. Being from a low socioeconomic class and having had previous unplanned visits to hospital also increase the risk for readmissions [11, 12, 14]. Moreover, the causes for readmission differ based on the specific patient population [15, 16]. Studies on surgery patients have identified risk factors for unplanned readmission that differ from medical patients [16]. Within the field of Otolaryngology – Head and Neck Surgery, the surgical procedures performed are diverse in nature. A single

* Correspondence: steve@sfhallmd.com
[2]Department of Otolaryngology – Head and Neck Surgery, Queen's Cancer Research Institute, Queen's University, 10 Stuart St, Level 2, Kingston, ON K7L 3N6, Canada
Full list of author information is available at the end of the article

readmission rate is not representative of the specialty as a whole, and can range from 2 to 8% depending on the subspecialty focus [17, 18]. Patients who undergo head and neck surgery (HNS) have been shown to have higher rates of 30-day ED utilization and readmission as IPs [18–20].

Causes for unplanned readmission following HNS have not been thoroughly identified within a Canadian population. Our objective was to analyze and characterize the rates and reasons for all-cause readmission as IP and visits to the ED within 30-days following HNS. The results may serve to potentially reduce readmission rates by acting on preventable causes.

Methods

Study design and population

Retrospective chart review was performed of patients who were readmitted as IP or visited the ED within 30-days following discharge post-HNS from a tertiary academic center from January 1, 2010 to May 31, 2015. Patients were identified using CIHI procedural codes from hospital-based datasets. Patient cases were separated based on the procedure performed, which were separated into procedural categories. Examples of surgeries performed with procedural categories are shown in Table 1. Procedures pertaining to the nasal cavity, paranasal sinuses, skull base, ears, tonsils, adenoids or skin were not included.

Definition and study variables

We defined 30-day readmission as an IP admission to hospital for any cause, regardless of assignment under the Department of Otolaryngology – Head and Neck Surgery or another clinical service, within 30-days following initial post-HNS discharge. ED utilization was

defined as any visit to the ED within 30-days following post-HNS discharge.

The primary outcome measure was causes for 30-day IP readmission, extracted as the primary diagnosis from electronic hospital discharge summaries. Secondarily, we evaluated causes for ED utilization, extracted from ED charts as the final diagnosis. If more than one ED visit or IP admission was noted within the 30-day period following surgery, only the first readmission/visit was recorded.

Additionally, patient demographics including age and sex were captured. The American Society of Anesthesiologists (ASA) score, admission date, procedure date, initial discharge date, and return date were also included. Patient comorbidities were captured using the Cumulative Illness Rating Scale (CIRS), which is a validated summative index aimed at quantifying the overall physical impairment of the patient through 13 independent organ system domains, with higher scores indicating greater comorbid illness [21].

Statistical analysis

All statistical analyses were performed using Prism (v7.0, GraphPad, La Jolla, CA, USA) and statistical significance was set to $\alpha = 0.05$. Results are reported as mean ± standard deviation (SD). Standard descriptive statistics were used to characterize causes for readmission. Patient information including age, gender, sex, comorbidities, ASA score were also described using descriptive statistics. Student's t-tests were performed to compare differences in ASA and CIRS among IPs and ED patients.

Results

Of the 1281 patients who underwent HNS during the study period, 120 (9.37%) patients returned to hospital within 30-days of discharge. In total, there were 41 (3.20%) IP readmissions and 108 (8.43%) ED visits. There were 29 patients who were admitted as IPs through the ED. Patient demographics are summarized in Table 2.

Table 1 Included procedural categories

Procedure Categories	Example
Major Head and Neck with No Flap	Laryngectomy without flap reconstruction
Major Head and Neck with Pedicled Flap	Oropharyngeal resection with pectoralis myocutaneous rotation flap reconstruction
Major Head and Neck with Free Flap	Excision of oropharynx with radial forearm free flap reconstruction
Open Airway	Tracheostomy
Limited Oral Cavity	Marginal mandibulectomy
Limited Neck	Branchial cleft cyst resection
Neck Dissection Only	Cervical lymph node dissection
Salivary Gland	Parotidectomy
Thyroid/Parathyroid	Total thyroidectomy

Table 2 Baseline Patient Characteristics

Variable	Included (n = 120)
Age (mean ± SD years)	57.5 ± 20.7
Male (n, %)	78, 65%
Length of stay (mean ± SD days)	7.58 ± 17.1
CIRS (mean ± SD)	5.15 ± 3.44
ASA (mean ± SD)	2.82 ± 0.83
Previous radiotherapy (n, %)	9, 7.5%
Previous chemotherapy (n, %)	2, 1.7%
Previous chemoradiation therapy (n, %)	7, 5.8%

*SD – standard deviation

Table 3 Rates and causes of in-patient admissions

Causes	Numbers	Rates
Infection: UTI, sepsis	11	26.83%
Respiratory: COPDE, dyspnea	7	17.07%
Pain: surgical/graft site	7	17.07%
Systemic: dehydration	7	17.07%
Neurologic: seizures	3	7.31%
Bleeding: surgical site	3	7.31%
Exacerbation of chronic condition	2	4.87%
Cardiac: chest pain	1	2.43%

*UTI – urinary tract infection; COPDE; chronic obstructive pulmonary disease exacerbation

Causes for readmission to hospital as IPs are listed in Table 3. The single most common reason for IP readmission was for infection (26.8%), which included sepsis, surgical site infection, and urinary tract infection. Reasons for visiting the ED are listed in Table 4, with the most common cause being pain at the surgical site (31.5%).

The CIRS comorbidity score in patients who were readmitted as IPs (6.29 ± 3.27) were significantly higher than patients who visited the ED (4.56 ± 3.39), $p = 0.004$. This was similarly seen with the ASA score, with readmitted IPs (3.12 ± 0.64) having significantly higher scores compared to patients visiting the ED (2.66 ± 0.88), $p = 0.002$. A simple linear regression of ASA and CIRS scores revealed a significant positive correlation between the measures, $F(1,118) = 73.37$, $p < 0.001$, with an $r^2 = 0.383$.

Discussion

This descriptive study highlighted the rates and causes of 30-day readmission following HNS for benign and malignant causes within a Canadian tertiary academic center. Although 30-day readmission rates have been

Table 4 Rates and causes of Emergency Department visits

Causes	Numbers	Rates
Pain: surgical/graft site	34	31.48%
Bleeding: surgical/graft site	19	17.59%
Infection: surgical/graft site, UTI	16	14.81%
Equipment: nasogastric tube, tracheostomy tube, surgical drain	8	7.41%
Cardiac: chest pain, syncope	7	6.48%
Respiratory: dyspnea	7	6.48%
Gastrointestinal: nausea/vomit, constipation	6	5.56%
Neurologic: seizure, weakness	5	4.63%
Exacerbation of chronic condition	4	3.70%
Psychiatric: delirium	2	1.85%

*UTI – urinary tract infection

used as a quality metric for hospital care, there are limitations to its use. While potentially preventable causes for readmission exist, there are factors which are non-modifiable that can contribute to patient readmission and hospital utilization. These factors include patient gender, race, socioeconomic status, and comorbidities [15]. Causes of readmission also differ based on the specific patient population. Therefore, by examining a sub-specialty population such as patients who underwent HNS, the specific needs of that group may be identified. Although truly preventable causes of 30-day readmission are low given various non-modifiable factors, this study ultimately identified common reasons for hospital visits such as pain and infection, which we believe may be preventable with changes made to discharge planning and improved patient education.

The rate of IP readmission among post-HNS patient was found to be 3.20% within our cohort. This is below the 5.1–14.5% readmission rate currently reported for HNS patients in the United States [19, 20, 22]. Compared to the study by Bur et al. who examined risk factors and causes for readmissions within HNS for malignant causes, our IP readmission numbers were lower [19]. This may be due to the incorporation of patients undergoing HNS for benign causes within our study. Similar causes for readmissions were noted within our cohort, with infection being the most common, followed by respiratory causes and dehydration [19]. In terms of risk factors, Bur et al. noted the presence of medical comorbidities such as diabetes and dyspnea at baseline were associated with increased readmission [19]. Although we did not capture specific comorbidities, we noted that increased ASA and CIRS were higher for IP readmitted patient as compared with patients who visited the ED only. Together, our results reaffirm that infectious and respiratory symptoms are common causes for readmission, and that readmitted IPs patients have increased baseline disease burden and comorbidities. Furthermore, our results revealed potentially preventable causes for readmission such as dehydration, which may be linked to altered diets, inadequate pain control, and/or poor oral intake, all of which may be optimized prior to discharge.

Literature surrounding ED utilization have mainly focused on specific procedures, not HNS as a whole. One study reported ED utilization after thyroidectomy and parathyroidectomy to be 11.22%, with common causes being paresthesia and wound complications [23]. Within our cohort, we noted an ED utilization rate of 8.43%, with the most common cause due to pain. To us, this represented a preventable cause of hospital utilization that may be better improved with discharge planning and patient education. As discharge is a transition time from hospital to home, many patients may feel inadequately prepared based on the information received in hospital [24]. Specific interventions including early discharge planning and individualized education can potentially reduce readmissions and ED utilization by 75% [25–27]. Moreover, noting the pain trajectories and addressing those patients with high pain levels prior to discharge may help to further decrease ED utilization [28]. Ultimately, systems analysis of discharge planning can be used to identify various steps associated with patient discharge including the delivery of information, and the type and amount of information that is delivered to the patient, in order to optimize the process.

ASA status has been reported to have a significant positive associated with higher readmission rates, and was among the variables strongly associated with predicting readmissions [13]. CIRS has also been used among HNS patients, with higher scores reflective of worsening health burden for an individual [21, 29]. This suggested that IPs were sicker and had increased health burden at baseline, which may have predisposed them to more frequent and serious medical complications requiring in-hospital admission. Often, procedures within HNS involve the resection of head and neck cancers. It is known that head and neck cancer patients have more medical comorbidities, often resulting from chronic exposures to risk factors such as tobacco and alcohol [30–33]. Therefore, it is not surprising that with potential increases in risk factor exposure that we noted higher ASA and CIRS scores among patients who were readmitted as IPs.

Currently, the distinction between surgical and medical causes for post-operative complications is still unclear. Even for surgical complications, there is still no agreed upon definition [34]. Common methods for categorizing post-operative complications, including the Clavien-Dindo Classification, makes no distinction made between medical and surgical causes [35]. There have been attempts to separate readmission based on surgical complications (bleeding, wound dehiscence, and surgical site infection) from other medical complications [36]. However, the inherent limitation of this approach is that the exacerbation of medical comorbidities, or development of new medical conditions, may be a result of the surgical stress. The standardization of post-operative complications will be helpful in distinguishing between complications as a result of the surgical procedure versus an exacerbation of a pre-existing medical condition due to the general stresses of surgery. This will be important for eliciting preventable surgical causes aimed at decreasing the overall readmission rate.

This study has potential limitations. First, inherent to retrospective chart reviews, there exists the possibility of selection bias. A preliminary list of patients who returned to hospital within 30-days following head and neck surgery was generated automatically through the hospital's centralized patient information database. To ensure validity of the extracted data, individual chart review was conducted by the study author (V.W.) only after extensive training on the electronic medical record. The senior author (S.F.H.) oversaw the data extraction with periodic reviews. Additionally, information was not extracted for patients who did not have a 30-day readmission or ED visit, thereby preventing risk assessment and comparisons being drawn between this group and patients who had a readmission. Moreover, data was not available for the rates of ED and IP readmission in regional hospitals for the same procedures, precluding the ability to compare readmissions rates outside of our academic center. Our sample size was limited by some of these factors, and as such, an increased study size can potentially address some of this study's limitations. Future prospective studies can also aim to account for these potential limitations and utilize additional metrics for hospital and patient quality of care including patient-reported outcomes and length of stay.

Conclusion

The 30-day IP readmission rate for post HNS patients was 3.20% and the ED utilization rate was 8.43%. Pain and infection represented common causes for returns to hospital. Discharge planning may be improved to target common causes for post-surgical readmission as potential steps in decrease hospital readmission and ED visit rates.

Abbreviations
ASA: American Society of Anesthesiologists; CIHI: Canadian Institute for Health Information; CIRS: Cumulative Illness Rating Scale; COPD: Chronic obstructive pulmonary disease; ED: Emergency Department; HNS: Head and neck surgery; IP: In-patient; SD: Standard deviation

Acknowledgements
1. This study was presented as a podium presentation at the Canadian Society of Otolaryngology – Head and Neck Surgery annual meeting in Charlottetown, Prince Edward Island, 2016.
2. The authors would like to thank David Barber, Decision Support, Kingston General Hospital, for generating the patient list.
3. The authors would like to thank Susan Rohland, Cancer Care and Epidemiology, Queen's University, for coordinating the study.

Funding
This research was funded by the Department of Otolaryngology – Head and Neck Surgery, Queen's University, Kingston, Ontario.

Authors' contributions
All authors were involved with the conception and design of the study, analysis and interpretation of data, revision of the manuscript, and have approved the final manuscript.

Competing interests

The authors declare that they have no competing interests.

Author details

[1]School of Medicine, Faculty of Health Sciences, Queen's University, 80 Barrie St, Kingston, ON K7L 3J8, Canada. [2]Department of Otolaryngology – Head and Neck Surgery, Queen's Cancer Research Institute, Queen's University, 10 Stuart St, Level 2, Kingston, ON K7L 3N6, Canada.

References

1. Jencks SF, Williams MV, Coleman EA. Rehospitalizations among patients in the Medicare fee-for-service program. N Engl J Med. 2009;360:1418–28.
2. Soeken KL, Prescott PA, Herron DG, Creasia J. Predictors of Hospital Readmission: A Meta-Analysis. Eval Health Prof. 1991;14(3):262–81.
3. Vest JR, Gamm LD, Oxford BA, Gonzalez MI, Slawson KM. Determinants of preventable readmissions in the United States: a systematic review. Implement Sci. 2010;5:88.
4. Anderson GF, Steinberg EP. Hospital readmissions in the Medicare population. N Engl J Med. 1984;311(21):1349–53.
5. Frankl SE, Breeling JL, Goldman L. Preventability of emergent hospital readmission. Am J Med. 1991;90(6):667–74.
6. All-cause readmission to acute care and return to the emergency department. Ottawa: Canadian Institute for Health Information; 2012.
7. Clarke A. Are Readmissions Avoidable? BMJ. 1990;301(6761):1136–8.
8. Graham H, Livesley B. Can readmissions to a geriatric medical unit be prevented? Lancet. 1983;1(8321):404–6.
9. Halfon P, Eggli Y, van Melle G, Chevalier J, Wasserfallen JB, Burnand B. Measuring potentially avoidable hospital readmissions. J Clin Epidemiol. 2002;55(6):573–87.
10. Oddone EZ, Weinberger M, Horner M, Mengel C, Goldstein F, Ginier P, et al. Classifying general medicine readmissions: are they preventable? Veterans affairs cooperative studies in health services group on primary care and hospital readmissions. J Gen Intern Med. 1996;11(10):597–607.
11. van Walraven C, Dhalla IA, Bell C, Etchells E, Stiell IG, Zarnke K, et al. Derivation and validation of an index to predict early death or unplanned readmission after discharge from hospital to the community. CMAJ. 2010; 182(6):551–7.
12. Boult C, Dowd B, McCaffrey D, Boult L, Hernandez R, Krulewitch H. Screening elders for risk of hospital admission. J Am Geriatr Soc. 1993;41(8): 811–7.
13. Merkow RP, Ju MH, Chung JW, Hall BL, Cohen ME, Williams MV, et al. Underlying reasons associated with hospital readmission following surgery in the United States. JAMA. 2015;313(5):483–95.
14. Weissman JS, Stern RS, Epstein AM. The impact of patient socioeconomic status and other social factors on readmission: a prospective study in four Massachusetts hospitals. Inquiry. 1994;31(2):163–72.
15. Benbassat J, Taragin M. Hospital readmissions as a measure of quality of health CareAdvantages and limitations. Arch Intern Med. 2000;160(8):1074–81.
16. Kassin MT, Owen RM, Perez S, Leeds I, Cox JC, Schnier K, et al. Risk factors for 30-day hospital readmission among general surgery patients. J Am Coll Surg. 2012;215:322–30.
17. Graboyes EM, Liou TN, Kallogjeri D, Nussenbaum B, Diaz JA. Risk factors for unplanned hospital readmission in otolaryngology patients. Otolaryngol Head Neck Surg. 2013;149(4):562–71.
18. Jain U, Chandra RK, Smith SS, Pilecki M, Kim JY. Predictors of readmission after outpatient otolaryngologic surgery. Laryngoscope. 2014;124(8):1783–8.
19. Bur AM, Brant JA, Mulvey CL, Nicolli EA, Brody RM, Fischer JP, Cannady SB, Newman JG. Association of clinical risk factors and postoperative complications with unplanned hospital readmission after head and neck cancer surgery. JAMA Otolaryngol Head Neck Surg. 2016;142(12):1184–90.
20. Offodile AC, II, Pathak A, Wenger J, Orgill DP, Guo L. Prevalence and patient-level risk factors for 30-day readmissions following free tissue transfer for head and neck Cancer. JAMA Otolaryngol Head Neck Surg. 2015;141(9):783–789.
21. Linn BS, Linn MW, Gurel L. Cumulative illness rating scale. J Am Geriatr Soc. 1968;16(5):622–6.
22. Dziegielewski PT, Boyce B, Manning A, Agrawal A, Old M, Ozer E, Teknos TN. Predictors and costs of readmissions at an academic head and neck surgery service. Head Neck. 2016;38(Suppl 1):E502–10.
23. Young WG, Succar E, Hsu L, Talpos G, Ghanem TA. Causes of emergency department visits following thyroid and parathyroid surgery. JAMA Otolaryngol Head Neck Surg. 2013 Nov 1;139(11):1175–80.
24. Zeng-Treitler Q, Kim H, Hunter M. Improving patient comprehension and recall of discharge instructions by supplementing free texts with pictographs. AMIA Annu Symp Proc. 2008;2008:849–53.
25. Evans RL, Hendrick RD. Evaluating hospital discharge planning: a randomized clinical trial. Med Care. 1993;31:358–70.
26. Jack BW, Chetty VK, Anthony D, Greenwald JL, Sanchez GM, et al. A reengineered hospital discharge program to decrease rehospitalization: a randomized trial. Ann Intern Med. 2009;150:178–87.
27. Coleman EA, Parry C, Chalmers S, Min S. The care transitions intervention: results of a randomized controlled trial. Arch Intern Med. 2006;166:1822–8.
28. Hernandez-Boussard T, Graham LA, Desai K, Wahl TS, Aucoin E, Richman JS, et al. The fifth vital sign: postoperative pain predicts 30-day readmissions and subsequent emergency department visits. Ann Surg. 2017;266(3):516–24.
29. Castro MA, Dedivitis RA, Ribeiro KC. Comorbidity measurement in patients with laryngeal squamous cell carcinoma. ORL J Otorhinolaryngol Relat Spec. 2007;69(3):146–52.
30. Hashibe M, Brennan P, Benhamou S, Castellsague X, Chen C, Curado MP, et al. Alcohol drinking in never users of tobacco, cigarette smoking in never drinkers, and the risk of head and neck cancer: pooled analysis in the international head and neck Cancer epidemiology consortium. J Natl Cancer Inst. 2007;99(10):777–89.
31. Blot WJ, McLaughlin JK, Winn DM, Austin DF, Greenberg RS, Preston-Martin S, et al. Smoking and drinking in relation to oral and pharyngeal cancer. Cancer Res. 1988;48(11):3282–7.
32. Hashibe M, Boffetta P, Zaridze D, Shangina O, Szeszenia-Dabrowska N, Mates D, et al. Evidence for an important role of alcohol- and aldehyde-metabolizing genes in cancers of the upper aerodigestive tract. Cancer Epidemiol Biomark Prev. 2006;15(4):696–703.
33. Gandini S, Botteri E, Iodice S, Boniol M, Lowenfels AB, Maisonneuve P, et al. Tobacco smoking and cancer: a meta-analysis. Int J Cancer. 2008;122(1):155–64.
34. Sokol DK, Wilson J. What is a surgical complication? World J Surg. 2008; 32(6):942–4.
35. Dindo D, Demartines N, Clavien PA. Classification of surgical complications: a new proposal with evaluation in a cohort of 6336 patients and results of a survey. Ann Surg. 2004;240(2):205–13.
36. Graboyes EM, Kallogjeri D, Saeed MJ, Olsen MA, Nussenbaum B. 30-day hospital readmission following otolaryngology surgery: analysis of a state inpatient database. Laryngoscope. 2017;127(2):337–45.

27

Auditory effects of autologous fat graft for TORP stabilization in the middle ear: a cadaveric study

Margaret Aron[1,4]*[iD], Thomas G. Landry[2] and Manohar Bance[3]

Abstract

Background: Total ossicular replacement prostheses (TORP) are often used to re-establish ossicular coupling of sound in an ear lacking a stapes supra-structure. The use of TORPs, however, is associated with a 2/3 five year failure rate due to their anatomic instability over time in the middle ear. The use of autologous fat to try and stabilize TORPs may improve long-term results with this challenging ossicular reconstruction technique.

Methods: A cadaveric temporal bone model was developed and laser Doppler vibrometry was used to measure and record round window membrane vibration in response to sound stimulation under the following conditions: normal middle ear, middle ear filled with fat, normal middle ear with TORP prosthesis, TORP prosthesis with fat around its distal end and TORP prosthesis with fat filling the middle ear. Fourteen temporal bones were used.

Results: There was a significant decrease in round window membrane velocity after filling the middle ear with fat in both the normal middle ear (− 8.6 dB; $p < 0.0001$) and prosthesis conditions (− 13.7 dB; $p < 0.0001$). However, there was no significant drop in round window membrane velocity associated with using fat around the distal end of the TORP prosthesis as compared to the prosthesis without fat condition ($p > 0.05$).

Conclusions: Autologous fat around the distal end of a TORP prosthesis may not be associated with any additional hearing loss, as demonstrated in this cadaveric model. The additional hearing loss potentially caused by using fat to completely surround the prosthesis and fill the middle ear is probably not clinically acceptable at this time, especially given the unknown way in which the fat will atrophy over time in this context.

Keywords: TORP, Autologous fat graft, Middle ear prosthesis stabilization, Laser Doppler vibrometry

Background

Re-establishing ossicular coupling of sound in an ear lacking a stapes supra-structure can be quite a challenge. Alloplastic prostheses, intended to be placed onto the intact footplate on one end and either the tympanic membrane (TM) or malleus handle on its other end, are often used to re-establish ossicular coupling in these cases. These prostheses, otherwise known as total ossicular replacement prostheses (TORP) have variable clinical results and have been disappointing in many cases. Despite being lightweight

and biocompatible, these reconstructions tend to lack stability, with 2/3 of TORPs failing after 5 years [1] as demonstrated by a recurrent increase in the air bone gap on audiologic testing. Prosthesis displacement or tilting are the major causes of unsatisfactory hearing after this type of surgery [2–4]. Re-exploration of these failed reconstructions most often reveals a prosthesis having been displaced from its original position on the footplate. Factors such as recurrent middle ear fluid, tympanic membrane retraction, scar formation/fibrosis, and atelectasis of the tympanic membrane may displace a perfectly placed prosthesis. Unfortunately, many of these factors cannot be controlled [5]. As surgeons, we must try to maximize prosthesis stability to allow it to withstand these displacing forces.

Our experience with fat in the middle ear largely comes from its use in fat graft myringoplasty where it

* Correspondence: maggiearon@gmail.com
[1]Division of Otolaryngology-Head and Neck Surgery, Université de Sherbrooke, Sherbrooke, QC, Canada
[4]Centre Hospitalier Université de Sherbrooke, Service d'Otorhinolaryngoloie et Chirurgie Cervicofaciale, Site Hôtel-Dieu, 580 rue Bowen Sud, Sherbrooke, QC J1G 2E8, Canada
Full list of author information is available at the end of the article

helps guide inflammatory cells to heal perforations. In this context, bulky fat grafts are dumb-belled through a tympanic membrane perforation. With healing, the bulkiness of the graft is lost, leaving a thickened and healed ear drum behind [6, 7]. We hypothesize that if we use fat to stabilize the TORP prosthesis intra-operatively it may offer stability during the healing period of the middle ear, helping resist displacement forces on the prosthesis and then may atrophy with time, leaving a ventilated middle ear space. In fact, the senior author (MB) uses this method clinically. The effect on hearing of using fat in the middle ear in this context, however, has not been studied. The objective of this study was to evaluate the effect on round window membrane vibration of autologous fat deposited into the middle ear under various conditions including that of using the fat to stabilize a TORP prosthesis.

Methods

In order to evaluate round window membrane vibration a temporal bone model was designed on which we could use a laser Doppler vibrometer (LDV) to record and compare round window membrane (RWM) movement in response to acoustic tone stimulation in several conditions. The model and measuring technique are detailed below. Ethics review board approval was obtained from the Dalhousie Research Ethics Committee for this study.

Temporal bone preparation

Fresh frozen cadaver temporal bones were used ($n = 14$) (Anatomy Gifts Registry, Hannover, USA) since inner ear fluid and soft tissue quality is preserved in these specimens. Soft tissue such as skin and muscle were removed from the lateral temporal bones and a canal wall up mastoidectomy was performed, as well as a posterior tympanotomy to expose the oval and round windows. The use of LDV to measure RWM movement requires a clear view of the entire RWM and thus the

facial nerve was sacrificed as necessary to obtain optimal exposure of the RW. The round window niche was then drilled off as needed to have a direct view of the entire RWM. Finally, holes were drilled into the lateral bony external auditory canal (EAC) for an ER-3A speaker tip and an ER-7C microphone probe tube (Etymotic, Elk Grove Village, USA) (Fig. 1a). These were glued to the EAC wall for stabilization and the Er-7C microphone tip as ensured to be within 2 mm of the TM. The EAC was sealed by modeling clay during the experiments.

In order to obtain reliable LDV measurements, reflective polystyrene tape containing microbeads (3 M, Minneapolis, MN, USA) was placed on the RWM via the posterior tympanotomy to serve as a reflective target (Fig. 1b).

Conditions under which RWM vibrations were recorded using laser Doppler vibrometry

Baseline (termed "Normal_NF"): Baseline LDV measurements of RWM movement in response to acoustic stimuli were measured with all native ossicles intact and the middle ear left ventilated.

Middle ear cavity filled with fat (termed "Normal_-MEF"): we harvested fat from the temporalis fat pad and used it to fill the middle ear. Over-filling was avoided in order to prevent placing excessive pressure on the TM and ossicles. We ensured that fat surrounded all of the ossicles as well as the air containing middle ear space, including the epitympanum. Only the RWM was left uncovered and in view for LDV measurements. This condition was chosen to simulate the maximal dampening effect possible by replacing the entire middle ear air space with fat.

TORP without fat (termed "Pros_NF"): After disarticulating and removing the incus as well as the stapes suprastructure through the posterior tympanotomy, a titanium TORP prosthesis (TTP-VARIAC Total Prosthesis, Kurz, Dusslingen, Germany) was measured up using the sizing template and placed between the footplate and the posterosuperior TM.

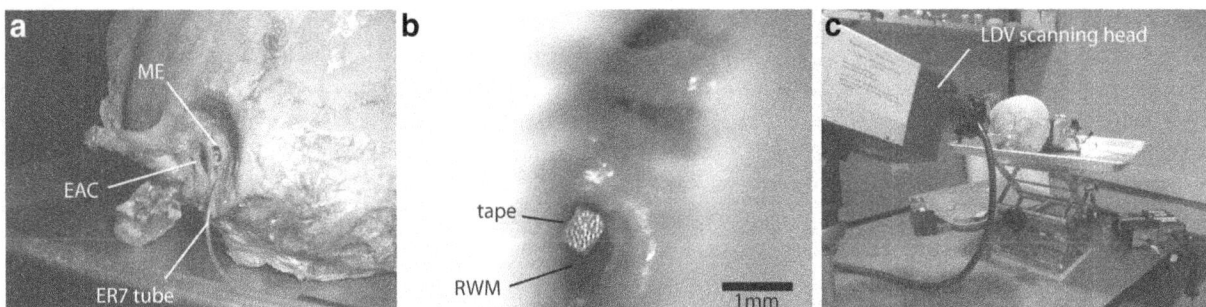

Fig. 1 a Temporal bone with posterior tympanotomy to access middle ear. Custom holes drilled into the bony EAC for an ER-3A speaker tip (not shown) and an ER-7C microphone probe tube. **b** RWM exposed through the posterior tympanotomy with reflective tape on it. **c** Experiment setup in the soundproof booth with temporal bone and scanning head supported by a stability table to dampen floor vibrations

TORP with fat around the footplate (termed "Pros_FPF"): the fat harvested from the temporalis fat pad was used to surround the prosthesis shaft on the stapes footplate. In all cases the distal bulged end of the TORP was completely covered by fat resulting in complete coverage of the oval window in all cases. This condition was chosen to predict the amount of dampening of sound one might expect when using fat to stabilize the distal end of the TORP on the footplate.

TORP with fat filling the middle ear (termed "Pros_MEF"): the conditions for "Normal_MEF" were repeated with the TORP in place.

Laser Doppler vibrometer setup and recording software

A LDV (PSV-400 scanning head, OFV-5000 controller, Polytec PI, Tustin, CA, USA) and software (Polytec Scanning Vibrometer version 8.7) were used to measure and record movement of the RWM.

Settings of the software system:

- Average of 4 trials per point
- 640 ms recordings window with a sample frequency of 25.6 kHz
- Acoustic stimulation used was constant sine waves at the following frequencies: 250, 500, 1000, 2000, 3000, 4000, 6000, 8000 Hz
- Sound was presented in the EAC using the ER-3A speaker at 100 dB SPL (or to a maximum of 4 V input if 100 dB could not be attained). This intensity was confirmed with the ER-7C microphone.

Physical setup for LDV measurements: (Fig. 1c)

- The bone was placed in a soundproof booth.
- The temporal bone specimen and scanning head were supported by a stability table to dampen floor vibrations.
- Modeling clay was used to seal the lateral EAC and the holes around the ER-3A and ER-7C to provide an air-tight seal in order to attain the desired sound pressure levels within the EAC. Air-tight closure was confirmed when sound pressure emitted by the ER-3 into the EAC was measured to be at 100 dB SPL by the ER-7.
- The bone was oriented to have a direct full-on view on the RWM in order to most accurately measure its vibration velocity with the LDV.
- 5–7 points were arbitrarily placed over the entire area of reflective tape on the RWM.
- Where visibly possible (all conditions other than "fat filling ME" condition) 2–3 points were also chosen along the stapes or prosthesis, depending on the condition.

  ◦ Setup did not provide the optimal angle for this measurement in every case but, when possible, measurement was completed for phase comparison with RWM movement. In all comparisons, the stapes and RWM were about 180° out of phase at low frequencies.
- The vibration velocity of the RWM and TORP/stapes, when possible, were measured by the laser in response to acoustic stimulation delivered through the EAC.

Data analysis

RWM vibration velocities were normalized to sound pressure (m/s/Pa), converted to dB re:1 µm/s/Pa and analyzed using SPSS 23 software (IBM, Armonk, USA). A two-way repeated measures analysis of variance (ANOVA) was performed with Greenhouse-Geisser corrections for three different condition groupings: 1) Normal-NF vs Normal_MEF; 2) Normal_NF vs Pros_NF; and 3) Pros_NF vs pros_FPF vs Pros_MEF. The within-subject factors that were considered were condition and frequency, with post hoc contrasts for condition being simple type (reference of Normal_NF for tests 1 and 2, Pros_NF for test 3). The middle ear has a known frequency response curve. Therefore, any significant frequency main effects are not important results. However, significant condition × frequency interactions are more relevant effects, indicating frequency-specific differences between conditions. The three different ANOVAs were performed rather than just one containing all conditions in order to better interpret any potential frequency interaction effects and because different reference conditions were desired for examining different contrasts. This approach allowed us to only examine effects which were most relevant post hoc, avoiding having to perform 40 (5 conditions × 8 frequencies) comparisons, which would have increased the probability of a type I error. Type I error rate for the three ANOVAs was reduced to 0.05/3 = 0.0167.

Results

Fourteen temporal bones were dissected. Because of technical issues during dissection (ex: TM perforation, accidental footplate removal with stapes suprastructure excision), some bones were unable to be used for certain conditions. Figure 2 details which bones had data available for each condition.

Normal_NF vs Normal_MEF ($n = 9$) (Fig. 3)

The ANOVA showed that there was a significant decrease of 8.6 dB in RWM velocity when the middle was filled with fat ($F(1,7) = 47.386$, $p < 0.0001$). There was also a significant effect of frequency ($F(2.281,15.965) = 23.355$, $p <$

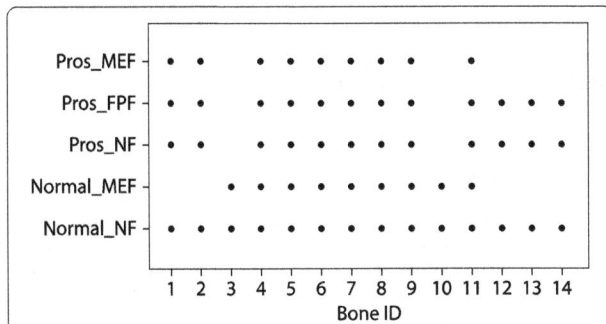

Fig. 2 Number of temporal bones used for each experimental condition

0.0001) on RWM velocity, but there was no significant condition × frequency interaction ($p > 0.05$).

Normal_NF vs Pros_NF ($n = 12$) (Fig. 3)

The ANOVA showed that there was a significant decrease of 13.7 dB in RWM velocity with the prosthesis in place compared to baseline ($F(1,9) = 18.095$, $p = 0.002$). There was also a significant frequency effect ($F(1.476,13.285) = 9.914$, $p = 0.005$) on RWM velocity, but no significant interaction ($p > 0.05$).

Pros_NF vs Pros_FP fat vs Pros_MEF ($n = 9$) (Fig. 3)

The ANOVA showed that there was a significant effect of middle ear condition ($F(1.904,13.329) = 23.405$, $p < 0.0001$) and frequency ($F(1.984,13.887) = 6.849$, $p = 0.009$), but there was no significant interaction ($p > 0.05$). Contrasts showed there was no difference in RWM velocity with placement of fat only around the prosthesis footplate compared to the prosthesis alone (Pros_NF) ($p > 0.05$). There was, however, a significant 7.1 dB loss when fat was used to fill the entire middle ear with the prosthesis (Pros_MEF), as compared to the prosthesis with no fat (Pros_NF) ($p < 0.0001$).

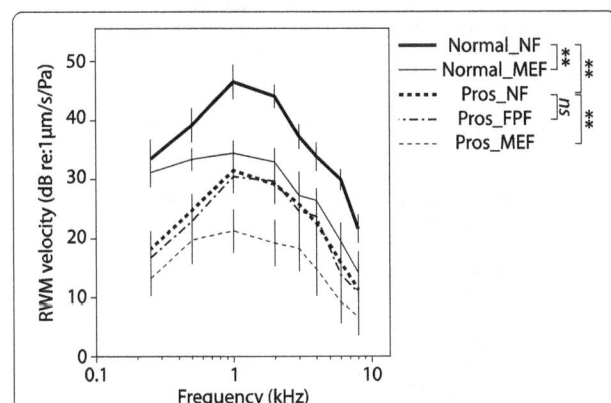

Fig. 3 Round window membrane velocity as a function of frequency for all tested conditions. (ns = not significant. ** = statistically significant)

Discussion

Ossicular reconstruction in the absence of a stapes super-structure can be quite frustrating. Despite intra-operative satisfaction with prosthesis stability, long-term success rates (maintenance of air-bone gap < 20 dB) for TORP prosthesis have been estimated to be as low as 38% [1].

To improve TORP stability on the stapes footplate, and thus minimize its chances of displacing post-operatively, surgeons have tried many different techniques. The use of cartilage between the prosthesis head and TM has been described to not only reduce extrusion rates, but also to improve lateral stability of the prosthesis [8]. Efforts have also been made to stabilize the medial, shaft portion of the prosthesis using a fenestrated cartilage "shoe" placed onto the footplate within which the TORP would stand [9]. Fisch and May suggested placing a small spike at the end of the TORP shaft which would be placed into a fenestration in the footplate [10]. A titanium shoe has also been used to try and stabilize the medial end of the prosthesis onto the stapes footplate [11]. Recently, a "two-point stabilization" technique was described combining prosthesis head stabilization with cartilage combined with an areolar tissue graft between the prosthesis and footplate. Although this latter study demonstrated good post-operative audiologic outcomes, the mean follow-up was 8 months making conclusions about long-term stability difficult to draw [12].

Autologous fat could be a good choice of tissue to use for TORP stabilization given its biocompatibility and ease of harvest in otologic surgery. To better understand the use of fat to stabilize prosthesis position in the middle ear we conducted this study to evaluate the effect on sound transmission to the inner ear of putting variable amounts of fat in the middle ear and measuring RWM velocity in response to sound delivered to the tympanic membrane.

Firstly, our model seems to be appropriate given the 13.7 dB loss in RWM velocity when the virgin middle ear condition (Normal_NF) was compared to the condition with prosthesis alone (Pros_NF). In the literature, an air-bone gap of < 20 dB is generally considered a success for TORP prosthesis [13]. The 13.7 dB loss in our study falls into this range. The fact that the loss is a slightly less than that seen with clinical use of TORP probably reflects the fact that the rest of the middle ear in our cadaver study was completely normal, as opposed to the changes seen in chronic otitis media where TORP prostheses are most often used clinically.

In our study, adding fat around the footplate/distal end of the TORP, did not cause any significant additional hearing loss when compared to the unsupported TORP, and thus can presumably be used intra-operatively to stabilize the prosthesis without dampening sound transmission. However, clearly there are scarring effects and biological changes in the fat in real life that cannot be mimicked in a cadaveric study. We cannot easily predict what these would be, but given that even large amounts of fat in the middle ear have been used for fat myringoplasty [14], and that these must surround the ossicles by necessity, if the fat did indeed cause scar-related fixation of the ossicles we would expect a significant dampening effect on their vibration and an associated hearing loss in these cases. Clinical studies, however, show hearing results from these studies to be quite good [14], making it unlikely that fat has a severe long term effect on middle ear vibration after post-surgery biological changes.

Under the conditions of this study, however, filling the middle ear with fat both in intact middle ears and prosthesis conditions did seem to dampen sound transmission in a significant way, adding about another 8 dB loss. The dampening effect of fat filling the ear makes physiologic sense. Firstly, the fat pushing up against the TM mass loads the drum, similar to fluid in the middle ear [15]. Secondly, by reducing the middle ear air volume, the compliance of the middle ear is decreased, resulting in increased mechanical impedance to sound. As in the comparison of virgin middle ear (Normal_NF) vs prosthesis alone (Pros_NF), we may assume that the additional loss with middle ear fat in our model is likely somewhat underestimated given the absence of chronic middle ear changes in our model. Adding this hearing loss to the hearing loss already associated with having a TORP prosthesis is probably clinically unacceptable. But given the known tendency of fat grafts to atrophy significantly [16], we question whether the hearing loss associated with middle ear fat would be permanent or not. If the fat did atrophy in the middle ear over time, it could serve its potential advantage of TORP stabilization during the healing period. Once the prosthesis becomes fibrosed in place, the atrophy of the fat in the middle ear can then allow for more liberal vibration of the TM and ossicles making the actual reduction in hearing less than what has been measured in this study. Additional work would, however, be needed to evaluate how much fat atrophies as well as its pattern of atrophy in the middle ear and over what time frame to justify its use in this way.

Conclusion

Fat is an easily available, biocompatible autologous graft material. Its use to stabilize the distal end of a TORP prosthesis on the footplate would not likely be associated with any additional hearing loss, as suggested by our cadaver model results. The additional hearing loss caused by using the fat to completely surround the prosthesis and abut the TM is probably not clinically acceptable at this time given the unknown way in which it will atrophy over time in this context.

Abbreviations

EAC: External auditory canal; LDV: Laser Doppler vibrometry; RWM: Round window membrane; TM: Tympanic membrane; TORP: Total ossicular reconstruction prosthesis

Funding

Financial support was provided by the Department of Surgery, Dalhousie University Research Fund. The funding body played no role in the study design, collection/analysis/interpretation of data or manuscript writing.

Authors' contributions

MB contributed to study design, aided in cadaver model preparation and data collection, contributed to data analysis and interpretation as well as manuscript writing. TL contributed to LDV use and set-up, data collection, analysis and interpretation as well as manuscript writing. MA contributed to cadaver model development, data collection, analysis and interpretation as well as manuscript writing. All authors read and approved the final manuscript.

Competing interests

The authors declare that they have no competing interests.

Author details

[1]Division of Otolaryngology-Head and Neck Surgery, Université de Sherbrooke, Sherbrooke, QC, Canada. [2]Division Otolaryngology-Head and Neck Surgery, Nova Scotia Health Authority, Dalhousie University, Halifax, NS, Canada. [3]Division Otolaryngology-Head and Neck Surgery, Nova Scotia Health Authority, Dalhousie University, Halifax, NS, Canada. [4]Centre Hospitalier Université de Sherbrooke, Service d'Otorhinolaryngoloie et Chirurgie Cervicofaciale, Site Hôtel-Dieu, 580 rue Bowen Sud, Sherbrooke, QC J1G 2E8, Canada.

References

1. Yung M. Long-term results of ossiculoplasty: reasons for surgical failure. Otol Neurotol. 2006;27(1):20–6.
2. Huttenbrink KB. Surgical treatment of chronic otitis media. III: middle ear reconstruction. HNO. 1994;42:701–18.
3. Katzke D, Steinbach E, Schodermaier C. The evaluation of allogenous incus transplants removed during revision tym- panoplasty. Arch Otorhinolaryngol. 1982;235:525–8.
4. Smyth GDL. TORPS: how have they fared after five years? J Laryngol Otol. 1983;97:991–3.
5. Huttenbrink KB. Biomechanical aspects of middle ear reconstruction. In: Jahnke K, editor. Current topics in otolar- yngology - head and neck surgery. Middle ear surgery: recent advances and future directions. Stuttgart: Thieme; 2004. p. 23–51.
6. Gold SR, Chaffoo RA. Fat myringoplasty in the guinea pig. Laryngoscope. 1991;101(1 Pt 1):1–5.
7. Alzahrani M, Saliba I. Hyaluronic acid fat graft myringoplasty vs fat patch fat graft myringoplasty. Eur Arch Otorhinolaryngol. 2015;272(8):1873–7.
8. Slater PW, Rizer FM, Schuring AG, et al. Practical use of total and partial ossicular replacement prostheses in ossiculoplasty. Laryngoscope. 1997;107(9):1193–8.
9. Beutner D, Luers JC, Huttenbrink KB. Cartilage 'shoe': a new technique for stabilisation of titanium total ossicular replacement prosthesis at centre of stapes footplate. J Laryngol Otol. 2008;122(7):682–6. Epub 2008 May 19
10. Fisch U, May J. Tympanoplasty, mastoidectomy and stapes surgery. Stuttgart, New York: Thieme; 1994.
11. Mantei T, Chatzimichalis M, Sim JH, et al. Ossiculoplasty with total ossicular replacement prosthesis and omega connector: early clinical results and functional measurements. Otol Neurotol. 2011;32(7):1102–7.
12. Berenholz L, Burkey J, Lippy W. Total ossiculoplasty: advantages of two-point stabilization technique. Int J Otolaryngol. 2012;2012:346260.
13. O'Connell BP, Rizk HG, Hutchinson T, et al. Long-term outcomes of titanium ossiculoplasty in chronic otitis media. Otolaryngol Head Neck Surg. 2016; 154(6):1084–92.
14. Saliba I. Hyaluronic acid fat graft myringoplasty: how we do it. Clin Otolaryngol. 2008;33(6):610–4.
15. Ravicz ME, Rosowski JJ, Merchant SN. Mechanisms of hearing loss resulting from middle-ear fluid. Hear Res. 2004;95(1–2):103–30.

28

Secretory carcinoma: the eastern Canadian experience

David Forner[1]* ⓘ, Martin Bullock[2], Daniel Manders[2], Timothy Wallace[1,3], Christopher J. Chin[1,4], Liane B. Johnson[1], Matthew H. Rigby[1], Jonathan R. Trites[1], Mark S. Taylor[1] and Robert D. Hart[1]

Abstract

Background: Secretory Carcinoma (SC) is a recently described malignancy affecting salivary glands of the head and neck, with a paucity of evidence regarding the natural history, morbidity, and mortality. This study aimed to investigate the current treatment options utilized for SC, as well as its presentation and outcomes.

Methods: This study is a retrospective case series and includes patients diagnosed with SC at four Maritime Canadian institutions. Literature review of patient outcomes following treatment of SC is also included.

Results: Thirteen patients were identified. Parotid was the most common subsite (69%), followed by minor salivary gland (23%) and submandibular gland (8%). All patients were S100 positive and had at least one additional positive confirmatory stain, including mammaglobin, CK7, or vimentin. Two patients had N2b disease. All patients were treated with primary surgery, and four were offered adjuvant radiotherapy. There was one instance of locoregional recurrence, and one of metastasis. Three patients displayed perineural invasion on pathology, and one patient displayed lymphovascular invasion.

Conclusion: Secretory Carcinoma remains understudied regarding its natural history, presentation, and treatment options. This study is the largest single case series in Canada, and highlights the young age and possible aggressiveness of SC. As well, we provide the most comprehensive literature review to date, with a focus on treatment and outcomes for this disease entity.

Keywords: Secretory carcinoma, Canada, Salivary gland, ETV6-NTRK3 mutation, Diagnostics

Background

Secretory Carcinoma (SC) is a recently described malignancy affecting salivary glands of the head and neck. Originally named Mammary Analogue Secretory Carcinoma (MASC), the World Health Organization has proposed the unifying title of SC [1]. The salivary glands share many similar features to the breast, including an identical ductulo-acinar architecture [2]. Indeed, MASC was identified due to its morphological and immunohistochemical similarity to the breast tumor Secretory Carcinoma. Further investigation has recently revealed that a subset of salivary gland tumors originally identified as Acinic Cell Carcinoma (AciCC) are actually the disease entity now known as SC.

Secretory Carcinoma has been shown to express the translocation mutation t (12;15) (p13;q25), which results in the fusion gene ETV6-NTRK3[2]. It was the lack of this mutation in AciCC and its subsequent positivity in SC that ultimately lead to the discovery of SC as a distinct disease entity [3]. In fact, the ETV6-NTRK3 mutation is specific to SC among salivary gland neoplasms [4].

The most common updated diagnoses where SC was identified were those originally diagnosed as AciCC, cystadenocarcinoma (not otherwise specified; NOS), adenoid cystic carcinoma, and low-grade carcinoma NOS. Of these, AciCC was by far the most common initial diagnosis[5].

The diagnosis of SC originally relied upon identification of the ETV6-NTRK3 fusion gene through fluorescence in-situ hybridization (FISH). As additional data has been added to the SC literature, identification of a common morphological and immunohistochemistry

* Correspondence: david.forner@dal.ca
[1]Division of Otolaryngology – Head & Neck Surgery, Department of Surgery, Dalhousie University, 5820 University Ave. 3rd Floor Dickson Bldg, Halifax, NS B3H 2Y9, Canada
Full list of author information is available at the end of the article

pattern has been identified, including strong positivity for vimentin, S100, and mammaglobin.

As it is now realized that some neoplasms previously identified as AciCC are actually SC, differences in the natural history of the diseases have been investigated. The evidence is lacking in this comparison, as is data regarding morbidity and mortality related to SC. It has been found that SC may present with cervical lymph node metastasis more commonly than AciCC. This may drive a decrease in both disease-free survival and overall survival[6]. As well, SC may more commonly develop local recurrence and distant metastasis [6]. Despite these findings, many authors have considered SC to generally be non-aggressive, analogous to AciCC.

Given the paucity of studies investigating SC treatment options and patient outcomes, we investigated a series of these patients in four Canadian institutions. Our outcomes are compared to a literature review presented here, the first to focus on secretory carcinoma outcomes. In addition, diagnostic methods for identification of SC were also investigated. To date, this study is the largest salivary gland SC cohort reported in Canada.

Methods
Patient selection and study design
All patients currently diagnosed with SC in the Canadian Maritime provinces were included in this study, including those with an alternative original diagnosis. Patients were identified using an institutional pathology database at the Queen Elizabeth II Health Science Center in Halifax, Nova Scotia; as well as from the consultation files of MJB. There were no exclusion criteria overall for the study. Particular patients were excluded if chart information was lacking, and are identified appropriately in the results section.

Retrospective chart review was carried out on all patients and included review of initial consultations, follow up reports, operative reports, and pathology review.

Diagnosis
Diagnosis was made by immunohistochemistry and histopathology with or without confirmation of the diagnostic ETV6-NTRK3 fusion gene via fluorescence in situ hybridization (FISH). Confirmatory FISH was performed at the Molecular Diagnostics Laboratory, University of Nebraska Medical Center.

Staging was by the American Joint Committee on Cancer Seventh Edition.

Statistics and research approval
Statistical analysis was completed using the commercially available software SPSS (v21; IBM, Chicago, Illinois). Overall survival and locoregional control rates were determined using Kaplan-Meier curves. Overall survival was calculated with events being considered any cause of patient death, with patients alive at time of last follow-up being censored. Local and locoregional control rates were calculated with events being considered either local or regional recurrences, and patients with no previous recurrence at time of last follow-up, or at time of death, being censored.

The Nova Scotia Research Ethics Board and Quality Improvement & Patient Safety Committee has approved this study as a Quality Assurance/Delivery of Care Initiative under Article 2.5 of the Tri-Council Policy Statement 2.

Literature review
Literature review was carried out in a non-systematic manner. Both MEDLINE/PubMed and Google Scholar searches were completed with the following search terms: "mammary analogue secretory carcinoma," and "secretory carcinoma AND salivary gland." English language articles between 2010 and 2018 were included. Citation lists of included articles were also reviewed for possible missing references. Articles were excluded only if they did not identify patient outcomes.

Results
Clinicopathological features
In total, 13 patients were identified. Patient demographics are presented in Table 1. There was no gender predominance and patients were young overall (mean age 54 years). The majority of patients were considered smokers. This series includes the youngest described patient in the current literature, a 6-year-old male with a parotid tumor.

Staging is presented in Table 1. Tumors were considered small in the majority of cases (T1 or T2), with the majority of patients having no nodal involvement. In those with nodal involvement, both were N2b due to the involvement of multiple ipsilateral lymph nodes. The majority of tumors were parotid in origin. Minor salivary gland subsites included hard palate and lower lip (Table 1).

Cytology and pathology
Cytological investigations and their results are presented in Table 2. The majority of patients had a fine needle aspirate performed, none of which yielded a diagnosis of SC. Warthin's tumor and AciCC were the most common diagnoses on FNA.

Two patients were originally diagnosed as AciCC, and one was originally diagnosed as adenocarcinoma NOS on initial pathology. Both of these patients were diagnosed prior to the recognition of SC as a distinct tumor entity in 2010. The remaining patients were identified as SC. Three patients were diagnosed on the basis of immunohistochemistry and morphology alone, while the remainder of diagnoses were confirmed with FISH for

Table 1 Patient demographics and TNM Staging

Variable	Value
Male Gender	7 (54)
Age	54 (6–84)
Smoker	6 (54)[a]
TNM	
T1	6
T2	3
T3	3
T4	1
N0	11
N1	0
N2a	0
N2b	2
N2c	0
N3	0
M0	13
M1	0
Subsites	
Parotid	9
Submandibular	1
Minor Salivary	0
Hard Palate	2
Lip	1

[a] 11 patients had known smoking history
Gender = number of patients (%), Age = median year (range years), Smoker = number of patients (%), TNM = number of patients

Table 2 Fine Needle Aspirate results

Patient	FNA Result
001	Benign appearing with appearance of oncocytes and lymphocytes suggestive of Warthin's Tumor
002	Few groups of epithelioid cells in a background of lymphocytes suggestive of Warthin's Tumor
003	No FNA performed
004	Mildly atypical cells arranged singly and in sheets with abundant, vacuolated, finely granular cytoplasm suggestive of acinic cell carcinoma vs oncocytic neoplasm
005	Suspicious for malignancy
006	No FNA performed
007	Negative for malignancy
008	No FNA performed
009	No FNA performed
010	Sheets of atypical cells with focally glandular spaces, suggestive of adenocarcinoma vs acinic cell carcinoma vs salivary duct carcinoma
011	Abnormal appearance, suggestive of papillary cystadenoma vs intraductal papilloma, cannot exclude low grade mucoepidermoid
012	Equivocal S100 staining, positive for vimentin and CK7; negative for TTF-1, thyroglobulin, and CD10; suggestive of adenocarcinoma
013	Few malignant cells, positive for AE1 and AE3; negative for LCA and S100; suggestive of poorly differentiated adenocarcinoma

the ETV6-NTRK3 rearrangement. In the two patients without FISH testing, tumors exhibited characteristic morphological features of SC and were therefore not tested. One patient had negative FISH testing but morphological and IHC features were strongly indicative of SC.

Three patients displayed perineural invasion on pathology, and one patient displayed lymphovascular invasion. All patients had immunohistochemistry reporting available, of which all were positive for S100 staining. All patients had at least one additional confirmatory stain that was positive beyond S100, with 11 patients having two additional stains. Additional confirmatory stains included vimentin, mammaglobin, or CK7. Figure 1 displays representative histology and immunohistochemistry patterns obtained from the six-year-old patient. Table 3 lists staining patterns.

Morbidity and mortality

Treatment details, complications, and mortality information is presented alongside patient details in Table 4. All patients were treated with primary surgery, with a minority receiving adjuvant radiotherapy. All nine patients with SC originating in the parotid gland received a parotidectomy, seven of which received a neck dissection. One patient with a minor salivary gland tumor underwent extensive resection and free flap reconstruction.

Complications related to treatment included radiation toxicity, marginal mandibular weakness, velopharyngeal insufficiency requiring surgical correction, and pharyngocutaneous fistula.

The five-year locoregional control rate was 83% (Additional file 1: Figure S1), with one patient having recurrence to the posterior triangle, as well as pulmonary metastasis. The five-year overall survival was 85.7%. There was only one death, in a patient that died secondary to metastatic thyroid cancer unrelated to their diagnosis of SC.

Case details of metastatic secretory carcinoma

A 48-year-old female presented with a 3.7 × 1.9 cm mass deep to the deep lobe of the parotid gland, with extension into the parapharyngeal space. Fine needle aspirate (FNA) of the lesion revealed malignant cells, but without a specific diagnosis. Surgical excision was carried out in the form of a transmandibular approach to facilitate subtotal parotidectomy, neck dissection, and resection of tumor at the skull base.

The tumor demonstrated a high-grade carcinoma with extensive perineural invasion and positive neck nodes. Original pathological diagnosis was of adenocarcinoma NOS of salivary gland origin. Thus, the patient underwent adjuvant radiotherapy in the form of 60 Gy in 30

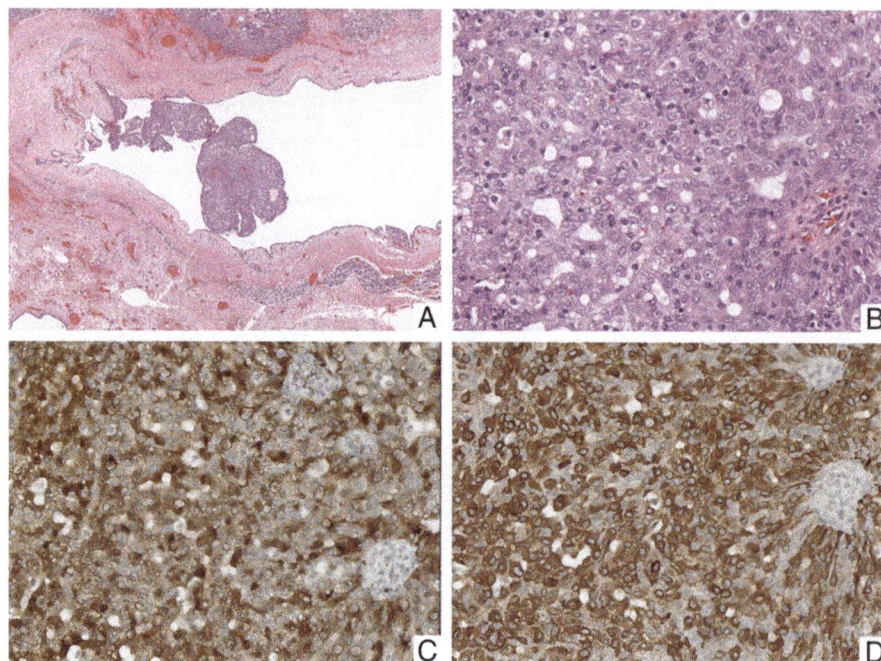

Fig. 1 Low power view of the cystic tumor (**a**). High power view demonstrating microcystic and solid architecture (**b**). The tumor cells exhibit strong nuclear staining for S100 (**c**). The tumor cells demonstrate cytoplasmic expression of mammaglobin (**d**)

fractions to the tumor bed, retropharyngeal lymph nodes, and left neck. An additional 10 Gy over five fractions was administered to the tumor bed and retropharyngeal nodes.

Four years following initial treatment, the patient returned to the otolaryngology clinic with a peri-incisional lesion originally thought to be a traumatic neuroma. Excisional biopsy was performed and revealed malignant cells. Immunohistochemistry was in keeping with her previous parotid cancer, confirming regional metastasis. Secretory

Table 3 Immunohistochemistry staining patterns by patient

Patient	S100	Vimentin	Mammaglobin	CK7
001	+	+	?	+
002	+	+	?	+
003	+	+	?	+
004	+	+	?	+
005	+	+	+	+
006	+	+	+	+
007	+	+	+	+
008	+	?	+	?
009	+	+	+	+
010	+	?	+	?
011	+	+	?	?
012	+	+	?	+
013	+	+	?	+

?: stain not used or not reported

carcinoma was suspected and subsequently confirmed by FISH analysis.

During this same time period, surveillance CT revealed a 0.7 cm lung nodule. This lesion would unfortunately expand to 0.9 cm in size. The patient underwent microcoil guided thoracoscopic wedge resection. Pathology of this lesion demonstrated metastatic SC, with negative margins but positive for vascular invasion. Serial surveillance CT scans were chosen in lieu of systemic chemotherapy. The patient has done well following metastasectomy, with no further evidence of recurrence or metastasis, now ten years from her original diagnosis and 5.5 years from her metastasectomy.

Literature review

Literature review was carried out to investigate patient outcomes following treatment for secretory carcinoma. In total, 37 studies investigating patient outcomes were identified since the original description of secretory carcinoma in 2010 (Table 5) [2, 6–41]. The included studies totaled 227 patients, of which 218 had reliable follow-up for all variables examined in this literature review. Twenty-two studies were case reports or small case series, with only one to four patients. The majority were single patient case reports. The largest study was 36 patients.

The most common primary tumor site was the parotid gland (73%). Of the remaining patients, 43 (19%) primarily involved the minor salivary glands, and 15 involved the submandibular gland (7%). Initial nodal disease was

Table 4 Clinical history, treatment, and complications

Patient	Clinical History	Treatment	Complications
001	84 years old; Not recorded	Submandibular gland excision	Right marginal mandibular nerve weakness
002	72 years old; Two to three months of gradually increasing parotid mass	Parotidectomy	Transient facial nerve weakness
003	54 years old; Ulcerative lesion posterior to last molar on right maxilla with large odontogenic cyst	Partial maxillectomy, partial soft palate excision, selective neck dissection (Levels II-III), radial forearm free flap, split thickness skin graftAdjuvant radiotherapy (60Gy in 30 fractions)	Minor radiation toxicities
004	55 years old; Ten year history of firm, superficial, round mass in the preauricular area on the left side, increasing in size, with mild ternderness on jaw clench	Superficial parotidectomy, selective neck dissection (level IIA), sternocleidomastoid rotational flap	Mild xerostomia
005	44 years old; Parotid mass present for more than one year	Superficial parotidectomyAdjuvant radiotherapy	None
006	65 years old; Six month history of subcutaneous parotid nodule, stable in size and nontender	Excision of mass, followed by:Superficial parotidectomy, selective neck dissection (Level II)	None
007	6 years old; Fourth month history of stable preauricular mass	Superficial right parotidectomy, selective neck dissection (Level IIA)Adjuvant radiotherapy (60 Gy)Left superficial parotidectomy	Radiation dermatitis
008	43 years old; Slowly growing lesion on lower lip mucosa with central ulceration, present for over one year	Excisional biopsy followed by wide local excision	None
009	27 years old; Slowly growing papillomatous lesion of the hard palate for five years	Local excision	None
010	78 years old; Six month history of slowly growing parotid mass with intermittent sharp, stabbing pain	Subtotal parotidectomy, selective neck dissection (Level II to IV)	None
011	22 years old; Two year history of fluctuating parotid lump	Superficial parotidectomy	None
012	72 years old; Three month history of parotid tail or high cervical mass	Parotidectomy, selective neck dissectionAdjuvant radiotherapy (56 Gy in 33 fractions)	Pain, lymphedema
013	48 years old; Parapharyngeal space involvement, including pterygoid muscles	Transmandibular resection of parapharyngeal mass, subtotal parotidectomy, selective neck dissectionAdjuvant radiotherapy (70 Gy in 35 fractions)	Sacrifice of glossopharyngeal nerve, orocutaneous fistula, eustachian tube scarring requiring tympanostomy, esophageal stenosis requiring dilatation, velopharyngeal insufficiency requiring pharyngoplasty with Radiesse, radiation associated toxicities

uncommon, with only 11% of patients presenting with clinically evident lymph nodes or positive nodes after lymph node dissection.

The majority of patients underwent surgical resection (97%), which included a combination of wide local excision, superficial and partial parotidectomy, total parotidectomy and radical parotidectomy. Lymph node dissection was relatively uncommon, as was adjuvant therapy. In total, 17% of patients underwent lymph node dissection of some form, while 26% of patients received adjuvant radiotherapy. Interestingly, one case report examined the possibility of tyrosine kinase inhibitors for the treatment of secretory carcinoma. Several patients did not undergo treatment.

Outcomes were generally favorable. Overall locoregional recurrence was 16%, which included both local recurrence, as well as lymph node metastasis. Distant metastasis was uncommon, with only nine describe reports (4%). In those patients with information available for analysis, mean time to distant metastasis development was 30 months. Four patients with distant metastasis had lung or pleural involvement, two had bone involvement, and two had disseminated disease. The overall survival was 93%, with mean time to death of 38 months after initial treatment. Of those deaths described, 87% were directly due to disease progression.

In those patients that died due to disease, five died due to distant metastasis, with the remainder dying as a result of aggressive locoregional recurrence, including several instances of temporal bone invasion. Skalova's group, in three separate studies, described the greatest number of deaths, including one paper focused on high

Table 5 Literature review

Study	Number of Patients	Tumor Location n (%)	Treatment n (%)	Initial Nodal Disease[b], n (%)	Survival % (cause; timing)	Recurrence n (%); timing	Regional metastasis n (%); timing	Distant metastasis n (%); location timing
Aizawa et al. 2016	1	Parotid: 1 (100)	Surgery: 1 (100)	0 (0)	100%	0 (0)	1 (100); 2 years	0 (0)
Baghai et al. 2017	10	Parotid: 9 (90) MSG: 1 (10)	Surgery: 10 (100) LND: 3 (30) ART: 4 (40) ACRT: 1 (10)	3 (30)	66% (DOD; 24 months, 18 months)	3 (30); 3, 5, 120 months	0	1 (10); bone 15 months
Balanza et al. 2015	1	Parotid: 1 (100)	Surgery: 1 (100)	0 (0)	100%	0 (0)	0 (0)	0 (0)
Boon et al. 2018	31	Parotid: 18 (58) SMG: 1 (3) MSG: 12 (39)	Surgery: 31 (100) LND: 4 (13) ART: 15 (48)	1 (3)	97% (DOC; 48 months)	1 (3); 50 months	0 (0)	0 (0)
Chiosea et al. 2012	36	Parotid: 26 (72) SMG: 3 (10) MSG: 7 (24)	Surgery: 36 (100)LND: 18 (50)ART: 5 (14)ACRT: 2 (6)	4 (11)	97% (DOD; time unknown)	3 (8); time unknown	0 (0)	1 (3); unknown
Cipriani et al. 2017	1	MSG: 1 (100)	Surgery: 1 (100)	0 (0)	0% (DOD; 3 months)	0 (0)	0 (0)	1 (100); lungs 2 months
Cooper et al. 2013	2	MSG: 2 (100)	Surgery: 2 (100)	0 (0)	100%	0 (0)	0 (0)	0 (0)
Din et al. 2016	11	Parotid: 7 (64)SMG: 3 (27)MSG: 1 (9)	Surgery: 10 (91)ART: 2 (18)ACRT: 2 (18)	2 (18)	91% (DOD; 5 years)	3 (38)[a], time unknown	0 (0)	0 (0)
Drilon et al. 2016	1	Parotid: 1 (100)	Surgery: 1 (100)ART: 1 (100)Revision Surgery: 3 procedureCrizotinibEntrectinib	0 (0)	100%	0 (0)	0 (0)	1 (100); lungs 5.5 years
Fakhoury et al. 2016	1	Parotid: 1 (100)	Surgery: 1 (100)	0 (0)	100%	0 (0)	0 (0)	0 (0)
Griffith et al. 2013	6	Parotid: 4 (67)SMG: 1 (17)MSG: 1 (17)	Surgery: 5 (83)LND: 3 (50)No treatment: 1 (17)	1 (17)	100%	0 (0)	0 (0)	0 (0)
Helkamaa et al. 2015	1	MSG: 1 (100)	Surgery: 1 (100)	0 (0)	100%	0 (0)	0 (0)	0 (0)
Higuchi et al. 2014	7	Parotid: 6 (86)SMG: 1 (14)	Surgery: 7 (100)ART: 1 (14)	0 (0)	100%	0 (0)	0 (0)	0 (0)
Hijazi et al. 2014	1	Parotid: 1 (100)	Surgery: 1 (100)	0 (0)	100%	0 (0)	0 (0)	0 (0)
Hwang et al. 2014	1	Parotid: 1 (100)	Surgery: 1 (100)	0 (0)	100%	0 (0)	0 (0)	0 (0)
Inaba et al. 2015	1	Parotid: 1 (100)	Surgery: 1 (100)	0 (0)	100%	0 (0)	0 (0)	0 (0)
Ito et al. 2015	14	Parotid: 9 (64)SMG: 1 (7)MSG: 4 (29)	Surgery: 14 (100)	2 (14)	100%	1 (20)[a], 90 months	0 (0)	0 (0)
Jackson et al. 2017	1	Parotid: 1 (100)	Surgery: 1 (100)	0 (0)	100%	0 (0)	0 (0)	0 (0)

Table 5 Literature review (Continued)

Study	Number of Patients	Tumor Location n (%)	Treatment n (%)	Initial Nodal Disease[b], n (%)	Survival % (cause; timing)	Recurrence n (%); timing	Regional metastasis n (%); timing	Distant metastasis n (%); location timing
Jung et al. 2013	13	Parotid: 11 (85)Unknown: 2 (15)	Surgery: 13 (100)ART: 2 (15)	0 (0)	100%	3 (23); 10–101 months (mean 44)	0 (0)	0 (0)
Jung et al. 2015	9	Parotid: 9 (100)	Unknown	Unknown	Unknown	3 (33); time unknown	0 (0)	0 (0)
Kratochvil et al. 2012	2	MSG: 2 (100)	Surgery: 2 (100)	0 (0)	100%	0 (0)	0 (0)	0 (0)
Laco et al. 2013	2	Parotid: 1 (50)SMG: 1 (50)	Surgery: 2 (100)	0 (0)	100%	0 (0)	0 (0)	0 (0)
Levine et al. 2014	1	Parotid: 1 (100)	Surgery: 1 (100)	0 (0)	100%	0 (0)	0 (0)	0 (0)
Luk et al. 2015	9	Parotid: 9 (100)	Surgery: 9 (100)LND: 1 (11)ART: 1 (11)	1 (11)	89% (DOD; 13 months)	0 (0)	1 (11); 12 months	0 (0)
Luo et al. 2014	1	MSG: 1 (100)	Surgery: 1 (100)ART: 1 (100)	1 (100)	100%	0 (0)	0 (0)	0 (0)
Majewska et al. 2015	7	Parotid: 6 (86)MSG: 1 (14)	Surgery: 7 (100)LND: 2 (29)ART: 2 (29)	3 (43)	71% (DOD; 20 months, 79 months)	2 (29); 4 months, 10 months	1 (14); 48 months	0 (0)
Mossinelli et al. 2018	1	Parotid: 1 (100)	Surgery: 1 (100)	0 (0)	100%	0 (0)	0 (0)	0 (0)
Ngouajio et al. 2017	1	Parotid: 1 (100)	Surgery: 1 (100)LND: 1 (100)	0 (0)	100%	0 (0)	0 (0)	0 (0)
Oza et al. 2016	3	Parotid: 3 (100)	Surgery: 3 (100)	0 (0)	100%	0 (0)	0 (0)	0 (0)
Rastatter et al. 2012	1	Parotid: 1 (100)	Surgery: 1 (100)LND: 1 (100)	1 (100)	100%	0 (0)	0 (0)	0 (0)
Salat et al. 2015	2	Parotid: 2 (100)	Surgery: 2 (100)LND: 1 (50)ART: 2 (100)	0 (0)	100%	0 (0)	0 (0)	0 (0)
Serrano-Arevalo et al. 2015	4	Parotid: 1 (25)SMG: 1 (25)MSG: 2 (50)	Surgery: 2 (50)Nothing: 2 (50)ART: 1 (25)	1(25)	100%	0 (0)	0 (0)	0 (0)
Shah et al. 2015	1	Parotid: 1 (100)	Surgery: 1 (100)	0 (0)	100%	0 (0)	0 (0)	0 (0)
Skalova et al. 2010	16	Parotid: 13 (81)MSG: 3 (19)	Surgery: 16 (100)ART: 7 (44)LND: 1 (6)	1 (6)	94% (DOD; 6 years)	3 (19); 6 months, 2 years, 6 years	1 (6); 86 months	1 (6); lungs 2 years
Skalova et al. 2014	3	Parotid: 3 (100)	Surgery: 3 (100)ART: 2 (67)LND: 1 (33)	0 (0)	0% (3 DOD; 20 months, 4 years, 6 years)	2 (66); 2 years, 6 years	2 (67); 20 months, 4 years	2 (67); disseminated 20 months, 4 years
Skalova et al. 2018	10	Parotid: 7 (70)SMG: 2 (20)MSG: 1 (10)	Surgery: 9 (90)LND: 1 (10)ART: 1 (10)ACRT: 1 (10)Nothing: 1 (10)	1 (10)	78% (1 DOD; 2 years. 1 DOC; 3 years)[a]	0 (0)	1 (11); time unknown	1 (11); bone 15 months

Table 5 Literature review (Continued)

Study	Number of Patients	Tumor Location n (%)	Treatment n (%)	Initial Nodal Disease[b], n (%)	Survival % (cause; timing)	Recurrence n (%); timing	Regional metastasis n (%); timing	Distant metastasis n (%); location timing
Stevens et al. 2015	14	Parotid: 9 (64)Thyroid: 1 (7)SMG: 1 (7)MSG: 3 (21)	Surgery: 12 (88)Nothing: 2 (14)ART: 3 (21)	2 (14)	100%	1 (7); 4 years	0 (0)	1 (7);lungs 4 years
Total	227	Parotid: 166 (73)Other: 61 (27)	Surgery: 211 (97)[c]LND: 37 (17)ART: 56 (26)	24 (11)	93% (13 DOD, 2 DOC)[c]Mean time: 38 months[d]	26 (12)	8 (4)	9 (4)Mean time: 30 months[c], [d]

ART adjuvant radiotherapy, *ACRT* adjuvant chemoradiotherapy, *LND* lymph node dissection, *MSG* minor salivary gland, *SMG* submandibular gland, *DOD* died of disease, *DOC* died of other causes
[a]study includes patients lost to follow up, [b]: category includes patients with clinically evident nodes, or those that had lymph node dissection, [c]: Jung et al. 2014 not included, [d]: Mean time dos not include Chiosea et al

grade transformation, and another series that includes one patient demonstrating high grade transformation. All of these patients died due to their disease. Excluding patients with high grade transformation, only nine patients died due to disease, giving a disease-specific survival of 98%.

Discussion

Secretory carcinoma is a recently described malignancy affecting the salivary glands of the head and neck. It expresses the translocation mutation t (12;15) (p13;q25), which results in the fusion gene ETV6-NTRK3 [2], a characteristic it shares with breast carcinoma of the same name. While several other chromosomal translocations have recently been described in salivary gland tumors, such as EWSR1-ATF1 in hyalinizing clear cell carcinoma and PRKD1–3 gene translocations in cribiform adenocarcinomas of the minor salivary glands [39], there remains a paucity of data surrounding the natural history, diagnosis, treatment, and outcomes of this relatively rare disease.

The initial presentation of SC seems to be mostly uniform. The majority of patients in our series presented with slowly growing, painless masses of the parotid, neck or oral cavity. The minority presented with more rapid growth, aggressive involvement of deep structures, or pain. This is similar to the largest series to date, presented by Chiosea and colleagues, in which 94% of patients presented with a painless mass [6]. Despite a relatively uniform presentation, the age of presentation varied substantially, with the youngest patient being only six years of age. This is amongst the youngest patient described to date [21]. The extremity of this patients age made treatment decisions initially difficult, given there was no data to guide these choices. As with other studies, the most common subsite for presentation in our study was the parotid gland, followed by minor salivary glands, and finally the submandibular gland was involved in a single patient. However, as evidenced by the metastatic SC in this case series, there is potential for aggressive presentations of this disease.

Interestingly, 75% of patients were originally diagnosed with SC in our study. In the three patients initially diagnosed as AciCC or adenocarcinoma NOS, each was diagnosed prior to the initial description of SC. Unfortunately, FNA was not particularly helpful in diagnosis of SC, with no patients receiving this diagnosis by FNA alone. Only 4 of 9 aspirates were correctly diagnosed as either malignant or suspicious for malignancy. The most common diagnoses by FNA were Warthin tumor and AciCC. Generally, the accuracy of fine needle aspiration for salivary gland tumors is good. However, certain diagnoses are relatively easy to make (e.g. benign mixed tumor, Warthin tumor, and high grade malignancies) while other diagnoses are

difficult because many salivary malignancies (including SC) have low grade cytological features and there is overlap between benign and malignant. The cytopathology community has been working to address these issues by developing a classification similar to the Besthesda thyroid classification, in which salivary gland cytopathology specimens are stratified into diagnostic categories with inherent rates of malignancy (Rossi et al. 2018). The cytological features of SC are not well known due to its only recent description (especially when diagnoses in this study were made) and its still unfamiliarity to most cytopathologists. However, the ability to prospectively diagnosis SC with cytology has been previously described [16]. In the study by Griffith and colleagues, SC was found to form papillary groups on cytology, with abundant, prominent or multivacuolated cytoplasm. Both AciCC and SC have similar cellular arrangement on cytology smears. However, SC tends to have increased extracellular and intracellular mucin compared to AciCC, and a greater variation in the size of the cytoplasmic vacuoles found.

Of those patients with FISH data available, there was a high correlation between positivity for an ETV6 rearrangement and varying combinations of S100, vimentin, and mammaglobulin staining. One study demonstrated a 95% correlation between combined morphologic and immunohistochemical features of SC, and the presence of the defining rearrangement [38]. Eleven patients in our series underwent testing with FISH, with ten showing the characteristic translocation. One case showed no evidence of an ETV6 rearrangement, but morphologically and immunohistochemically it was a classic SC. The case was referred for an outside pathology consultation and the consultant agreed with the diagnosis of SC. It is now apparent that in some cases of SC, alternative gene rearrangements are possible, such as ETV6 rearrangements with yet discovered partners (ETV6-X), atypical fusion junctions with NTRK [42], as well as ETV6-RET fusion [43]. All patients in our study had S100 immunohistochemistry available, and all were positive. Additionally, all patients had at least one other positive confirmatory stain. Two other cases were not sent for FISH testing but were consistent by IHC and morphology as described below.

In all cases, the IHC results and morphological features were consistent with the diagnosis of SC (see below), although the staining panels used differed slightly from case to case, largely because they were diagnosed at different times while knowledge of the IHC patterns evolved. Some cases were given a different diagnosis initially because the SC entity was newly described and not widely known. There are many salivary gland tumors with characteristic translocations in which proving the presence of a translocation is not required for the diagnosis (e.g. adenoid cystic carcinoma). The same is *now* true of SC because we are becoming more familiar with the typical morphology and IHC. Basically, at our institution, we would require: typical morphology (as described below), positivity for S100 and another confirmatory stain, and lack of PAS-positive zymogen granules (to exclude acinic cell ca). Confirmatory FISH is currently preferred, but not required by some expert pathologists, especially in cases with typical features.

Characteristic morphological features of SC, include lobulated and/or cystic architecture with tumor cells having fairly abundant, eosinophilic vacuolated cytoplasm, bubbly secretory material, mucin production and low grade vesicular nuclei. Immunohistochemical staining patterns consistent with SC include strong S100 positivity, as well as CK7, vimentin, mammaglobin, and GATA3. They should not be positive for basal/myoepithelial markers, such as p63, nor should they display significant numbers of PAS-positive zymogen granules, which excludes acinic cell carcinoma.

Oncological characteristics and outcomes were similar to previous studies. Tumors were more advanced in our study compared to Chiosea et al., in which 81% were T1 or T2, compared to only 69% in our study. Two had positive lymph nodes (15%). Our patients tended to have more advanced nodal disease (15% N2b, versus 6%). This rate of regional lymph node involvement is overall slightly less than that reported by Chiosea and colleagues, but remains higher than the rate found in ACiCC [6, 44]. Only one patient in our series was found to have locoregional recurrence, and this patient also had distant metastasis (7.7%). This rate of recurrence is similar to Chiosea and colleagues, while the rate of metastasis is higher in our series. Although the 5-year control rate is not reported in Chiosea et al's study, extrapolating from their Kaplan-Meier curve shows eight of 28 patients recurred, five of which were within the first five years (18% recurrence rate before five years). In a study by Jung and colleagues, three of nine patients had recurrence of disease, with a median time to recurrence of 44 months. The only death in our series was unrelated to the diagnosis of SC. It is recognized that both our case series and that by Chiosea and colleagues have small sample sizes and smaller still event rates.

Literature surrounding treatment and outcomes for SC of the salivary glands is somewhat limited. Only 218 patients, over 36 studies, could be reliably included in all variables examined in our literature review, and several key factors could not accurately be examined. Notably, TNM staging, extent of surgical resection, pathology results, radiotherapy intensity, and chemotherapy details were not examined and would offer key pieces of information in deciding future treatment. As well, given that the majority of included patients were identified retrospectively, information applicable to treatment decision making is limited. Yet another limitation is length of followup, with the majority of studies being well below five

years for most patients. Of course, this is owing to SC only recently being described. However, it seems clear that aside from patients with high grade transformation, long term survival is favorable.

The vast majority of SC are considered to be histologically or cytologically "low grade", even when the correct diagnosis is not made initially. This is evident in the fact that many fine needle aspirates are diagnosed as benign lesions, such a Warthin's tumor. In one case in our series, the patient with lung metastases initially was diagnosed as "high grade adenocarcinoma-NOS" and only recognized as SC once it had recurred (and following the initial recognition of the entity). This case was chosen to highlight the possible aggressive nature that SC may display, and documents one of the few cases of distant metastasis in SC, including one of the only patients to survive. The diagnosis of a high-grade adenocarcinoma was based on increased nuclear atypia and mitotic activity. Thus, there is a spectrum of atypia in SC, from morphologically bland to those tumors with more obvious malignant features.

Although the above case was not considered to be an example, many salivary gland carcinomas, such as acinic cell carcinoma, adenoid cystic carcinoma and epithelial-myoepithelial carcinoma, can undergo "high grade transformation" in which the tumor is transformed to a high-grade malignancy that is different from the original tumor [45]. Secretory carcinoma with high-grade transformation resulting in recurrence, metastasis, and cancer related death has been previously described in three cases by Skalova and colleagues [40]. In their report, the first descriptions of high-grade SC morphology were provided. In all three cases, the patients presented with recurrence and died within two to six years following initial treatment.

As has been previously suggested elsewhere, patients in this case series were managed similar to AciCC [3]. All patients underwent primary surgery. Four patients were offered adjuvant radiotherapy. Complications were primarily related to radiation toxicity, and included esophageal stenosis, skin reactions, mucositis, and dysphagia. However, patients did also experience complications related to surgery, including prolonged marginal mandibular nerve weakness, pharyngocutaneous fistulas, and velopharyngeal insufficiency requiring operative intervention.

Further investigations should be completed across multiple institutions in order to bolster the population sizes examined. Despite being more common than originally suspected, SC remains rare overall. In order to accrue patients required to elucidate optimal management, multiple institutions would likely be required.

Conclusion

In summary, SC is a recently described disease entity affecting the head and neck salivary glands. Diagnosis may occur through typical immunohistochemistry and morphological patterns, and should be confirmed in most cases by detection of the ETV6-NTRK3 fusion gene. Patients generally fair well, although the rates of regional lymph node involvement are higher than AciCC. The currently presented series is the largest set of Canadian patients, the only to focus purely on Canadian patients, and amongst the largest series overall. As well, we provide the most comprehensive literature review to date, with a focus on treatment and outcomes for this disease entity.

Abbreviations
AciCC: Acinic Cell Carcinoma; FISH: Fluorescence in situ hybridization; FNA: Fine Needle Aspiration; NOS: Not Otherwise Specified; SC: Secretory Carcinoma

Funding
There are no funding sources to declare.

Authors' contributions
DF completed data gathering, data analysis, manuscript preparation, and approved the final draft of the manuscript. MB assisted in conception of the project, assisted in data gathering, offered expert opinion, manuscript review, and approved the final draft of the manuscript. DM provided imaging, manuscript review, and approved the final draft of the manuscript. TW offered expert opinion, manuscript review, and approved the final draft of the manuscript. CC offered expert opinion, manuscript review, and approved the final draft of the manuscript. LJ offered expert opinion, manuscript review, and approved the final draft of the manuscript. MH offered expert opinion, manuscript review, and approved the final draft of the manuscript. JT offered expert opinion, manuscript review, and approved the final draft of the manuscript. MT offered expert opinion, manuscript review, and approved the final draft of the manuscript. RH assisted in conception of the project, offered expert opinion, manuscript review, and approved the final draft of the manuscript.

Competing interests
The authors declare that they have no competing interests.

Author details
[1]Division of Otolaryngology – Head & Neck Surgery, Department of Surgery, Dalhousie University, 5820 University Ave. 3rd Floor Dickson Bldg, Halifax, NS B3H 2Y9, Canada. [2]Department of Pathology, Dalhousie University, Halifax, NS, Canada. [3]Division of Otolaryngology – Head & Neck Surgery, Department of Surgery, Cumberland Regional Health Care Center, Amherst, NS, Canada. [4]Division of Otolaryngology – Head & Neck Surgery, Department of Surgery, Saint John Regional Hospital, Saint John, NB, Canada.

References
1. Seethala RR, Stenman G. Update from the 4th edition of the World Health Organization classification of head and neck Tumours: tumors of the salivary gland. Head neck pathol. 2017;11(1):55–67.
2. Skálová A, Vanecek T, Sima R, Laco J, Weinreb I, Perez-Ordonez B, Starek I, Geierova M, Simpson RH, Passador-Santos F. Mammary analogue secretory carcinoma of salivary glands, containing the ETV6-NTRK3 fusion gene: a hitherto undescribed salivary gland tumor entity. Am J Surg Pathol. 2010; 34(5):599–608.
3. Stevens TM, Parekh V. Mammary analogue secretory carcinoma. Arch Pathol Lab Med. 2016;140(9):997–1001.
4. Skalova A. Mammary analogue secretory carcinoma of salivary gland origin: an update and expanded morphologic and immunohistochemical spectrum of recently described entity. Head neck pathol. 2013;7(Suppl 1):S30–6.
5. Bishop JA, Yonescu R, Batista D, Eisele DW, Westra WH. Most non-parotid "Acinic cell carcinomas" represent mammary analogue secretory carcinomas. Am J Surg Pathol. 2013;37(7):1053–7.
6. Chiosea SI, Griffith C, Assaad A, Seethala RR. Clinicopathological characterization of mammary analogue secretory carcinoma of salivary glands. Histopathology. 2012;61(3):387–94.
7. Aizawa T, Okui T, Kitagawa K, Kobayashi Y, Satoh K, Mizutani H. A case of mammary analog secretory carcinoma of the lower lip. Journal of Oral and Maxillofacial Pathology. 2016;28(3):277–82.
8. Baghai F, Yazdani F, Etebarian A, Garajei A, Skalova A. Clinicopathologic and molecular characterization of mammary analogue secretory carcinoma of salivary gland origin. Pathol-Res Pract. 2017;213(9):1112–8.
9. Balanzá R, Arrangoiz R, Cordera F, Muñoz M, Luque-de-León E, Moreno E, Toledo C, González E. Mammary analog secretory carcinoma of the parotid gland: a case report and literature review. Int J Surg Case Rep. 2015;16:187–91.
10. Boon E, Valstar M, van der Graaf W, Bloemena E, Willems S, Meeuwis C, Slootweg P, Smit L, Merkx M, Takes R. Clinicopathological characteristics and outcome of 31 patients with ETV6-NTRK3 fusion gene confirmed (mammary analogue) secretory carcinoma of salivary glands. Oral Oncol. 2018;82:29–33.
11. Cipriani NA, Blair EA, Finkle J, Kraninger JL, Straus CM, Villaflor VM, Ginat DT. Salivary gland secretory carcinoma with high-grade transformation, CDKN2A/B loss, distant metastasis, and lack of sustained response to crizotinib. Int J Surg Pathol. 2017;25(7):613–8.
12. Cooper D, Burkey B, Chute D, Scharpf J. Mammary analogue secretory carcinoma of the soft palate: a report of two cases. International Journal of Otolaryngology and Head & Neck Surgery. 2013;2(05):174.
13. Din NU, Fatima S, Kayani N. Mammary analogue secretory carcinoma of salivary glands: a clinicopathologic study of 11 cases. Ann Diagn Pathol. 2016;22:49–53.
14. Drilon A, Li G, Dogan S, Gounder M, Shen R, Arcila M, Wang L, Hyman D, Hechtman J, Wei G. What hides behind the MASC: clinical response and acquired resistance to entrectinib after ETV6-NTRK3 identification in a mammary analogue secretory carcinoma (MASC). Ann Oncol. 2016; 27(5):920–6.
15. Fakhoury E, Abbasi S, Trinh S, Connolly M, Pope RJ. Surgical excision of a rare case of mammary analogue secretory carcinoma: a case review. Journal of Current Surgery. 2016;6(1):30–2.
16. Griffith CC, Stelow EB, Saqi A, Khalbuss WE, Schneider F, Chiosea SI, Seethala RR. The cytological features of mammary analogue secretory carcinoma. Cancer cytopathology. 2013;121(5):234–41.
17. Helkamaa T, Rossi S, Mesimäki K, Suomalainen A, Tarkkanen J, Leivo I, Skalova A, Hagström J. Mammary analog secretory carcinoma of minor palatal salivary glands: a case report and review of the literature. Journal of Oral and Maxillofacial Pathology. 2015;27(5):698–702.
18. Higuchi K, Urano M, Takahashi RH, Oshiro H, Matsubayashi J, Nagai T, Obikane H, Shimojo H, Nagao T. Cytological features of mammary analogue secretory carcinoma of salivary gland: fine-needle aspiration of seven cases. Diagn Cytopathol. 2014;42(10):846–55.
19. Hijazi N, Rahemtulla A, Zhou C, Thomson T. An FNA pitfall: mammary analog secretory carcinoma mistaken for acinic cell carcinoma due to cytoplasmic granules. Human Pathology. 2014;1(4):58–61.
20. Hwang MJ, Wu PR, Chen C-M, Chen C-Y, Chen C-J. A rare malignancy of the parotid gland in a 13-year-old Taiwanese boy: case report of a mammary analogue secretory carcinoma of the salivary gland with molecular study. Medical molecular morphology. 2014;47(1):57–61.
21. Inaba T, Fukumura Y, Saito T, Yokoyama J, Ohba S, Arakawa A, Yao T. Cytological features of mammary analogue secretory carcinoma of the

parotid gland in a 15-year-old girl: a case report with review of the literature. Case Reports in Pathology. 2015;2015:656107.

22. Ito Y, Ishibashi K, Masaki A, Fujii K, Fujiyoshi Y, Hattori H, Kawakita D, Matsumoto M, Miyabe S, Shimozato K. Mammary analogue secretory carcinoma of salivary glands. Am J Surg Pathol. 2015;39(5):602–10.

23. Jackson B, Pratt T, Van Rooyen A. Mammary analogue secretory carcinoma: a rare salivary gland tumour. S Afr Med J. 2017;107(4):304–6.

24. Jung MJ, Kim SY, Nam SY, Roh JL, Choi SH, Lee JH, Baek JH, Cho KJ. Aspiration cytology of mammary analogue secretory carcinoma of the salivary gland. Diagn Cytopathol. 2015;43(4):287–93.

25. Jung MJ, Song JS, Kim SY, Nam SY, Roh J-L, Choi S-H, Kim S-B, Cho K-J. Finding and characterizing mammary analogue secretory carcinoma of the salivary gland. Korean journal of pathology. 2013;47(1):36.

26. Kratochvil FJ III, Stewart JC, Moore SR. Mammary analog secretory carcinoma of salivary glands: a report of 2 cases in the lips. Oral Surg Oral Med Oral Pathol Oral Radiol. 2012;114(5):630–5.

27. Laco J, Švajdler M Jr, Andrejs J, Hrubala D, Hácová M, Vaněček T, Skálová A, Ryška A. Mammary analog secretory carcinoma of salivary glands: a report of 2 cases with expression of basal/myoepithelial markers (calponin, CD10 and p63 protein). Pathol-Res Pract. 2013;209(3):167–72.

28. Levine P, Fried K, Krevitt LD, Wang B, Wenig BM. Aspiration biopsy of mammary analogue secretory carcinoma of accessory parotid gland: another diagnostic dilemma in matrix-containing tumors of the salivary glands. Diagn Cytopathol. 2014;42(1):49–53.

29. Luk PP, Selinger CI, Eviston TJ, Lum T, Yu B, O'Toole SA, Clark JR, Gupta R. Mammary analogue secretory carcinoma: an evaluation of its clinicopathological and genetic characteristics. Pathology. 2015;47(7):659–66.

30. Luo W, Lindley SW, Lindley PH, Krempl GA, Seethala RR, Fung K-M. Mammary analog secretory carcinoma of salivary gland with high-grade histology arising in hard palate, report of a case and review of literature. Int J Clin Exp Pathol. 2014;7(12):9008.

31. Majewska H, Skálová A, Stodulski D, Klimková A, Steiner P, Stankiewicz C, Biernat W. Mammary analogue secretory carcinoma of salivary glands: a new entity associated with ETV6 gene rearrangement. Virchows Arch. 2015; 466(3):245–54.

32. Mossinelli C, Pigni C, Sovardi F, Occhini A, Preda L, Benazzo M, Morbini P, Pagella F. Synchronous parotid (mammary analog) secretory carcinoma and Acinic cell carcinoma: report of a case. Head neck pathol. 2018:1–6.

33. Ngouajio AL, Drejet SM, Phillips DR, Summerlin D-J, Dahl JP. A systematic review including an additional pediatric case report: pediatric cases of mammary analogue secretory carcinoma. Int J Pediatr Otorhinolaryngol. 2017;100:187–93.

34. Oza N, Sanghvi K, Shet T, Patil A, Menon S, Ramadwar M, Kane S. Mammary analogue secretory carcinoma of parotid: is preoperative cytological diagnosis possible? Diagn Cytopathol. 2016;44(6):519–25.

35. Rastatter JC, Jatana KR, Jennings LJ, Melin-Aldana H. Mammary analogue secretory carcinoma of the parotid gland in a pediatric patient. Otolaryngol Head Neck Surg. 2012;146(3):514–5.

36. Salat H, Mumtaz R, Ikram M, Din NU. Mammary analogue secretory carcinoma of the parotid gland: a third world country perspective—a case series. Case reports in otolaryngology. 2015;2015:4.

37. Serrano-Arévalo ML, Mosqueda-Taylor A, Domínguez-Malagón H, Michal M. Mammary analogue secretory carcinoma (MASC) of salivary gland in four Mexican patients. Medicina oral, patologia oral y cirugia bucal. 2015;20(1):e23.

38. Shah AA, Wenig BM, LeGallo RD, Mills SE, Stelow EB. Morphology in conjunction with immunohistochemistry is sufficient for the diagnosis of mammary analogue secretory carcinoma. Head neck pathol. 2015;9(1):85–95.

39. Skálová A, Stenman G, Simpson RH, Hellquist H, Slouka D, Svoboda T, Bishop JA, Hunt JL, Nibu K-I, Rinaldo A. The role of molecular testing in the differential diagnosis of salivary gland carcinomas. Am J Surg Pathol. 2018;42(2):e11–27.

40. Skálová A, Vanecek T, Majewska H, Laco J, Grossmann P, Simpson RH, Hauer L, Andrle P, Hosticka L, Branžovský J. Mammary analogue secretory

carcinoma of salivary glands with high-grade transformation: report of 3 cases with the ETV6-NTRK3 gene fusion and analysis of TP53, β-catenin, EGFR, and CCND1 genes. Am J Surg Pathol. 2014;38(1):23–33.

41. Stevens TM, Kovalovsky AO, Velosa C, Shi Q, Dai Q, Owen RP, Bell WC, Wei S, Althof PA, Sanmann JN, et al. Mammary analog secretory carcinoma, low-grade salivary duct carcinoma, and mimickers: a comparative study. Modern pathology. 2015;28(8):1084–100.

42. Skálová A, Vanecek T, Simpson RHW, Laco J, Majewska H, Baneckova M, Steiner P, Michal M. Mammary analogue secretory carcinoma of salivary glands: molecular analysis of 25 ETV6 gene rearranged tumors with lack of detection of classical ETV6-NTRK3 fusion transcript by standard RT-PCR Report of 4 Cases Harboring ETV6-X Gene Fusion. Am J Surg Pathol. 2016;40(1):3–13.

43. Skalova A, Vanecek T, Martinek P, Weinreb I, Stevens TM, Simpson RH, Hyrcza M, Rupp NJ, Baneckova M, Michal M Jr. Molecular profiling of mammary analog secretory carcinoma revealed a subset of tumors harboring a novel ETV6-RET translocation: report of 10 cases. Am J Surg Pathol. 2018;42(2):234–46.

44. Chiosea SI, Griffith C, Assaad A, Seethala RR. The profile of acinic cell carcinoma after recognition of mammary analog secretory carcinoma. Am J Surg Pathol. 2012;36(3):343–50.

45. Costa AF, Altemani A, Hermsen M. Current concepts on dedifferentiation/ high-grade transformation in salivary gland tumors. Pathol Res Int. 2011; 2011:325965.

29

The impact of chronic airway disease on symptom severity and global suffering in Canadian rhinosinusitis patients

Kimberly Luu[1]*(iD), Jason Sutherland[2], Trafford Crump[3], Giuping Liu[2] and Arif Janjua[1]

Abstract

Background: Patients with Chronic Rhinosinusitis (CRS) can suffer from a significant decline in their quality of life. CRS patients have a high prevalence of comorbid conditions and it is important to understand the impact of these conditions on their CRS-related quality of life. This study measures the impacts of chronic pulmonary comorbidities on quality of life, pain, and depression scores among patients with CRS awaiting Endoscopic Sinus Surgery (ESS).

Methods: This study is based on cross-sectional analysis of prospectively collected patient-reported outcome data collected pre-operatively from patients waiting for ESS. Surveys were administered to patients to assess sino-nasal morbidity (SNOT-22), depression and pain. The impact of pulmonary comorbidity on SNOT-22 scores, pain and depression was measured.

Results: Two hundred fifthy-three patients were included in the study, 91 with chronic pulmonary comorbidity. The mean SNOT-22 scores were significantly higher among patients with chronic pulmonary comorbidities than among patients without (37 and 48, respectively). This difference is large enough to be clinically significant. Patients with chronic pulmonary comorbidities reported slightly higher depression scores than those without.

Conclusions: This study found that among CRS patients waiting for ESS, chronic pulmonary comorbidities are strongly associated with significantly higher symptom burden.

Keywords: Endoscopic sinus surgery, Comorbidities, Quality of life, Unified airway

Background

At least 5 % of Canadians suffer from Chronic Rhinosinusitis (CRS) [1, 2]. Patients with CRS may experience significant facial pain, nasal congestion, nasal discharge and, or a reduction in their sense of smell [3]. Relative to other chronic diseases, it is estimated that the quality-of-life burden of patients with CRS is comparable to diseases such as congestive heart failure, chronic obstructive pulmonary disease (COPD), angina, and back pain [4]. This decrease in quality of life is the reason patients seek treatment and the goal of treatment is to decrease this symptom burden. In order to better triage and treat CRS patients, we need to identify and explore what factors negatively affect these patients' quality of life.

Patients with CRS are known to have a significantly higher prevalence of comorbid conditions [5], most commonly asthma and chronic pulmonary diseases [1]. Additionally, the concept of a united airway theory connects disorders of the lower and upper respiratory tract, prompting clinicians to consider the impact of respiratory pathology when managing CRS [6]. It is therefore likely that lower airway diseases will have an effect on the symptomatology of CRS patients. It is important to elaborate on the effect that lower respiratory conditions have on CRS patients, so that identification of these comorbidities will prompt clinicians to treat these patients appropriately and thoroughly.

There is evidence that correlates lower airway disease severity with radiological CRS severity [7]. However, radiologic evidence does not correlate well with clinical

* Correspondence: kimberlyluu@gmail.com
[1]Division of Otolaryngology – Head & Neck Surgery, University of British Columbia, Gordon and Leslie Diamond Health Care Centre, DHCC, Vancouver General Hospital, 4th. Floor Rm. 4299B 2775 Laurel Street, Vancouver, BC V5Z 1M9, Canada
Full list of author information is available at the end of the article

symptoms, thus cannot necessarily be used as an indication of symptom burden. Clinical management of CRS is based on disease symptoms and not physical or radiologic findings. Presently, although generally assumed, we do not have much evidence that lower airway disease impacts quality of life, pain, sinonasal symptoms, or depression in CRS patients. Thus, the primary objective of this study is to measure the relationship between chronic pulmonary comorbidities and patients' sino-nasal symptom severity, pain and depression prior to Endoscopic Sinus Surgery (ESS).

Research on CRS is underrepresented in the literature when taking into account the clinical burden of disease compared to other chronic illnesses such as asthma or diabetes [8]. Dissemination of this information will provide a better understanding of this relationship and thus a more holistic understanding of CRS patients. This information will help inform all aspects of patient management, including: involvement of multidisciplinary teams, identification and management of specific symptoms, and triage decisions about patients who may most benefit from ESS.

Methods

This study is a prospective cross sectional analysis of patient reported outcomes. Consecutive new patients diagnosed with chronic rhinosinusitis by two tertiary care rhinologists in the Vancouver Coastal Health Authority were prospectively identified. To target patients with quality of life impact from CRS, the patients who failed medical management and consented for endoscopic sinus surgery were recruited for the study. Data collection was initiated in September 2012 and ended April 2016. This study is approved by the University of British Columbia's Behavioural Research Ethics Board.

Surveys were administered to the enrolled patients through mail or online methods, depending on the preferences of the patient. Response was encouraged through a maximum of three follow-up telephone calls. The survey package included questions regarding patients' demographic characteristics, such as age and gender. Additional demographic data, including comorbidities, medications, and past surgical history were additionally obtained from the patients through surgical intake forms. Patient reported outcomes data was obtained via instruments for CRS-specific symptoms, depression, and pain. All instruments utilized are validated and widely used in measuring and reporting health-related quality of life outcomes.

Instruments: SNOT-22, PHQ-9, PEG-3

The Sino-Nasal Outcome Test-22 (SNOT-22) was the instrument used to measure CRS-specific symptoms. The SNOT-22 is a common and well-validated instrument [9, 10], that includes twenty-two items associated with sino-nasal health. Each item is ranked using a Likert scale ranging from 1 (no problem) to 5 (problem as bad as it can be). The rankings are aggregated into a global score that ranges from 22 (best health) to 110 (worst health). A nine-point change in the SNOT-22 global score has demonstrated to be clinically meaningful [9].

Depression was measured using the Patient-Health Questionnaire-9 (PHQ-9) [11]. The PHQ-9 uses nine items to measure domains of depressive symptoms and functional impairment. Each items is ranked from zero (not at all bothered) to three (bothered nearly every day). The rankings are aggregated into a global score that ranges from zero to 27. Higher PHQ-9 scores are associated with more severe depression symptoms, and scores above nine are associated with clinically significant depression [12].

Pain was measured using the PEG-3 instrument [13]. This is a three-item instrument measuring domains of pain intensity and interference. Each item in the PEG-3 is ranked from zero (no pain) to 10 (highest level of pain). The overall score is determined by averaging the items' rankings, thus ranging from zero to 10. An overall score above three is associated with clinically significant pain [14].

Analysis

Using the chart review comorbidity data, patients were categorized into one of two groups. The first group was defined as having a chronic pulmonary comorbidity if there was documentation of the following comorbidities: asthma, emphysema, or chronic bronchitis. The second group did not have documentation of any chronic pulmonary comorbidity.

Differences between the two groups in terms of their demographic characteristics were evaluated using Pearson's chi-square tests. Differences between the two groups in terms of their overall SNOT-22, PHQ-9, and PEG-3 scores were tested using t-tests.

The research question being answered was whether chronic pulmonary comorbidity was associated with poorer health-related quality-of-life. To do this, three multivariate linear regression models were developed to measure the association between a chronic pulmonary comorbidity and the SNOT-22, PHQ-9, and PEG-3 scores, respectively. In the linear models, the effects of age group (defined in 10-year increments), gender, and the number of other comorbid conditions (defined as 0, 1, or ≥ 2, comorbidities other than chronic pulmonary comorbidities) were adjusted for.

Tests of significance of individual variables were evaluated and reported at the 5% level. All variables were retained in the regression models, irrespective of their significance.

Results

Overall, 34% of eligible CRS patients waiting for elective ESS in VCH returned their survey. Among the study's patients, 36% reported a chronic pulmonary comorbidity. Table 1 shows that patients in both groups were comparable in terms of distribution of age. Women were much more likely to report a chronic pulmonary comorbidity than men. Patients with a chronic pulmonary comorbidity were somewhat more likely to report hypertension, arthritis, diabetes and kidney disease, though somewhat less likely to report heart failure, though the differences were not statistically significant.

As reported in Table 2, there were a number of significant differences between patients with and without chronic pulmonary comorbidities. Based on the bivariate results, patients with a chronic pulmonary comorbidity had significantly higher SNOT-22, PHQ-9 and PEG-3 scores, than those without a chronic pulmonary comorbidity. The difference in mean SNOT-22 scores between the two groups was greater than the minimal clinically important difference of nine points.

When age, gender, and the presence of other comorbidities were controlled for in the multivariate linear models, only the differences in the SNOT-22 scores remained significant between those with a chronic pulmonary comorbidity and those without. As detailed in Table 3, age and the presence of other comorbidities eliminated the effect of having a chronic pulmonary comorbidity on the differences between either the PHQ-9 or PEG-3 scores. Although, the results for the PHQ-9 scores were on the threshold of statistical significance ($p = 0.06$).

Discussion

This study set out to examine the association between chronic pulmonary conditions and the quality of life in CRS patients. We observed that patients with asthma, emphysema or chronic bronchitis reported significantly more severe CRS-specific symptoms compared to those who did not report having these conditions.

The concomitant relationship between lower airway disease and upper airway symptoms suggests a mechanism of inflammation that targets all respiratory mucosa and elevates the patient's overall inflammatory load. Previous studies examining this relationship report comparable results [15, 16]. Alobid et al. looked at the specific relationship between in asthma, aspirin sensitivity and CRS patients with nasal polyposis and found that asthmatic patients with nasal polyps had worse quality of life than non-asthmatic patients [17]. Other authors have found the severity of CRS is correlated with the presence of Asthma [18]. More recent studies have investigated the relationship between asthma and CRS in further detail. Multiple authors have found that severity of asthma, as measured by a validated score or number of exacerbations, is correlated with severity of CRS symptoms. This suggests that the clinical status of asthma, not merely the presence of asthma, impacts CRS severity [19, 20].

Additionally, data from the respiratory literature examines this 'unified airway phenomenon' from a lower

Table 1 Summary statistics of CRS patients

	CRS patients without Chronic Pulmonary Comorbidities		CRS patients with Chronic Pulmonary Comorbidities	
	N	%	N	%
Overall	162	100	91	100
Gender				
Female	71	43.8%	55	60.4%
Male	91	56.2%	36	39.6%
Age				
< 40	27	16.7%	13	14.3%
40–49	29	17.9%	19	20.9%
50–59	46	28.4%	25	27.5%
60–69	35	21.6%	25	27.5%
70+	25	15.4%	9	9.9%
Other Chronic Health Conditions (Top 5)				
Hypertension	42	25.9%	26	28.6%
Arthritis	42	25.9%	28	30.8%
Diabetes	20	12.4%	12	13.2%
Heart failure	14	8.6%	6	6.6%
Kidney or renal disease	8	4.9%	6	6.6%

Table 2 Average scores of the SNOT-22, PHQ-9, and PEG-3, comparing patients with chronic pulmonary comorbidities to those without

	Without Chronic Pulmonary Comorbidities	With Chronic Pulmonary Comorbidities	P-Value
Instrument	Mean (SD)	Mean (SD)	T-Test
SNOT-22	37.7 (21.6)	48.6 (21.9)	< 0.001
Depression (PHQ-9)	4.3 (4.7)	6.2 (6.0)	0.010
Pain (PEG-3)	2.5 (2.6)	3.4 (2.9)	0.009

airway perspective, showing that patients with moderate to severe COPD also have higher SNOT 20 scores, compared with those with mild COPD [21]. When assessing overall quality-of-life metrics, the literature suggests that both upper and lower airway symptoms substantially impact quality of life [22, 23]. The results reported in this study add to this knowledge, encompassing CRS patients with and without nasal polyposis and a larger class of lower airway diseases. What is still unclear is whether the association between the upper and lower airway disease is an additive or synergistic effect.

The results from this study also suggest a complex relationship between upper and lower respiratory disease and depression. While the results were not statistically significant, this study's use of a sensitive instrument for depression found that depression scores were higher among patients with a chronic pulmonary comorbidity. This finding is supported by other studies that examine

the relationship between chronic conditions and depression. It has been observed that the prevalence of depression is higher among patients with COPD and asthma [24, 25]. Anxiety has also been shown to occur in higher prevalence in CRS patients and results in worse quality of life, as well as reduced improvement following ESS [26].

Since the rate of depression among people with CRS reportedly exceeds 30% [27], the findings of this study are potentially relevant given that, in the VCH region, wait times for elective ESS can exceed 6 months. The results from this study should draw attention to potential gaps in mental health interventions for patients with CRS awaiting surgery. Targeted interventions could be used to improve the mental health of these patients. These opportunities are particularly salient for CRS patients with a chronic pulmonary comorbidity where this study showed a much higher symptom burden, but only modestly higher depression scores.

There are a number of limitations of this study. The presence of asthma, emphysema, or chronic bronchitis was patient-reported, and not clinically verified. We believe that this reflects the predominant way in which this data is obtained during a clinical encounter, and thus it is a reasonable surrogate marker. If the evidence is based on data that can be simply obtained on history, this information can be used for practical point of care management, such as increased symptom management, referral and surgical triage. Patients with Aspirin

Table 3 Multivariate regression results of the SNOT-22, PEG-3 and PHQ-9 scores among CRS patients waiting for ESS, evaluating the impact of at least one chronic pulmonary comorbidity

Model Effect	SNOT-22 Score			PEG-3			PHQ-9		
	Estimate	SE	P-Value	Estimate	SE	P-Value	Estimate	SE	P-Value
Intercept	18.3	4.5	< 0.001	0.53	0.15	< 0.001	1.03	0.17	< 0.001
Gender									
Female	4.7	2.6	0.070	0.16	0.09	0.056	−0.07	0.10	0.472
Male (Ref.)									
Age									
< 40	13.9	5.0	0.005	0.49	0.17	0.003	0.46	0.19	0.015
40–49	19.9	4.7	< 0.001	0.47	0.16	0.003	0.52	0.18	0.003
50–59	13.5	4.4	0.002	0.48	0.15	0.001	0.39	0.17	0.020
60–69	12.9	4.4	0.003	0.21	0.15	0.150	0.16	0.17	0.358
70+ (Ref.)									
Chronic Pulmonary Comorbidity									
Yes	8.1	2.7	0.002	0.14	0.09	0.127	0.20	0.11	0.065
No (ref.)									
Other Comorbidity Count									
0 (Ref.)									
1	2.0	3.3	0.547	0.29	0.11	0.007	0.32	0.13	0.013
2 or more	13.6	3.2	< 0.001	0.64	0.11	< 0.001	0.76	0.12	< 0.001

Exacerbated Respiratory Disease (AERD) were not excluded from the chronic comorbidity group. There is evidence that this unique group of patients has worse CRS related symptomatology and their inclusion may increase the differences observed between our two groups. Finally, it is possible that the findings' generalizability was undermined by the response rate among potential study participants; and although we did not detect noticeable differences between respondents and non-respondents, it was possible that there were some unmeasured sources of bias attributable to response rate.

The respiratory diseases were pooled, precluding sub-group analysis. Future research could provide insight into whether, individually, these conditions were associated with differential CRS symptom burden. In addition, the next study could add disease severity measures, such as pulmonary function tests, to isolate sources of variability among sub-groups' levels of self-reported health.

Conclusion

This study found that among CRS patients waiting for ESS, chronic pulmonary comorbidities are strongly associated with significantly higher symptom burden. Patients with asthma, emphysema, or chronic bronchitis reported significantly higher SNOT-22 scores than compared to those who did not report having these conditions. The difference in SNOT-22 scores was over nine, indicative of clinical significance.

Abbreviations

COPD: Chronic obstructive pulmonary disease; CRS: Chronic rhinosinusitis; ESS: Endoscopic sinus surgery; PEG-3: Pain outcome test; PHQ-9: Patient Health Questionnaire-9; SNOT-22: Sino-Nasal Outcome Test-22

Funding

This study was partially funded by the Canadian Institutes for Health Research (CIHR) and in-kind contributions from Vancouver Coastal Health authority (VCH). Sutherland is a Scholar of the Michael Smith Foundation for Health Research (MSFHR). CIHR, MSFHR and VCH had no role in developing the methods, analyzing the data, or interpreting the results.

Authors' contributions

Dr. KL drafted the project concept and proposal and the majority of the manuscript. Drs. TC and JS contributed to project concept, data analysis and manuscript drafting. Dr. GL performed the majority of the data analysis. Dr. AJ oversaw the project conception, data analysis, and write up. All authors read and approved the final manuscript.

Competing interests

The authors declare that they have no competing interests.

Author details

[1]Division of Otolaryngology – Head & Neck Surgery, University of British Columbia, Gordon and Leslie Diamond Health Care Centre, DHCC, Vancouver General Hospital, 4th. Floor Rm. 4299B 2775 Laurel Street, Vancouver, BC V5Z 1M9, Canada. [2]UBC Centre for Health Services and Policy Research, Vancouver Campus, 201-2206 East Mall, Vancouver, BC V6T 1Z3, Canada. [3]University of Calgary, 2500 University Dr. NW, Calgary, AB T2N 1N4, Canada.

References

1. Habib ARR, Javer AR, Buxton JA. A population-based study investigating chronic rhinosinusitis and the incidence of asthma. Laryngoscope. 2015:17–20. https://doi.org/10.1002/lary.25831.
2. Macdonald M, McNally D, Massoud E. The health and resource utilization of Canadians with chronic rhinosinusitis. Laryngoscope. 2009;119:184–9.
3. Chen Y, Dales R, Lin M. The epidemiology of chronic rhinosinusitis in Canadians. Laryngoscope. 2003;113(7):1199–205.
4. Gliklich R, Metson R. The health impact of chronic sinusitis in patients seeking otolaryngologic care. Otolaryngol Head Neck Surg. 1995;113(1):104–9.
5. Chung S, Chen P, Lin H, Al E. Comorbidity profile of chronic rhinosinusitis: a population-based study. Laryngoscope. 2014;124:1536–41.
6. Feng C, Miller M, Simon R. The united allergic airway: connections between allergic rhinitis, asthma, and chronic sinusitis. Am J Rhinol Allergy. 2012;26(3):187–90.
7. Lin D, Chandra R, Bruce K, Al E. Association between severity of asthma and degree of chronic rhinosinusitis. Am J Rhinol Allergy. 2011;25(4):205–8.
8. Hopkins C, Gillett S, Slack R, Lund VJ, Browne JP. Psychometric validity of the 22-item Sinonasal outcome test. Clin Otolaryngol. 2009;34:447–54. https://doi.org/10.1111/j.1749-4486.2009.01995.x.
9. Rudmik L, Soler ZM, Mace JC, Deconde AS, Schlosser RJ, Smith TL. Using preoperative SNOT-22 score to inform patient decision for endoscopic sinus surgery. Laryngoscope. 2015;125(7):1517–22. https://doi.org/10.1002/lary.25108.
10. Martin A, Rief W, Klaiberg A, Al E. Validity of the brief patient health questionnaire mood scale (PHQ-9) in the general population. Gen Hosp Psychiatry. 2006;28:171–7.
11. Kroenke K, Spitzer RL, Williams JB. The PHQ-9: validity of a brief depression severity measure. J Gen Intern Med. 2001;16(9):606–13. http://www.pubmedcentral.nih.gov/articlerender.fcgi?artid=1495268&tool=pmcentrez&rendertype=abstract. Accessed 12 Feb 2013
12. Krebs E, Lorenz K, Bair M, et al. Development and initial validation of the PEG, a three-item scale assessing pain intensity and interference. J Gen Intern Med. 2009;24(6):733–8. https://doi.org/10.1007/s11606-009-0981-1.
13. Miller K, Combs S, van Puymbroeck M, et al. Fatigue and pain: relationships with physical performance and patient beliefs after stroke. Top Stroke Rehabil. 2013;20(4):347–55. https://doi.org/10.1310/tsr2004-347.
14. Ragab S, Scadding G, Lund V. Treatment of chronic rhinosinusitis and its effect on asthma. Eur Respir J. 2006;28:68–74.
15. Dunlop G, Scadding G, Lund V. The effect of endoscopic sinus surgery on asthma: management of patients with chronic rhinosinusitis, nasal polyposis, and asthma. Am J Rhinol Allergy. 1999;14(4):261–5.
16. Alobid I, Benitez P, Bernal-Sprekelsen M, et al. The impact of asthma and aspirin sensitivity on quality of life of patients with nasal polyposis. Qual Life Res. 2005;14:789–93.
17. Banoub RG, et al. Relationship between chronic rhinosinusitis exacerbation frequency and asthma control. Laryngoscope. 2017;128:1033–8.
18. Campbell AP, et al. Association between asthma and chronic rhinosinusitis severity in the context of asthma control. Otolaryngol Head Neck Surg. 2018;158(2):386–90.
19. Hurst J, Wilinson T, Donaldson G, Wedzicha J. Upper airway symptoms and quality of life in chronic obstructive pulmonary disease (COPD). Respir Med. 2004;98(8):767–70.
20. Guatt GH, Berman LB, Townsend M, et al. A measure of quality of life for clinical trials in chronic lung disease. Thorax. 1987;42:773–8.
21. Birch DS, Saleh HA, Wodehouse T, et al. Assessing the quality of life for patients with chronic rhinosinusitis using the "rhinosinusitis disability index". Rhinology. 2001;39(4):191–6.
22. Moussas G, Tselebis A, Karkanias A, et al. A comparative study of anxiety and depression in patients with bronchial asthma, chronic obstructive pulmonary disease and tuberculosis in a general hospital of chest diseases. Ann General Psychiatry. 2008;7(1):7.
23. Di Marco F, Verga M, Reggente M, et al. Anxiety and depression in COPD patients: the roles of gender and disease severity. Respir Med. 2006;100: 1767–74.

24. Steele T, Mace J, Smith T. Does comorbid anxiety predict quality of life
     outcomes in patients with chronic rhinosinusitis following endoscopic sinus
     surgery? Int Forum Allergy Rhinol. 2015;5:829–38.
25. Brandsted R, Sindwani R. Impact of depression on disease-specific
     symptoms and quality of life in patients with chronic rhinosinusitis. Am J
     Rhinol Allergy. 2007;21:150–4.
26. Rudmik L. Chronic rhinosinustis: an under-researched epidemic.
     J Otolaryngol Head Neck Surg. 2015;44:11.
27. Pearlman AN, Chandra RK, Chang D, et al. Relationships between severity of
     chronic rhinosinusitis and nasal polyposis, asthma, atopy. Am J Rhinol
     Allergy. 2009;23:145–8.

30

Efficacy of postoperative pain management in head and neck cancer patients

Ashley Hinther[1], Steven C. Nakoneshny[2], Shamir P. Chandarana[1,2], T. Wayne Matthews[1,2] and Joseph C. Dort[1,2*] (iD)

Abstract

Background: Our study quantifies the effectiveness of perioperative pain control in a cohort of patients undergoing major head and neck surgery with free flap reconstruction. Our long-term goal is to improve pain control and thereby increase mobility, decrease postoperative complications and decrease hospital stay.

Methods: A retrospective analysis was performed at a tertiary, academic head and neck surgical oncology program in Calgary, Alberta, Canada from January 1, 2015 – December 31, 2015. Pain scores were recorded prospectively. Primary outcomes were frequency of postoperative pain assessments and pain intensity using the numeric rating scale.

Results: The cohort included 41 patients. Analysis was limited to pain scores recorded from postoperative days 1–14. There was an average of 7.3 pain measurements per day (SD 4.6, range 1–24) with the most frequent monitoring on postoperative days 1–4.
Median pain scores ranged from 0 to 4.5 with the highest median score on postoperative day 6. The daily maximum pain scores recorded ranged from 8 to 10 with scores of 10 recorded on postoperative days 1, 2, 3, 5, 7, 8, and 10. Patients most frequently had inadequate pain control on postoperative days 1, 2, 4, and 5 with the majority occurring on postoperative day 1.

Conclusions: Postoperative pain control could be improved at our centre. The frequency of pain assessments is also highly variable. Ongoing measurement, audit, and feedback of analgesic protocol effectiveness is an excellent first step in improving perioperative pain management in patients undergoing major head and neck cancer surgery with free flap reconstruction.

Keywords: Postoperative pain management, Postoperative pain control, ERAS, Enhanced recovery after surgery, Head and neck cancer, quality improvement

Background

Adequate pain control is a key element in successful recovery after major head and neck surgery. Inadequate postoperative pain management has been correlated with poor functional recovery [1]. Furthermore, continuous unrelieved post-operative pain can activate the pituitary-adrenal axis leading to immunosuppression resulting in postsurgical wound infection and poor wound healing [2–4]. Inadequate pain control can also reduce patient mobility, which can lead to deep vein thrombosis,

pulmonary embolism, and pneumonia [5, 6]. Effective postoperative pain control can shorten hospital stay, improve short-term post-operative outcomes, and decrease morbidity [7]. Additionally, poorly managed acute postoperative pain is often associated with chronic pain [8]. Major head and neck cancer resections with free flap reconstruction are lengthy and complex procedures and patients often require nasogastric and tracheotomy tubes. These interventions have a major impact on postoperative patient comfort and can make pain management challenging.

Adequate pain control implies consistent assessment of pain status and reliable delivery of appropriate analgesic medication. Important components of the pain assessment include determining the location of the pain as well as any aggravating or alleviating factors. Self-reported pain

* Correspondence: jdort@ucalgary.ca
Presented at the 2017 AAO Meeting
[1]Department of Surgery, Section of Otolaryngology- Head and Neck Surgery, Cumming School of Medicine, University of Calgary, HRIC 2A02, 3280 Hospital Dr NW, Calgary, AB T2N 4Z6, Canada
[2]Ohlson Research Initiative, Arnie Charbonneau Cancer Institute, Cumming School of Medicine, University of Calgary, Calgary, AB, Canada

intensity is the most commonly assessed bedside pain dimension. Anderson et al. found that lack of pain assessment was a major barrier to achieving adequate pain control [9]. Optimal pain assessment requires standardization of schedule and format. Prior authors determined that greater than two pain assessments per day across 4 days is required to have an overall accurate assessment of patients' pain [10]. Ideally pain is reassessed after each intervention to not only determine the effectiveness of that intervention but also help determine what, if any, additional modifications are needed. Numerous pain intensity measures have been developed and validated. The numeric rating scale (NRS) uses a 0–10 scale to rate the intensity of pain with 10 being the most intense pain [10–13]. As defined by the WHO, poorly controlled pain, or breakthrough pain, is defined as any score on the NRS greater than 3 [14–16].

Pain is prevalent in over 50% of cancer patients with the highest prevalence in patients with head and neck cancer (70%) [17]. Orgill et al. reported that only 35% of post-laryngectomy patients received adequate and effective pain management [18]. Few studies have investigated the effectiveness of pain control in head and neck cancer patients. In most head and neck centers, narcotic analgesics form a major component of postoperative pain control regimens [19, 20]. In our center, similar to others, most patients are managed with intravenous patient controlled analgesia (PCA) for the first five postoperative days and subsequently switched to a combination of narcotic and non-narcotic analgesics (acetaminophen and / or ibuprofen); however, narcotic analgesics have numerous adverse effects that include nausea and vomiting, constipation, sedation, and impaired mobilization [21, 22]. Furthermore, overuse of narcotics in the perioperative period can lead to subsequent drug dependence and its resulting personal and societal impacts.

The objective of this study was to better understand the effectiveness of our current approach to pain management in patients undergoing major head and neck surgery with free flap reconstruction. The type and effectiveness of our drug regimes, and the consistency and reliability of pain evaluation were of particular interest. We hypothesized there would be considerable variability in the evaluation and effectiveness of our approach to pain management. We also believed there would be generalizable findings that would inform our, and others', practice of pain management in this complex patient population. This information is a critical first step toward improving the overall management of pain in this high-risk patient population.

Methods

We performed a retrospective study of all patients undergoing head and neck cancer surgery with free flap reconstruction at the Foothills Medical Centre in Calgary, Alberta,

Canada from January 1, 2015 – December 31, 2015. Pain assessment scores were collected from an in-hospital electronic medical record for the duration of inpatient stay. Patient demographics and treatment data were collected from a prospectively annotated head and neck cancer database. Primary outcomes were frequency of postoperative pain assessments and pain intensity using the NRS. Secondary outcomes were time to mobilization and length of hospital stay.

Table 1 Patient demographics and clinical characteristics

Characteristic	Number of subjects (%)
Gender	
Male	32 (78%)
Female	9 (22%)
Age (yrs)	
Mean (SD)	61.2 (12.3)
Range	23.6–82.0
Primary site	
Oral Cavity	23 (56%)
Oropharynx	3 (7%)
Larynx	4 (10%)
Paranasal Sinus	3 (7%)
Skin	3 (7%)
Salivary Gland	2 (5%)
Other Site	3 (7%)
pT Classification	
T0	3 (7%)
T1	6 (15%)
T2	13 (32%)
T3	3 (7%)
T4	11 (27%)
Tx	5 (12%)
pN Classification	
N0	23 (56%)
N1	4 (10%)
N2	7 (17%)
Nx	7 (17%)
Clinical Stage	
0	3 (7%)
I	5 (12%)
II	8 (20%)
III	7 (17%)
IV	13 (32%)
Not Stated	5 (12%)
Length of Stay (d)	
Mean (SD)	11.6 (5.5)
Range	4.0–29.0

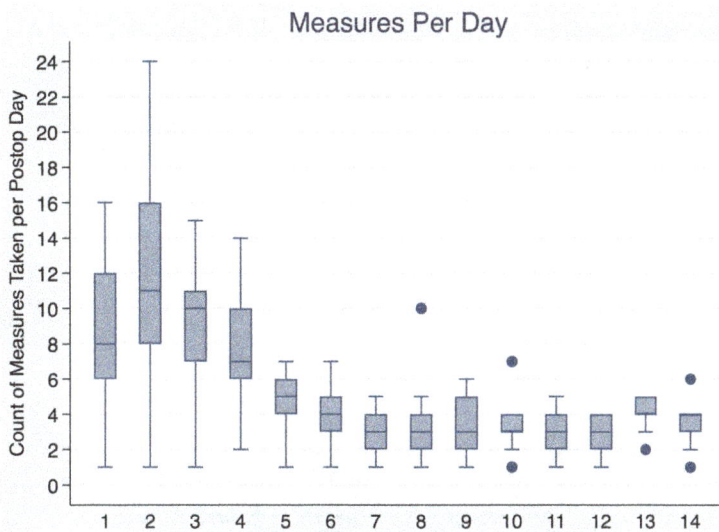

Fig. 1 Total number of pain assessments performed per postoperative day

Categorical variables are reported as proportions and continuous data are presented with means +/– standard deviation as appropriate. All data were analyzed using Stata version 15 (Stata Corp, College Station, Tx, USA).

The authors used A pRoject Ethics Community Consensus Initiative (ARECCI) framework to assess for and mitigate ethical risks, including the ARECCI Ethics Screening Tool and the ARECCI Ethics Guidelines. The project was deemed a quality improvement initiative with a minimal risk (ARECCI score = 1).

Results

Clinical characteristics of the cohort ($n = 41$) are found in Table 1. The mean age was 61.2 years with a range of

23–82 years. Pain scores, using the NRS, were analyzed from postoperative days (POD) 1–14.

The mean length of hospital stay was 11.6 days with a range of 4–29 days. By POD 2, 71% ($n = 29$) of patients were mobilized and 95% ($n = 39$) were mobilized by POD 5.

There was substantial variability in the number of daily pain assessments in the postoperative period (Fig. 1). On average, 7.3 pain measurements were performed daily (SD 4.6, range 1–24) with the most frequent monitoring taking place on PODs 1–4.

Figure 2 illustrates the proportion of patients receiving more than two pain assessments per day. Again, we found large variability in the number of pain assessments, with the greatest proportion of patients receiving more than

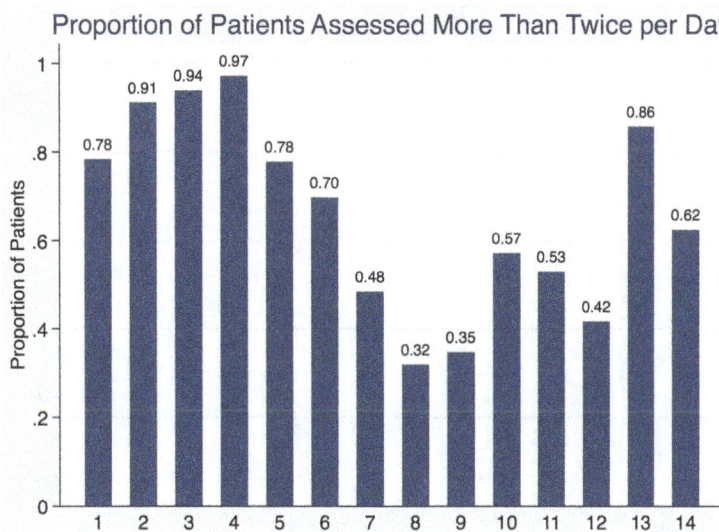

Fig. 2 Proportion of patients receiving > 2 pain assessments per postoperative day

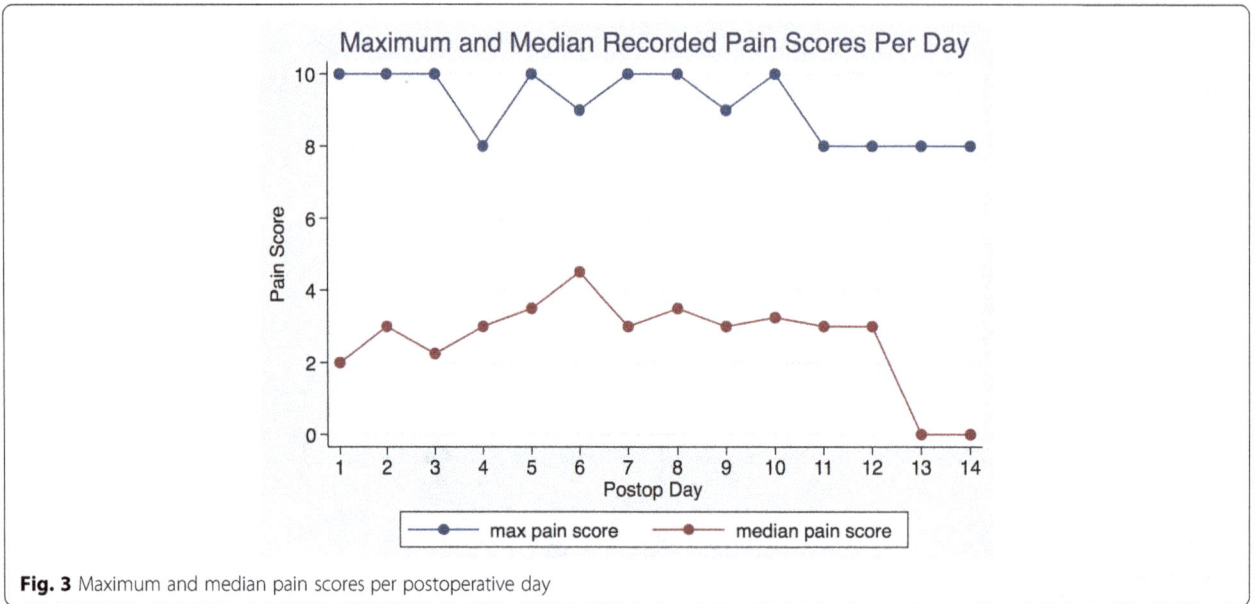

Fig. 3 Maximum and median pain scores per postoperative day

two assessments per day taking place on PODs 2, 3, 4, and 13. PODs 8 and 9 had the lowest proportion of patients receiving appropriate pain assessments with 32% and 35% of patients receiving greater than two pain assessments that day, respectively. At no time did all of the patients receive an adequate number of daily pain assessments.

Figure 3 shows the maximum and median daily pain scores for all patients. Median pain scores ranged from 0 to 4.5 with the highest median score on POD 6. The daily maximum pain scores recorded ranged from 8 to 10 with scores of 10 recorded on PODs 1, 2, 3, 5, 7, 8, and 10.

Figure 4 demonstrates the efficacy of pain control by indicating the proportion of daily pain scores greater than 3, reflecting poorly controlled pain. 31.5% (531/1684) of

the total recorded pain scores were 5 or greater (not shown), signifying moderate to severe pain for at least part of the postoperative period. High scores were observed in 35 of 41 patients, indicating this is a common problem. Poor pain control was most frequent on PODs 1, 2, 4, 5, and 11 with the highest proportion occurring on POD 1. The highest proportion of patients with adequate pain control occurred on POD 8, 9, and 14.

Discussion

In this study, we found considerable variation in the frequency of pain assessments and the efficacy of pain control. Despite the frequent use of narcotic-based PCA regimes, many of our patients had pain scores

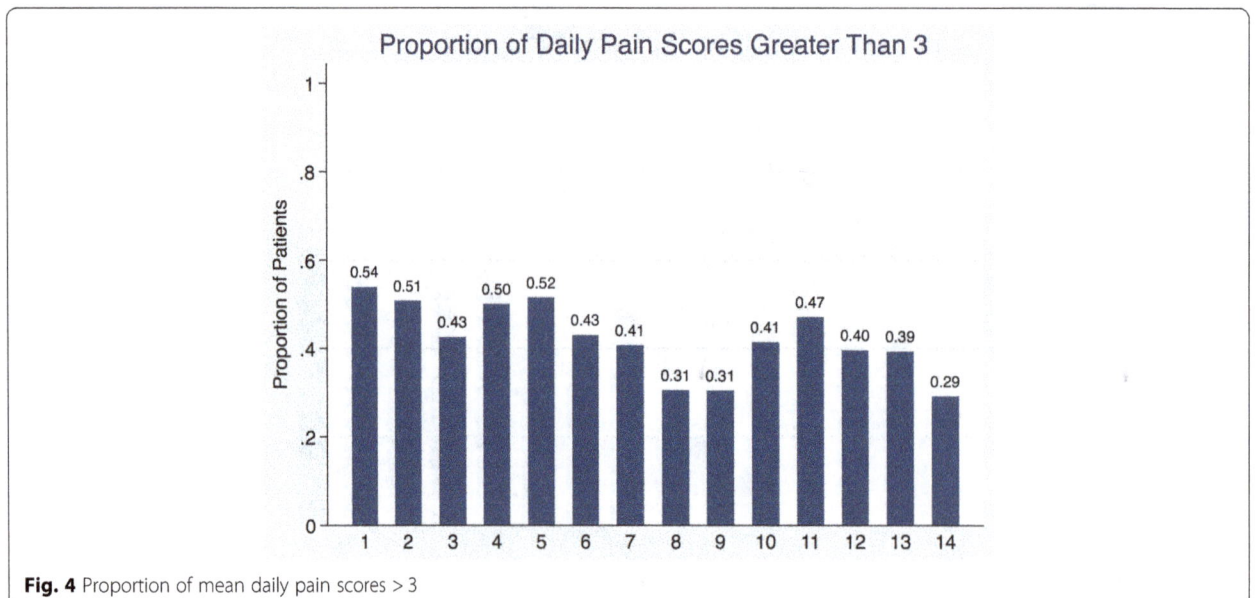

Fig. 4 Proportion of mean daily pain scores > 3

greater than 3 with 35 of 41 patients having scores greater than or equal to 5 for at least some part of their hospital stay. These results indicate that current pain management is inconsistent and often ineffective. This study demonstrates there is an opportunity to standardize both postoperative pain assessments and pain management.

Inadequate pain control is a major barrier to a patient's postoperative recovery and can be a factor in the development of postoperative complications. Appropriate pain control not only takes into account the type of analgesic employed, but also the adequacy of pain assessment in order to ensure the patient's pain is controlled. Previous studies suggest that despite the existence of guidelines for managing oncologic pain, pain is inadequately treated in nearly half of cancer patients. Head and neck cancer patients have the highest pain prevalence at 70% [14, 23]. These studies outline the importance of critically analyzing current pain management and addressing areas of weakness.

We are currently using the NRS for pain assessment. The NRS is a validated pain assessment tool that is easy to administer and record. Pain scores vary considerably throughout the day; therefore, the NRS must be administered frequently to adequately assess pain control. Jensen et al. demonstrated a minimum of three daily assessments per day should be performed for at least the first 4 postoperative days to provide a reliable pain assessment [24]. Although our results demonstrate a variable number of assessments throughout the day, we also determined there were no significant differences in average pain scores regardless if there were greater than two pain assessments per day (data not shown). We also found there is important inter-patient variability in the number of pain scores recorded per day and considerable intra-patient variability between the numbers of daily pain assessments. The WHO guidelines suggest poorly managed pain is any pain score on the NRS greater than 3 and scores of 5 or greater indicate moderate to severe pain. Figure 4 shows that a meaningful proportion of our patients are spending time in pain states of 3 or greater and our finding that 31.5% of total recorded pain scores were 5 or greater highlights that many patients (35 of 41) likely had less than optimal pain control.

Multimodal analgesic approaches used in other surgical populations minimize the use of narcotics and provide stable, reliable pain control, reduce postoperative nausea and vomiting, and improve ambulation for most patients [24–26]. The complex nature of head and neck cancer surgery suggests pain could be managed through a multimodal analgesic approach [20]. A 2014 randomized controlled study demonstrated decreased opioid requirements and length of hospital stay associated with pre-emptive intravenous paracetamol at the time of induction [27]. The French Oto-Rhino-Laryngology- Head and Neck Surgery Society published guidelines pertaining to the management of postoperative pain in head and neck cancer patients. The French guidelines recommend multimodal analgesia; however, this recommendation is not evidence-based and relies upon professional consensus alone [23, 25, 28]. We therefore believe multimodal analgesia protocols represent an important avenue for further research in the head and neck patient population.

A major challenge in implementing multimodal analgesia is patients' medical comorbidities, which may contraindicate the use of multimodal protocols. Specifically, any patient with past history of peptic ulcer disease, renal failure, or liver disease will limit the use of NSAIDs and paracetamol.

This study is limited by its retrospective design that prevented an assessment of narcotic-induced complications and side effects. The retrospective design also meant we could not control the nature and frequency of analgesic administration. However, our primary goal was to assess adequacy of pain management and it was apparent that our current approach needs improvement.

This study is strengthened by its use of high quality administrative data that was collected prospectively at the point of care. Such data are highly reliable and we are confident in its accuracy and reliability. Few studies of perioperative pain management in major head and neck cancer surgery with free flap reconstruction have been published. Studies that have been published show a high reliance on narcotic based pain control [8, 9]. We believe that multimodal analgesic protocols, as shown in other surgical disciplines, will reduce the need for postoperative narcotics in head and neck cancer patients and the complications that attend their use [16–18].

Conclusions

We conclude that in a tertiary academic head and neck surgical oncology program there is significant variation in the number of pain assessments and in the adequacy of pain control in patients undergoing major head and neck cancer surgery with free flap reconstruction. Our results suggest that ongoing measurement, audit, and feedback of analgesic protocol effectiveness is an excellent first step in improving perioperative pain management in patients undergoing major head and neck cancer surgery with free flap reconstruction.

Abbreviations
ARECCI: A pRoject Ethics Community Consensus Initiative; NRS: Numeric rating scale; PCA: Patient-controlled analgesia; POD: Postoperative day; WHO: World Health Organization

Acknowledgements
We gratefully acknowledge the Ohlson Research Initiative for supporting this project.

Funding
Funding support for this research was provided by a grant from the Ohlson Research Initiative. The funder had no role in study design, or collection, analysis, interpretation of data, or in the writing of the manuscript.

Authors' contributions
AH participated in data analysis, interpretation of the data, and participated in writing and preparation of the manuscript. JCD developed the study concept and design, acquired the data, was involved in the analysis and interpretation, and co-wrote and critically revised the manuscript. SCN assisted with study design, performed data analysis and interpretation of the data, and helped draft and critically revise the manuscript. SPC and TWM assisted in the interpretation of the data and critically revised the manuscript. All authors give final approval for the manuscript to be published and agree to be accountable for it.

Competing interests
The authors declare that they have no competing interests.

References
1. Capdevila X, Barthelet Y, Biboulet P, Ryckwaert Y, Rubenovitch J, d'Athis F. Effects of perioperative analgesic technique on the surgical outcome and duration of rehabilitation after major knee surgery. Anesthesiology. 1999;91(1):8–15.
2. Wells N, Paeroa C, McCaffery M. Chapter 17 improving the quality of care through pain assessment and management. In: Hughes RG, ed. Patient safety and quality: an evidence-based handbook for nurses: Rockville (MD): Agency for Healthcare Research and Quality (US); 2008.
3. Barr J, Boulind C, Foster JD, et al. Impact of analgesic modality on stress response following laparoscopic colorectal surgery: a post-hoc analysis of a randomised controlled trial. Tech Coloproctol. 2015;19(4):231–9.
4. Scott MJ, Baldini G, Fearon KC, et al. Enhanced recovery after surgery (ERAS) for gastrointestinal surgery, part 1: pathophysiological considerations. Acta Anaesthesiol Scand. 2015;59(10):1212–31.
5. Yeung JK, Dautremont JF, Harrop AR, et al. Reduction of pulmonary complications and hospital length of stay with a clinical care pathway after head and neck reconstruction. Plast Reconstr Surg. 2014;133(6):1477–84.
6. Yeung JK, Harrop R, McCreary O, et al. Delayed mobilization after microsurgical reconstruction: an independent risk factor for pneumonia. Laryngoscope. 2013;123(12):2996–3000.
7. Wick EC, Grant MC, Wu CL. Postoperative multimodal analgesia pain management with nonopioid analgesics and techniques: a review. JAMA Surg. 2017;152(7):691–7.
8. Kuo P-Y, Williams JE. Pain control in head and neck Cancer. In: Agulnik M, editor. Head and neck Cancer: InTech; 2012. p. 351–70.
9. Anderson KO, Mendoza TR, Valero V, et al. Minority cancer patients and their providers: pain management attitudes and practice. Cancer. 2000; 88(8):1929–38.
10. Jensen MP, McFarland CA. Increasing the reliability and validity of pain intensity measurement in chronic pain patients. Pain. 1993;55(2):195–203.
11. Hawker GA, Mian S, Kendzerska T, French M. Measures of adult pain: visual analog scale for pain (VAS pain), numeric rating scale for pain (NRS pain), McGill pain questionnaire (MPQ), short-form McGill pain questionnaire (SF-MPQ), chronic pain grade scale (CPGS), short Form-36 bodily pain scale (SF-36 BPS), and measure of intermittent and constant osteoarthritis pain (ICOAP). Arthritis Care Res (Hoboken). 2011;63(Suppl 11):S240–52.
12. Jensen MP, Karoly P, O'Riordan EF, Bland F Jr, Burns RS. The subjective experience of acute pain. An assessment of the utility of 10 indices. Clin J Pain. 1989;5(2):153–9.
13. Williamson A, Hoggart B. Pain: a review of three commonly used pain rating scales. J Clin Nurs. 2005;14(7):798–804.
14. Grond S, Zech D, Lynch J, Diefenbach C, Schug SA, Lehmann KA. Validation of World Health Organization guidelines for pain relief in head and neck cancer. A prospective study. Ann Otol Rhinol Laryngol. 1993;102(5):342–8.
15. Zech DF, Grond S, Lynch J, Hertel D, Lehmann KA. Validation of World Health Organization guidelines for cancer pain relief: a 10-year prospective study. Pain. 1995;63(1):65–76.
16. Organization WH. Cancer pain relief. 1996. http://apps.who.int/iris/bitstream/10665/37896/1/9241544821.pdf. Accessed May 2017.
17. van den Beuken-van Everdingen MH, de Rijke JM, Kessels AG, Schouten HC, van Kleef M, Patijn J. Prevalence of pain in patients with cancer: a systematic review of the past 40 years. Ann Oncol. 2007;18(9):1437–49.
18. Orgill R, Krempl GA, Medina JE. Acute pain management following laryngectomy. Arch Otolaryngol Head Neck Surg. 2002;128(7):829–32.
19. Bianchini C, Malago M, Crema L, et al. Post-operative pain management in head and neck cancer patients: predictive factors and efficacy of therapy. Acta Otorhinolaryngol Ital. 2016;36(2):91–6.
20. Bianchini C, Maldotti F, Crema L, Malago M, Ciorba A. Pain in head and neck cancer: prevalence and possible predictive factors. J BUON. 2014;19(3):592–7.
21. Tan M, Law LS, Gan TJ. Optimizing pain management to facilitate enhanced recovery after surgery pathways. Can J Anaesth. 2015;62(2):203–18.
22. Oderda GM, Evans RS, Lloyd J, et al. Cost of opioid-related adverse drug events in surgical patients. J Pain Symptom Manag. 2003;25(3):276–83.
23. Binczak M, Navez M, Perrichon C, et al. Management of somatic pain induced by head-and-neck cancer treatment: definition and assessment. Guidelines of the French Oto-rhino-laryngology–head and neck surgery society (SFORL). Eur Ann Otorhinolaryngol Head Neck Dis. 2014;131(4):243–7.
24. Khan SK, Malviya A, Muller SD, et al. Reduced short-term complications and mortality following enhanced recovery primary hip and knee arthroplasty: results from 6,000 consecutive procedures. Acta Orthop. 2014;85(1):26–31.
25. Kalogera E, Bakkum-Gamez JN, Jankowski CJ, et al. Enhanced recovery in gynecologic surgery. Obstet Gynecol. 2013;122(2 Pt 1):319–28.
26. Miller TE, Thacker JK, White WD, et al. Reduced length of hospital stay in colorectal surgery after implementation of an enhanced recovery protocol. Anesth Analg. 2014;118(5):1052–61.
27. Majumdar S, Das A, Kundu R, Mukherjee D, Hazra B, Mitra T. Intravenous paracetamol infusion: superior pain management and earlier discharge from hospital in patients undergoing palliative head-neck cancer surgery. Perspect Clin Res. 2014;5(4):172–7.
28. Espitalier F, Testelin S, Blanchard D, et al. Management of somatic pain induced by treatment of head and neck cancer: postoperative pain. Guidelines of the French Oto-rhino-laryngology–head and neck surgery society (SFORL). Eur Ann Otorhinolaryngol Head Neck Dis. 2014;131(4):249–52.

31

Carcinoembryonic antigen levels correlated with advanced disease in medullary thyroid cancer

Sena Turkdogan[1], Véronique-Isabelle Forest[2], Michael P. Hier[2], Michael Tamilia[3], Anca Florea[4] and Richard J. Payne[2,5*]

Abstract

Background: Medullary thyroid cancer (MTC) cells are capable of secreting various tumor markers including calcitonin and carcinoembryonic antigen (CEA). The purpose of this study is to determine whether abnormal CEA levels may be used as a tumor marker to predict the severity of disease in MTC.

Methods: A retrospective analysis was completed for 33 patients with MTC who had preoperative serum CEA levels. Univariate and multivariate analyses were used to quantify the relationship between serum CEA levels and tumor stage and prognosis.

Results: On multivariate analysis, elevated preoperative CEA levels were significantly associated with the size and stage of tumor, distant metastasis, decreased biochemical cure, and mortality. There was a significant association between tumor size greater than 37 mm and elevated CEA levels (> 271 ng/ml). There was also a positive correlation with increased cancer stage (> 377 ng/ml), distant metastasis (> 405 ng/ml), and contralateral compartment location of lymph node metastasis (> 162 ng/ml). When pre-operative CEA levels are > 500 ng/ml, patient mortality was 67%.

Conclusion: In this study, both pre-operative calcitonin and CEA levels were significantly correlated with the extent of disease in MTC. While calcitonin has a linear relationship with disease progression, abnormal CEA levels were a better indicator of advanced disease. CEA levels > 271 ng/ml are significant for advanced tumor size and staging, metastasis to the central compartment, and decreased chance of biochemical cure. CEA levels greater than 500 ng/ml are associated with significant patient mortality.

Keywords: Medullary thyroid carcinoma, Carcinoembryonic antigen, Tumor marker, Advanced disease, Mortality, Calcitonin

Background

Medullary thyroid cancer (MTC) is a neuroendocrine tumor of the parafollicular or C cells of the thyroid gland, and currently accounts for approximately 5 to 10% of all thyroid cancers [1, 2]. The clinical course of MTC can vary from an extremely indolent tumor that remains unchanged for years to an aggressive variant associated with a high mortality rate. The majority of MTCs are sporadic, but approximately 20% of MTCs are a result of a germline genetic gain-of-function mutation in the rearranged during transfection (RET) proto-oncogene. Hereditary MTC can be seen in isolation or as part of the multiple endocrine neoplasia (MEN) syndrome type 2A or 2B.

Because calcitonin is mainly produced by C cells of the thyroid gland, the measurement of calcitonin concentrations in blood reflects C cell activity and can therefore be used as a tumor marker for MTC [3]. However, there are many limitations to using calcitonin as a screening method. These limiting factors include problems of cost benefit, lab methods, false positives and low prevalence of MTC. Cost-benefit is a major concern; one cost-effective analysis has shown that the addition of calcitonin screening to current American Thyroid Association

* Correspondence: rkpayne@sympatico.ca
[2]Department of Otolaryngology-Head and Neck Surgery, Sir Mortimer B. Davis-Jewish General Hospital, Montreal, Canada
[5]Department of Otolaryngology-Head and Neck Surgery, McGill University Health Centre, Montreal, Canada
Full list of author information is available at the end of the article

guidelines for the evaluation of thyroid nodules would cost $11,793 per life years saved leading to a subsequent $1.4 billion societal fee [4]. Secondly, measurement of calcitonin levels can be challenging and variable depending on lab methods. Calcitonin is a hormone with molecular heterogeneity as it may exist in both bioactive and immature forms in serum and tumor tissue. This characteristic of calcitonin is one factor that can lead to measurements which vary widely as different assays exploit antiserum that recognize different epitopes of the hormone, leading to variable measurement values [5]. Lastly, false positives may occur frequently in both basal and stimulated measurements of calcitonin [6]. Benign pathologies causing an increase in calcitonin levels include benign hyperplasia of C cells, benign thyroid nodules, differentiated thyroid carcinoma and Hashimoto thyroiditis [7, 8].

Although carcinoembryonic antigen (CEA) has also been proposed as a tumor marker for MTC, it's trends after surgery and in correlation with calcitonin have not been thoroughly studied in the literature. The limiting factor of low incidence of MTC in the population has led to few studies evaluating CEA in the context of MTC tumor markers, biochemical cure and prognosis, and the ones that exist have shown conflicting results. Machens et al. have studied the implications of preoperative biomarkers including CEA levels on the management of MTC, and concluded that abnormal CEA levels heralds advanced disease, consisting of larger tumors and metastasis [9]. They also propose the addition of biochemical stratification of patients as part of a standardized approach to MTC in order to minimize surgical morbidity [10]. They conclude that further studies are necessary to confirm the effectiveness CEA measurements in risk-stratifying MTC patients. However, in contrast to their findings, Yip et al. discovered that only calcitonin, and not CEA, reflected the extent of disease [11]. They did not find any correlation between preoperative CEA levels and tumor size, lymph node metastasis, or extent of the operation performed.

The purpose of this study is to help clarify the discrepancies in the literature and determine whether abnormal CEA levels may be used as a tumor marker to predict the severity of disease in MTC in regards to size of tumor, stage of tumor, lymph node involvement, distant metastasis, surgical cure, and mortality. As CEA measurements are less costly to the system compared to calcitonin, we hypothesize that it could be a more cost-effective tool in monitoring MTC.

Methods

Study design and population

Our study is an analysis of MTC patients who underwent a total thyroidectomy with or without a selective or radical neck dissection at two tertiary surgical centers in Montreal, including the Jewish General Hospital and the Royal Victoria Hospital between the years of 2003–2016. The inclusion criteria included all MTC patients who had pre-operative and post-operative calcitonin and CEA levels, bloodwork which has become part of a routine workup in our institutions. Informed consent was obtained before each surgical procedure that represented standard practice of care.

Operative approach and histopathological examination

The extent of the primary surgery was at the discretion of the treating physician. Patients underwent either total thyroidectomy or total thyroidectomy with prophylactic central and/or lateral compartment lymphadenectomy. During the operation all thyroid specimens and neck dissections were oriented and marked in the operating room, and then sent for pathological analysis post-operatively. All tissue specimens were embedded in paraffin and subjected to histopathological examination and calcitonin immunohistochemistry. Histological diagnosis, tumor size, depth of invasion, margins, extra-capsular extension, lymphovascular invasion, C-cell hyperplasia and lymph node involvement was then examined by expert thyroid pathologists at our institution. When multiple MTC were present, the largest tumor dimension was considered. Distant metastasis was diagnosed with radiological evidence (ultrasonography, computed tomography, magnetic resonance imaging, positron emission tomography, or any combination thereof) and confirmed by tissue diagnosis when feasible. The American Joint Committee on Cancer 7th edition, TNM staging, was chosen for tumor staging.

Statistical approach

Various categorical variables were tested using a univariate analysis. In order to study dose effects, continuous variables such as primary tumor size were grouped in increments of 10 mm. Multivariate conditional logistic regression models were then fitted to identify histopathologic variables associated with an abnormal preoperative CEA test result. The level of significance was set at $p < .05$.

Results

The study included a total of 33 patients (21 females and 12 males) with an average age of 58. The general characteristics of our population were similar to those in other studies; including mean age at surgery = 58, sex ratio = 1 male: 1.75 female, stage I = 15.1%, stage II = 27.3%, stage III = 9.1%, and stage IV = 42.4%. All patients underwent surgery, and 54.5% of these patients were biochemically cured. Survival was 93.9% at 10 years. Multivariate analysis showed that age and stage were independent predictive factors of survival (Table 1).

Table 1 Multivariate logistic regression analysis - preoperative CEA levels and medullary thyroid cancer progression

	# of patients	Pre-Op CEA (ng/ml)	(95% CI)	P-value
Primary tumor size (mm)				
1–9	3	3.36	(1.7-10)	0.01
10–19	7	6.42		
20–29	5	16.54		
30–39	8	168.63		
40+	10	188.73		
Stage				
I	5	2.7	(3.8-130)	0.04
II	11	38.8		
III	3	15.7		
IVa	8	74.7		
IVb	1	128.1		
IVc	5	405.9		
Metastasis				
Locoregional	12	20.55	(−14.4–225.7)	0.08
Distant	6	405.83		
Location of lymph node metastasis				
Central	30	36.1		
Central + Lateral	18	120.1	(19–228)	0.02
Central + Lateral + Contralateral	12	162.31		
Biomedical Cure				
Yes	17	48.3	(8.5–244)	0.03
No	16	174.6		
Mortality				
Yes	2	74.9	(0.0006–0.0013)	< 0.001
No	31	583.7		

Tumor size

Univariate analysis demonstrates an exponential relationship between pre-operative CEA levels and the size of the tumor as displayed by graph / Table 2. This relationship demonstrates that CEA levels are normal to mildly elevated with small tumor sizes, the pre-operative CEA levels rises significantly once the tumor reaches a size greater than 30 mm (Fig. 1, Table 2).

Stage

A moderate increase in CEA levels is present with stage I, II and III disease, while the CEA levels rise significantly with stage IVC disease, reaching an average of 405.9 ng/ml (Fig. 2, Table 3).

Extent of surgery, metastasis and lymph node involvement

Out of our 33 patients who underwent total thyroidectomy, 30 had central compartment lymphadenectomy, 18 had central and ipsilateral neck dissections, while 12

underwent central and bilateral neck dissections (both ipsilateral and contralateral). The average pre-operative CEA for all patients was 94.4 ng/ml, which increased to 103.4 ng/ml for those who had central compartment dissections, 148.3 ng/ml for central and ipsilateral neck dissections, and 162.31 ng/ml for central and bilateral neck dissections. This represents a correlation between pre-operative CEA levels and the extent of the surgical procedure performed.

Table 2 Relationship between the size of the tumor and pre-operative carcinoembryonic antigen levels

Size of tumor (mm)	Pre-OP CEA (ng/ml)
1–9	3.36
10–19	6.42
20–29	16.54
30–39	168.63
40+	188.73

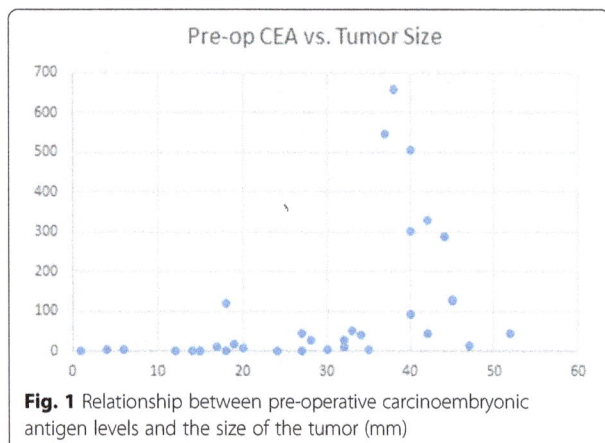

Fig. 1 Relationship between pre-operative carcinoembryonic antigen levels and the size of the tumor (mm)

Table 3 Relationship between stage of tumor and pre-operative carcinoembryonic antigen levels

Stage	Pre-op CEA (ng/ml)
Stage I	2.7
Stage II	38.8
Stage III	15.7
Stage IVA	74.7
Stage IVB	128.2
Stage IVC	405.9

In total, 18 had metastasis of their disease outside the thyroid gland. The metastasis was divided into locoregional vs. distant metastasis. Of the 18 patients with metastasis, 12 had locoregional and 6 had distant metastasis. These patients had average pre-operative CEA levels of 20.6 ng/ml and 405.8 ng/ml respectively. As with tumor size and staging, the pre-operative CEA levels were seen to be drastically increased in distant metastasis compared to that of locoregional disease (Table 4).

Presence of disease in the contralateral neck compartment was also associated with higher CEA level measurements. While presence of positive lymph nodes only in the central neck compartments were seen with an average pre-operative CEA of 103.39 ng/ml, lateral neck and contralateral neck lymph node findings were associated with a much higher CEA level at 120.1 ng/ml and 162.31 ng/ml respectively (Table 5).

Surprisingly, no correlation with the number of metastatic cervical lymph node involvement was seen. Both minimal lymph node involvement and extensive lymph node metastasis had the potential to correlate with high CEA levels (Fig. 3).

Biochemical cure

Chances of biochemical cure, defined as normal basal post-operative serum CEA and calcitonin levels, were greatly diminished in patients who had higher pre-operative CEA levels (Tables 6).

Mortality

In total, two patients succumbed from their disease. The pre-operative CEA levels of these patients were 659.9 and 507.4, representing the two patients in our population with the highest CEA levels and demonstrating that significantly increased CEA levels can be associated with mortality.

Calcitonin

Although not the focus of this study, pre-operative calcitonin levels were also compared to extent of medullary thyroid cancer progression in tumor size. Univariate analysis demonstrated a more linear relationship between pre-operative calcitonin levels and the size of the tumor compared to that of CEA as displayed by Fig. 4.

Discussion

MTC, a relatively rare type of thyroid malignancy, is associated with a poor survival when compared to other common thyroid cancers. Our cohort had a 93.9% 10-year survival rate which is similar to previous studies reporting survival rates ranging from 69 to 89% [12–14]. As with other studies, our current analysis is in agreement with previously identified clinical prognostic factors for MTC including age (> 45 years), tumor stage, presence of lymph node and distant metastasis.

MTC is known to produce many tumor markers, including calcitonin, CEA, and chromogranin A. These markers can be easily detected with blood levels and

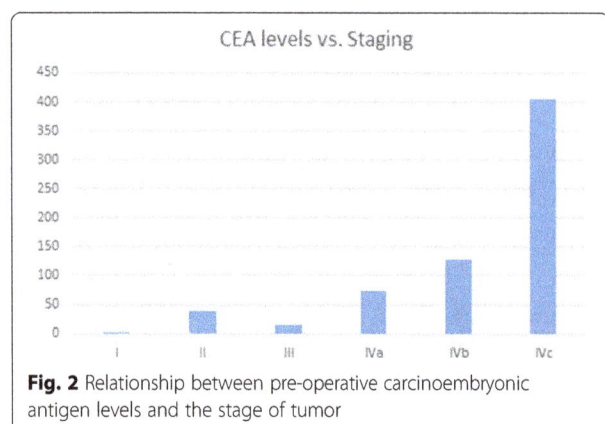

Fig. 2 Relationship between pre-operative carcinoembryonic antigen levels and the stage of tumor

Table 4 Relationship between metastatic medullary thyroid cancer (logoregional vs. distant) and pre-operative carcinoembryonic antigen levels

Metastasis	Pre-Op CEA (ng/ml)
Locoregional	20.55
Distant	405.83

Table 5 Relationship between location of lymph node metastasis and pre-operative carcinoembryonic antigen levels

Location of LN	Pre-Op CEA (ng/ml)
Central only	318.6
Central and lateral	100.3
Lateral only	91.1

Table 6 Relationship between biochemical cure and pre-operative carcinoembryonic antigen levels

Biochemical Cure	Pre-Op CEA (ng/ml)
Yes	48.3
No	174.6

immunohistological stains. Serum calcitonin is known to be a highly sensitive tumor biomarker, shown to be 100% predictive of MTC when basal levels are > 100 pg/ml or when stimulated levels with pentagastrin increase to > 1000 pg/ml [15]. Although these levels have been proven for calcitonin, a similar measure has not yet been proposed in the literature for CEA levels. CEA is a glycoprotein that was first detected by Gold et al. in 1965 in relation to colon cancer [16]. It is most commonly known as a tumor marker for gastrointestinal malignancies, frequently used to monitor tumor recurrence. In patients presenting with high CEA levels, tumors originating from the gastrointestinal tract should always be excluded using endoscopy, colonoscopy, and CT. CEA levels may also increase in benign disease, including inflammatory bowel disease and liver cirrhosis. Despite this, many cases have been noted in the literature in which elevated CEA levels with no other clinical findings may be the first and only finding of MTC [17].

It has been shown in the past that production of various tumor markers may differ between patients and that tumors with a high production of CEA alongside a low expression of calcitonin may be more aggressive [18]. It was postulated that this finding may reflect a degree of maturation block of tumor cells in patients with aggressive disease. However, this "flip-flop phenomenon" was not seen in our study, as the patients with the highest tumor burden (represented by presence of distant metastasis and mortality) also had the highest calcitonin levels in our cohort. While calcitonin is thought to have a linear relationship with disease progression, our analysis discovered that abnormal CEA levels were exponentially correlated with advanced disease. This suggests that CEA can be a better predictor of advanced disease and mortality, in agreement with previous studies suggesting CEA may be a sensitive marker for aggressive MTC [19]. CEA was consistently elevated in all cases with metastasis, whereas calcitonin may be normal or moderate with metastatic presence. This may suggest that using CEA levels in correlation with calcitonin may detect disease metastasis or recurrence earlier than calcitonin alone. Our results also demonstrate that CEA is a better detector of lateral and contralateral lymph node involvement, which may help in guiding surgical approaches.

Interestingly, the only variable in which we saw no correlation with disease severity was the number of metastatic cervical lymph nodes. Although the presence and location of metastasis was significant for advanced disease, the specific number of pathologically proven lymph nodes had no correlation with CEA levels. Previous research has proposed that the number of lymph nodes harboring metastasis can be used as an independent prognostic factor in differentiated thyroid cancer [20]. However, in keeping with our findings, these papers also concluded that although biomarker levels correlate closely with tumor mass, they often don't have as strong of a predictive value in the number of lymph node metastasis. Some theories include that while the tumor mass itself has excellent vascular supply and drainage, lymph node metastasis may exist in area of reduced perfusion thus correlating more poorly with pre-operative CEA and calcitonin levels. It is also contemplated that lymph node metastasis may have acquired additional somatic mutations rendering these cells less

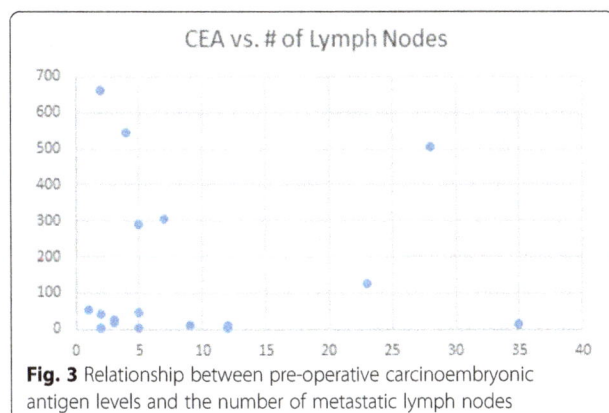

Fig. 3 Relationship between pre-operative carcinoembryonic antigen levels and the number of metastatic lymph nodes

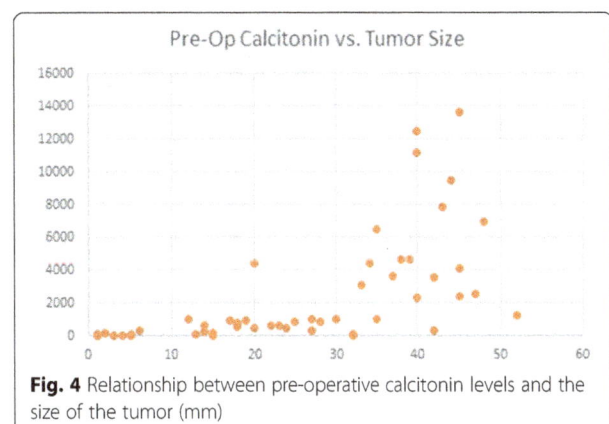

Fig. 4 Relationship between pre-operative calcitonin levels and the size of the tumor (mm)

differentiated than those of the primary tumor and thus leading to reduced correlation with serum levels.

Although often overlooked, there exists a significant importance on cost-comparison when considering additional screening tests. At our institutions, one serum calcitonin test costs approximately $30, compared to $4 for a serum CEA level, which theoretically could cut screening costs by 87%. Furthermore, it is also important to note that at many institutions CEA is analysed rapidly (comparable to the way blood glucose levels are analysed and resulted) whereas calcitonin levels are requested much less frequently requiring outsourcing and delays in receiving laboratory values.

This population-based study evaluating CEA tumor marker levels on MTC progression has several potential limitations. First, MTC is quite rare compared to other differentiated thyroid cancers, leading to small study population. Second, MTC occurs in both hereditary and sporadic forms. As sporadic forms tend to be more aggressive, this may confound our findings as our population consisted of 94% sporadic form of MTC. Lastly, as our institution is that of a tertiary center, the referral pattern may also lean towards a biased increase in patients with aggressive disease. Despite these limitations, the findings of our project have guided some new clinical applications in our practice. Currently, all patients with diagnosed MTC receive pre-operative and post-operative CEA levels. In instances of high pre-operative CEA levels, attention is given to counseling the patient on the invasiveness of the tumor and a discussion can take place for more aggressive surgical therapy. Similarly, if post-operative CEA levels are surprisingly high, closer surveillance for the patient may be considered.

Conclusion

In this study, both pre-operative calcitonin and CEA levels were significantly correlated with the extent of disease in MTC. While calcitonin has a linear relationship with disease progression, abnormal CEA levels were also correlated with advanced disease suggesting that it also may be a predictor of tumor size, central lymph node metastasis, and mortality. CEA levels greater than 271 ng/ml are significant for advanced tumor size, advanced tumor staging, metastasis to the contralateral neck compartment, and decreased chance of biochemical cure. CEA levels greater than 500 ng/ml are greatly associated with patient mortality.

Abbreviations
CEA: Carcinoembryonic antigen; CT: Omputed tomography; MEN: Multiple endocrine neoplasia; Mtc: Medullary thyroid cancer; RET: Rearranged during transfection

Authors' contributions
ST performed acquisition of data, analysis and interpretation, assisted on some surgical procedures and drafted the manuscript. VIF, MPH and RJP collectively performed all surgeries in the patient population. MT and AF followed the patient's endocrine results and pathology results, respectively. RJP supervised the entire project, carried out study conception and design, and edited the manuscript. All authors read and approved the final manuscript.

Competing interests
The authors declare that they have no competing interests.

Author details
[1]McGill University Health Center, Montreal, QC, Canada. [2]Department of Otolaryngology-Head and Neck Surgery, Sir Mortimer B. Davis-Jewish General Hospital, Montreal, Canada. [3]Department of Endocrinology and Metabolism, Sir Mortimer B. Davis-Jewish General Hospital, Montreal, Canada. [4]Department of Pathology, Sir Mortimer B. Davis-Jewish General Hospital, Montreal, Canada. [5]Department of Otolaryngology-Head and Neck Surgery, McGill University Health Centre, Montreal, Canada.

References
1. Parkin DM, Whelan SL, Ferlay J, Teppo L, Thomas DB. Cancer Incidence in Five Continents Vol. VIII. France: IARC Scientific Publication No. 155. 2002; 155:53.
2. Wells SA Jr, Asa SL, Dralle H, et al. American Thyroid Association guidelines task force on medullary thyroid carcinoma. Thyroid. 2015;25(6):567.
3. Bae YJ, Schaab M, Kratzsch J. Calcitonin as Biomarker for the Medullary Thyroid Carcinoma. Recent Results Cancer Res. 2015;204:117–37.
4. Cheung K, Roman SA, Wang TS, Walker HD, Sosa JA. Calcitonin measurement in the evaluation of thyroid nodules in the United States: a cost-effectiveness and decision analysis. J Clin Endocrinol Metab. 2008;93:62173–80.
5. Costante G, Durante C, Francis Z, Schlumberger M, Filetti S. Determination of calcitonin levels in C-cell disease: clinical interest and potential pitfalls. Nat Clin Pract Endocrinol Metab. 2009;5:35–44.
6. Karanikas G, Moameni A, Poetzi C, Zetting G, Kaserer K, Bieglmayer C, et al. Frequency and relevance of elevated calcitonin levels in patients with neoplastic and nonneoplastic thyroid disease and in healthy subjects. J Clin Endocrinol Metab. 2004;89:515–9.
7. Batista RL, Toscanini AC, Brandao LG, Cunha-Neto MB. False positive results using calcitonin as a screening method for medullary thyroid carcinoma. Indian J Endocrinol Metab. 2013;17(3):524–8.
8. Scheuba C, Kaserer K, Weinhäusl A, Pandev R, Kaider A, Passler C, et al. Is medullary thyroid cancer predictable? A prospective study of 86 patients with abnormal pentagastrin tests. Surgery. 1999;126:1089–95.
9. Machens A, Ukkat J, Hauptmann S, Dralle H. Abnormal carcinoembryonic antigen levels and medullary thyroid cancer progression; A multivariate analysis. Arch Surg. 2007;142(3):289–93. https://doi.org/10.1001/archsurg.142.3.289.
10. Andreas Machens, Henning Dralle; Biomarker-Based Risk Stratification for Previously Untreated Medullary Thyroid Cancer. J Clin Endocrinol Metabol. 2010;95(6):2655–63.
11. Yip DT, Hassan M, Pazaitou-Panayiotou K, et al. Preoperative basal calcitonin and tumor stage correlate with postoperative calcitonin normalization in patients undergoing initial surgical management of medullary thyroid carcinoma. Surgery. 2011;150(6):1168–77.
12. Utiger RD. Medullary thyroid carcinoma, genes, and the prevention of cancer. N Engl J Med. 1994;331:870–1.
13. Keminger K, Kokoschka R, Schmalzer E. Medullary thyroid cancer. Wein Klin Wochenschr. 1983;95:214–9.
14. Qu N, Shi R, Lu Z, et al. Metastatic lymph node ratio can further stratify risk for mortality in medullary thyroid cancer patients: a population-based analysis. Oncotarget. 2016;7(40):65937–45.
15. Phitayakorn R, McHenry CR. Incidental thyroid carcinoma in patients with graves' disease. Am I Surg. 2008;195(3):292–7.

16. Gold P, Freddman SO. Demonstration of tumor-specific antigens in human colonic carcinomata by immunological tolerance and absorption techniques. J Exp Med. 1965;121:439–62.

17. Akbulut S, Sogutcu N. A high level of carcinoembryonic antigen as initial manifestation of medullary thyroid carcinoma in a patient with subclinical hyperthyroidism. Int Surg. 2011;96:254–9.

18. Mendelsohn G, Wells SJ, Baylin S. Relationship of tissue carcinoembryonic antigen and calcitonin to tumor virulence in medullary thyroid carcinoma. An immunohistochemical study in early, localized, and virulent disseminated stages of disease. Cancer. 1984;54:657–62.

19. Rougier PH, Calmettes C, Laplanche A, et al. The values of calcitonin and carcinoembryonic antigen in the treatment and management of nonfamilial medullary thyroid carcinoma. Cancer. 1983;51:855–62.

20. Leboulleux S, Rubino C, Baudin E, et al. Prognostic factors for persistent or recurrent disease of papillary thyroid carcinoma with neck lymph node metastases and/or tumor extension beyond the thyroid capsule at initial diagnosis. J Clin Endocrinol Metab. 2005;90:5723–9.

32

An evaluation of in-office flexible fiber-optic biopsies for laryngopharyngeal lesions

Francisco Lee[1], Kristine A. Smith[1], Shamir Chandarana[1,2], T. Wayne Matthews[1,2], J. Douglas Bosch[1], Steven C. Nakoneshny[2] and Joseph C. Dort[1,2]*

Abstract

Background: Operative endoscopy and flexible fiber-optic in-office tissue biopsy are common techniques to assess suspicious laryngopharyngeal lesions.

Methods: The primary outcome was the delay to the initiation of treatment. Secondary outcomes were delay to biopsy, histopathological diagnosis, and assessment at a multidisciplinary oncology clinic. A retrospective analysis was performed to assess the relative delays between these approaches to biopsy of laryngopharyngeal lesions.

Results: There were 114 patients in the study cohort; 44 in-office and 70 operative endoscopic biopsies). The mean delay from consultation to biopsy was 17.4 days for the operative endoscopy group and 1.3 days for the in-office group. The mean delay from initial otolaryngology consultation to initiation of treatment was 51.7 days and 44. 6 days for the operative endoscopy and in-office groups, respectively.

Conclusion: In-office biopsy reduced the time from initial consultation to biopsy. The temporal gains via in-office biopsy did not translate into faster access to treatment. This outcome highlights the opportunity to improve access to treatment for patients with early diagnosis.

Keywords: Endoscopy, In-office biopsy, Larynx, Pharynx, Lesion

Background

Laryngopharyngeal lesions encompass a wide range of disease processes that includes benign lesions, local manifestations of systemic disease, inflammatory disorders and primary malignancies. In the United States, an estimated 61,700 new cases of oral cavity, pharynx, and larynx cancer will arise in 2016 and an estimated 13,190 deaths will occur from these cancers combined. [1] Given that early identification and treatment of head and neck cancers improves prognosis, [2–5] timely evaluation and diagnosis of suspicious lesions is important.

The larynx and lower pharynx are potentially challenging areas to assess and operative endoscopy is often necessary for thorough evaluation and biopsy of suspicious

lesions. Operative endoscopy requires operating room (OR) time and general anesthesia and uses costly healthcare resources such as operating rooms and OR personnel. Complications arising from rigid instrumentation and general anesthesia, although uncommon, do occur, especially in high-risk patients with comorbid conditions.

One alternative, flexible fiber-optic nasopharyngoscopy, offers excellent visualization of the aerodigestive tract in an awake patient with low risk of complications. Newer technologies such as high-definition distal-chip nasopharyngoscopes provide excellent image quality, and side channels facilitate tissue biopsy with diagnostic accuracy comparable to that of operative endoscopy [6]. In a study by Castillo Farias et al. (2014), in-office biopsy of suspicious laryngeal lesions under fiber optic visualization offered a specificity of 81% and sensitivity of 100% compared to direct laryngoscopy [7]. Moreover, by performing an in-office biopsy as a first-line diagnostic step, and avoiding anesthetic and OR expenses, the

* Correspondence: jdort@ucalgary.ca
[1]Section of Otolaryngology – Head and Neck Surgery, Department of Surgery, Cumming School of Medicine, University of Calgary, HRIC 2A02, 3280 Hospital Dr NW, Calgary, AB T2N 4Z6, Canada
[2]Ohlson Research Initiative, Arnie Charbonneau Cancer Institute, Cumming School of Medicine, University of Calgary, Calgary, Alberta, Canada

authors reported a cost savings of 80% when compared to an operative biopsy for all patients presenting with suspicious lesions.

In addition to cost savings, it is important to understand the impact on time to diagnosis of different diagnostic approaches. The time differences between in-office and operative approaches to the biopsy of suspicious laryngopharyngeal lesions remains relatively unknown. Furthermore, little is known about the impact of time to diagnosis on overall time to initiation of treatment. We therefore undertook a study to measure the differences in time to diagnosis and time to initiation of treatment in patients with laryngopharyngeal lesions who were undergoing operative endoscopy compared to a patient cohort undergoing in-office biopsy. Our hypothesis was that in-office biopsy would result in faster diagnosis and faster access to treatment.

Methods
Study design
We performed a retrospective case-control study comprising patients referred to a tertiary Head and Neck Oncology and Laryngology Clinic from January 1st, 2010 to December 31st, 2015. Cases were defined as patients undergoing in-office biopsies and the controls were defined as patients undergoing operative endoscopy requiring general anesthesia. This study was reviewed and approved by the Health Research Ethics Board of Alberta – Cancer Committee.

Patients
The study focused on patients presenting with oropharyngeal or laryngeal lesions requiring biopsy. These subsites were chosen because conventional access and biopsy of these lesions traditionally requires operative endoscopy. Patients older than 18 years of age with lesions visible on office endoscopy were eligible for inclusion. In-office biopsy patients were identified by review of billing codes and laryngology clinic records during the time period of interest and charts of potentially eligible patients were reviewed. Operative endoscopy patients were identified by querying a relational database (Otobase®, Seattle, WA) used to prospectively track all patients treated in our program. Patients with lesions accessible to a simple transoral biopsy without endoscopic assistance were not included. Patients unable to tolerate flexible endoscopy or who had a history of bleeding disorder were also ineligible for an in-office procedure. Patients with non-squamous cell carcinoma or a benign diagnosis were also excluded. The final cohort comprised 114 patients (44 in-office biopsy group and 70 operative endoscopy group) (Fig. 1).

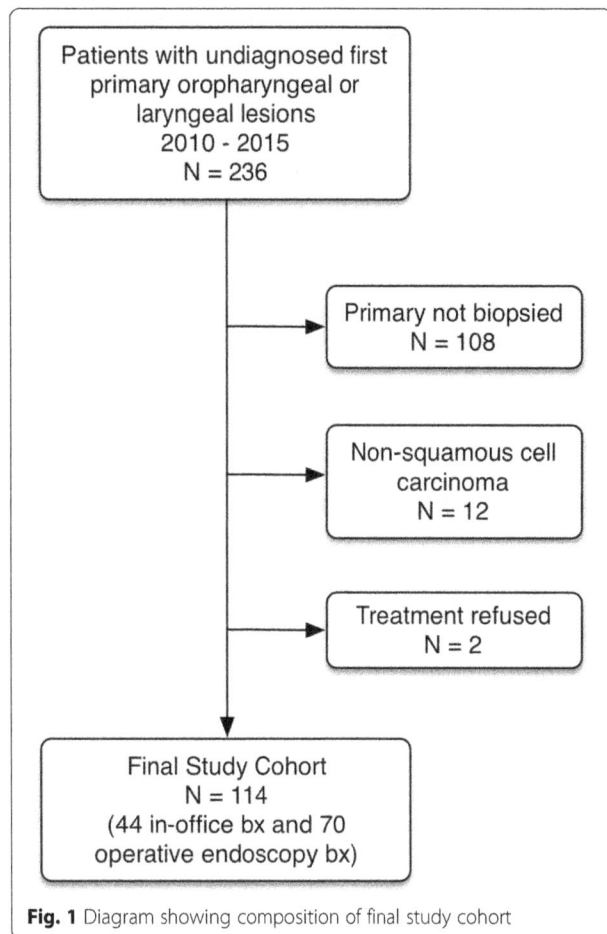

Fig. 1 Diagram showing composition of final study cohort

Outcomes
The primary outcome of interest was the time from the date of initial consultation by an otolaryngologist to the date of tissue biopsy. Secondary outcomes were the time from initial consultation to treatment, time from cancer diagnosis to multidisciplinary oncology consultation (MDOC), time from consultation to histopathological diagnosis and time from consultation to treatment.

Statistical analysis
Categorical variables were analyzed using either the Chi square or Fisher's exact test as appropriate. Continuous variables were analyzed using Students t-test or a Wilcoxon rank-sum test as appropriate. P-values of < 0.05 were considered statistically significant for all tests. Statistical analyses were performed using Stata 14.2 (StataCorp LP, College Station, Texas, USA).

Results
One hundred fourteen patients were eligible for inclusion in the study (Fig. 1). The operative endoscopy biopsy group had 70 patients while the in-office biopsy

group had 44 patients. Demographic information for the study population are summarized in Table 1.

Patient ages ranged from 37 to 87 years, with a mean age of 62.3 years (SD = 8.4). Patients were predominately male (88%) and presented most commonly with clinical stage IV disease (72%). The tongue base/vallecula were sampled most frequently (69%). Chemoradiation therapy was the commonest modality of treatment (68%). Subjects in the operative endoscopy biopsy group were younger, more likely to have a laryngeal primary and more likely to have fine needle aspiration (FNA) biopsy performed prior to biopsy of the primary cancer. There were no biopsy-related complications in either group.

Table 2 shows the time delays for different events. The mean time delay from consultation to biopsy was 17.4 days for the operative endoscopy biopsy group and 1.3 days for the in-office biopsy group ($p < 0.0001$). The time from consultation to tumor diagnosis was also significantly shorter in the in-office biopsy group (23 vs 7.5 days for the operative endoscopy biopsy and in-office biopsy groups respectively, $p < 0.0001$). There was no difference in the time taken to generate a pathology report between the 2 groups. There were no differences in lag times from initial consultation to MDOC, from MDOC to treatment or from initial consultation to treatment suggesting that access to MDOC and treatment is a challenge regardless of how quickly a histopathological diagnosis is made. Further analysis revealed that MDOCs are triggered by any diagnosis of cancer, including an FNA. Fifty three percent of operative endoscopy biopsy patients had an FNA compared to fewer than 10% of in-office biopsy patients (Table 1). Because FNA was often performed prior to biopsy of the primary lesion, FNA patients entered the queue for MDOC sooner than patients without an FNA, potentially confounding this result.

Discussion

Diagnosis of suspicious laryngopharyngeal lesions is usually managed by otolaryngologists. Often suspicious lesions can be seen, and accessed, by the transoral route and in those cases a simple transoral biopsy can be performed in the office. However, many patients have lesions that are not accessible transorally and in those cases biopsy in the operating room becomes necessary. The adoption of flexible fiber-optic nasopharyngoscopes has made the assessment, biopsy, and diagnosis of suspicious lesions comparable to that of operative endoscopy biopsy with minimal risk and discomfort [6, 8]. This technique, when used in suitable patients, avoids a general anesthetic, reduces the need for operative resources, and offers the potential for earlier diagnosis and treatment.

In our case series, patients were able to receive an in-office tissue biopsy 16 days earlier and a tumor tissue

Table 1 Demographics of the Study Population

Characteristic	Biopsy Group		p-value
	Operative Endoscopy	In-Office	
	$n = 70$	$n = 44$	
Age			**0.04**
Mean years [SD]	60.9 [8.2]	64.3 [8.6]	
Range	37.1–81.3	51.1–86.6	
Gender			ns
Male	64	36	
Female	6	8	
Clinical Stage			ns
In-situ	3	1	
I	4	4	
II	2	3	
III	5	4	
IVA	53	29	
IVB	3	3	
Biopsy Site			ns
Tongue base/vallecula	51	28	
Larynx	16	12	
Pharyngeal wall	3	2	
Other	0	2	
FNA Performed			**< 0.001**
Yes	37	4	
No	33	40	
Treatment			ns
Surgery alone	8	4	
RT alone	7	8	
Surgery and adjuvant RT	4	0	
CRT	48	30	
Surgery and adjuvant CRT	1	1	
Neoadjuvant CRT and surgery	2	1	

RT radiation therapy, *CRT* chemoradiation therapy, *ns* non-significant
Bold illustrates a statistically significant result

diagnosis 14.5 days sooner than a biopsy performed in the operating room. The availability of side-channel equipped office endoscopes makes in-office biopsy procedures feasible. Most patients are able to receive a tissue biopsy on the same day as their consultation or within a few days of presentation when side-channel forceps were needed. In addition to an earlier biopsy time, our data illustrate the safety of in-office endoscope-guided tissue sampling, with no procedure-related complications. This finding agrees with studies published elsewhere [6–9].

We were able to obtain tissue sufficient for histopathologic diagnosis in all cases where in-office biopsy was attempted. Analysis of healthcare costs avoided by in-

Table 2 Time Delays to Clinical Events

Event	Biopsy Group		p-value
	Operative Endoscopy	In-Office	
	n = 70	n = 44	
ENT Consultation to Biopsy			
Mean days (95% C.I.)	17.4 (13.5–21.3)	1.3 (−0.2–2.9)	**< 0.0001**
ENT Consultation to Diagnosis			
Mean days (95% C.I.)	23.0 (18.8–27.2)	7.5 (5.5–9.4)	**< 0.0001**
Pathology Delay (Biopsy to Diagnosis)			
Mean days (95% C.I.)	5.6 (4.9–6.4)	6.1 (4.9–7.3)	ns
ENT Consultation to MDOC			
Mean days (95% C.I.)	23.4 (19.4–27.4)	19 (16.0–22.0)	ns
MDOC to Treatment			
Mean days (95% C.I.)	33 (27.0–39.0)	32 (28.3–35.7)	ns
ENT Consultation to Treatment			
Mean days (95% C.I.)	51.7 (46.6–56.8)	49.6 (44.6–54.6)	ns

MDOC multidisciplinary oncology consultation, *95% C.I.* 95% confidence interval, *ns* non-significant
Bold illustrates a statistically significant result

office biopsy was beyond the scope of this study but other authors have reported cost outcomes. In a case series by Naidu et al. (2012), diagnostic in-office biopsy represented a 77% reduction in costs when compared to operative endoscopy biopsy for all patients presenting with laryngopharyngeal tumors [8]. Because all 44 patients in our in-office biopsy group received diagnostic biopsies, a referral to our pre-admission clinic for anesthesiology and internal medicine consultation, and scheduling for operative time and perioperative care were avoided. This likely resulted in an overall reduction in costs to our healthcare system.

Despite the shorter time delay to biopsy and potential for cost savings, some authors express concern regarding the diagnostic clarity of in-office tissue sampling. Richards et al. (2015) reported pathological variability between in-office and operative endoscopy biopsy of laryngeal lesions, with a relatively low sensitivity of 60% [9]. Of particular concern was the identification of invasive squamous cell carcinoma (SCC); just 15% of in-office biopsies proved positive for SCC on initial in-office evaluation. These authors therefore concluded that while in-office biopsies were a safe alternative to operative endoscopy biopsy, they were only moderately successful in identifying dysplastic lesions. Cohen et al. (2013) reported a similarly low sensitivity of 69% and false-negative rate of 33% when compared to direct

operative endoscopy biopsy [10]. These values were comparable to results published in a subsequent study of laryngeal biopsies [11]. The authors therefore recommended that suspicious lesions returned as benign pathology or carcinoma in-situ proceed directly to microlaryngoscopy for histopathological verification. While these study results contrast with other published reports [6–8], they nevertheless highlight that variables such as biopsy size, depth, and patient tolerance are potential causes of false negative results. These factors need to be considered in the context of the entire clinical picture when determining patient candidacy for in-office biopsy.

Our study found that the time delays from diagnosis to MDOC, MDOC to treatment, and overall time to treatment were equivalent. This is in contrast to Lippert et al. (2014), in which the authors reported an average time saving of 24.6 days to treatment for patients who received a successful in-office biopsy [6]. In our series the delays from diagnosis to MDOC and treatment were similar between the in-office and operative biopsy groups and the reasons for this are likely multifactorial.

First, patient referrals for MDOC at our cancer center are triggered by a histopathological diagnosis of cancer. Incoming referrals are triaged and reviewed weekly by the Head and Neck Tumor Group. Patients with a diagnosis of cancer on FNA are offered an MDOC even in the absence of a proven primary. Operative endoscopy biopsy can therefore occur after the MDOC and this explains why there were no differences in lag times between the 2 groups.

Second, patients requiring radiation therapy need dental consultation as well as subsequent appointments for fitting of a custom head and neck mold prior to the initiation of radiation. This can take up to 2 weeks, or longer, to complete adding further delay to the initiation of therapy. Third, because 37 of the 70 patients in the operative endoscopy biopsy group initially presented to the MDOC with an FNA biopsy positive for neck malignancy, referral bias is likely present within our population. We therefore believe that a combination of system factors and referral bias explains why we did not see significant reductions in treatment delay in the in-office biopsy group.

Our study has some limitations, primarily its retrospective design and the potential for referral bias as noted above. Despite these shortcomings, the impact on time to biopsy and diagnosis is large and, we believe, real.

Delays in the initiation of treatment for head and neck carcinoma may lead to worse oncologic outcomes therefore strategies that reduce temporal delays ought to be identified and adopted. Our study shows that in-office flexible fiber-optic endoscope-guided biopsy represents a statistically and clinically significant method to expedite the identification of suspicious laryngopharyngeal lesions when compared to operative endoscopy biopsy. However, the overall time to the initiation of treatment, was not significantly impacted by in-office biopsy. We believe further study will clarify these uncertainties and identify opportunities for efficiency. Further study on the economic impact of in-office biopsy will also be helpful in understanding the true benefit of this procedure.

Conclusions

Our results show that in-office biopsy significantly reduces the time from initial presentation to diagnosis in patients with suspicious laryngopharyngeal lesions presenting to otolaryngologists. The temporal gains via in-office biopsy did not translate into faster access to treatment and we believe that the reasons for this are multifactorial. Further study is needed to quantify the economic impact on healthcare resource utilization.

Abbreviations
FNA: Fine needle aspiration; MDOC: Multidisciplinary oncology consultation; OR: Operating room; SCC: Squamous cell carcinoma

Acknowledgements
We gratefully acknowledge the Ohlson Research Initiative for supporting this project.

Funding
Support for this research was provided by a grant from the Ohlson Research Initiative. The funder had no role in study design, or collection, analysis, interpretation of data, or in the writing of the manuscript.

Authors' contributions
FL and KS participated in data analysis, interpretation of the data, and participated in writing and preparation of the manuscript. JCD developed the study concept and design, acquired the data, was involved in the analysis and interpretation, and co-wrote and critically revised the manuscript. SCN assisted with study design, performed data analysis and interpretation of the data, and helped draft and critically revise the manuscript. SPC, TWM, and JDB assisted in the interpretation of the data and critically revised the manuscript. All authors give final approval for the manuscript to be published and agree to be accountable for it.

Competing interests
The authors declare that they have no competing interests.

References
1. SEER Cancer Stat Fact Sheet [http://seer.cancer.gov/statfacts/].
2. van Harten MC, Hoebers FJ, Kross KW, van Werkhoven ED, van den Brekel MW, van Dijk BA. Determinants of treatment waiting times for head and neck cancer in the Netherlands and their relation to survival. Oral Oncol. 2015;51:272–8.
3. Pitchers M, Martin C. Delay in referral of oropharyngeal squamous cell carcinoma to secondary care correlates with a more advanced stage at presentation, and is associated with poorer survival. Br J Cancer. 2006;94:955–8.
4. Stefanuto P, Doucet JC, Robertson C. Delays in treatment of oral cancer: a review of the current literature. Oral Surg Oral Med Oral Pathol Oral Radiol. 2014;117:424–9.
5. Jensen AR, Nellemann HM, Overgaard J. Tumor progression in waiting time for radiotherapy in head and neck cancer. Radiother Oncol. 2007;84:5–10.
6. Lippert D, Hoffman MR, Dang P, McCulloch TM, Hartig GK, Dailey SH. In-office biopsy of upper airway lesions: safety, tolerance, and effect on time to treatment. Laryngoscope. 2015;125:919–23.
7. Castillo Farias F, Cobeta I, Souviron R, Barbera R, Mora E, Benito A, Royuela A. In-office cup biopsy and laryngeal cytology versus operating room biopsy for the diagnosis of pharyngolaryngeal tumors: efficacy and cost-effectiveness. Head Neck. 2015;37:1483–7.
8. Naidu H, Noordzij JP, Samim A, Jalisi S, Grillone GA. Comparison of efficacy, safety, and cost-effectiveness of in-office cup forcep biopsies versus operating room biopsies for laryngopharyngeal tumors. J Voice. 2012;26:604–6.
9. Richards AL, Sugumaran M, Aviv JE, Woo P, Altman KW. The utility of office-based biopsy for laryngopharyngeal lesions: comparison with surgical evaluation. Laryngoscope. 2015;125:909–12.
10. Cohen JT, Safadi A, Fliss DM, Gil Z, Horowitz G. Reliability of a transnasal flexible fiberoptic in-office laryngeal biopsy. JAMA Otolaryngol Head Neck Surg. 2013;139:341–5.
11. Cohen JT, Benyamini L. Transnasal flexible Fiberoptic in-office laryngeal biopsies-our experience with 117 patients with suspicious lesions. Rambam Maimonides Med J. 2014;5:e0011.

33

Long term follow-up demonstrating stability and patient satisfaction of minimally invasive punch technique for percutaneous bone anchored hearing devices

Yaeesh Sardiwalla[1], Nicholas Jufas[2,3,4] and David P. Morris[1,2,5*] (iD)

Abstract

Objective: Minimally Invasive Ponto Surgery (MIPS) was recently described to facilitate the placement of percutaneous bone anchored hearing devices. As early adopters of this new procedure, we sought to perform a quality assurance project using our own small prospective cohort to justify this change in practice. We chose to examine device stability and to gauge our patients' perspective of the surgery and their overall satisfaction with the process.

Methods: A total of 12 adult patients who underwent MIPS between 2016 and 2017 with a minimum post-operative follow-up of 12 months were included in this study. A prospective MIPS research clinic was used to follow patients, assess the implant site soft tissue status and gather qualitative information through patient interviews and surveys.

Results: The mean (SD) soft tissue status score averages using the IPS Scale were low for inflammation 0.1 (0.1), pain 0.1 (0.1), skin height 0.2 (0.1) and total IPS score 0.4 (0.3) indicating minimal soft tissue changes. Patient experiences with MIPS were overwhelmingly positive in reports through the MIPS modified SSQ-8. All patients reported speedy recoveries and no long-term complications. There were zero device losses.

Conclusion: The series presented in this paper represents the first MIPS cohort with long term follow-up to be published to date in North America. Our findings conclude both device stability and patient satisfaction with no loss of fixtures. Consequently, we have adopted MIPS as our procedure of choice for the placement of all percutaneous BAHDs.

Keywords: Patient safety, Otologic surgical procedures, Bone conduction, Minimally invasive surgical procedures, Patient satisfaction, Quality improvement

Introduction

In 2011, Hultcrantz et al. described the Minimally Invasive Ponto Surgery (MIPS) procedure where a 5 mm dermal punch was used to remove the limited tract of soft tissue needed to accommodate the Ponto (Oticon, Copenhagen, Denmark) abutment [1]. The drilling procedure could then be completed in seconds through a cannula placed to protect the skin and soft tissues while holding cooling fluid. MIPS heralded a departure from the traditional "open approach" to percutaneous fixture placement. Soft tissue preservation and longer abutments placed in a few simple surgical steps marked a significant evolution of the original surgical procedure. While keen to adopt this simplified approach, we were equally vigilant to discover whether such changes were possible without compromise to patient care.

* Correspondence: dp.morris@dal.ca
[1]Faculty of Medicine, Dalhousie University, Halifax, NS, Canada
[2]Division of Otolaryngology – Head and Neck Surgery, Dalhousie University, Halifax, NS, Canada
Full list of author information is available at the end of the article

In our groups previously published direct cost analysis, we calculated that MIPS offered a saving of approximately $450 per operation when compared to open approaches [2]. The majority of this saving stems from the large time saving with MIPS procedure (0.10 h) versus the open approach (1.13 h) [2]. We were also able to move bone anchored hearing device (BAHD) surgery out of the main operating room (OR) with this transition, making valuable OR time accessible for other services [2].

In this follow-up study, we sought to investigate the long-term stability of the fixture/abutment in our single-center Halifax cohort. Early evidence from soft tissue preserving techniques for BAHD have already suggested favorable outcomes [3, 4]. To date, there have been few MIPS case series published. Bonilla et al. showed promising MIPS outcomes in their cohort, confirming a shorter procedure time and fewer skin complications one week after surgery when compared to the linear incision technique [5]. While details of other experiences are limited, there are mixed results reported [6]. The highly anticipated long-term, multi-centre MIPS outcomes data recently published showed no difference in inflammation compared to linear incisions [7–9]. There was improvement in skin sensation, sagging, cosmetic result and reduction of surgical time but a non-significant increase in implant extrusion rate that warrants further investigation [7–9].

Generally, it is accepted that osseointegration and implant stability occurs within 3 months for adults and 6 months for children [10–12]. This period has traditionally been used to guide the timing for loading the abutment. We reasoned that if the fixtures were to fail or have complications, they would do so early after surgery. We proposed a minimum follow-up period of 12 months to capture such failures.

As early adopters of this new procedure, we sought to perform a quality assurance project using our own small prospective cohort to justify this change in practice. As medical professionals, we balance the introduction of new techniques and intervention with patient safety, especially where large bodies of evidence do not yet exist [10]. We chose to examine device stability and to gauge our patients' perspective of the surgery and their overall satisfaction with the process.

Methods
Patient selection and surgery
Institutional permission from Nova Scotia Health Authority Research Ethics Board was obtained to conduct the quality assurance of the new MIPS technique. A total of 12 sequential adult patients who underwent MIPS between 2016 and 2017 with a minimum post-operative follow-up

of 12 months were prospectively enrolled in this study at the time of proceeding with surgery. All cases were performed or directly assisted and supervised by the same experienced consultant otologist. Specific training covering the MIPS procedure and novel drilling technique in both an animal and synthetic temporal bone model had been undertaken prior to the first real-time surgery. Exclusive MIPS cases were performed under local anesthetic. General anesthesia was reserved for those undergoing concomitant middle ear or mastoid surgery. Cases requiring general anesthesia were performed in the main OR. Most local anesthesia cases were performed in a minor procedures room conforming to Infection Prevention and Control standards. For an overview of the surgical technique and equipment required for MIPS, please review our groups previous article on this topic [2]. Sound processors were loaded at median of 6 weeks, with a range from 4 to 6 weeks. Table 1 shows complete demographic information.

The details of each surgical case, fixture/abutment specifications, external BAHD chosen and operating time was recorded. Each patient's surgical data is captured in Table 2. The MIPS operating time was calculated prospectively from the moment of skin punch, to the moment the healing cap was placed.

Research clinic
Follow-up was prospective. A coordinated MIPS research clinic was used to follow patients, assess implant sites and gather qualitative information through patient interviews and surveys. Soft tissue status around the implant was evaluated independently by three different assessors (staff otologist, otology fellow and senior medical student) using the eight point Inflammation, Pain, Skin Height (IPS) Scale proposed by Kruyt [13]. The IPS scale was designed to assess long-term wound healing at the bone conduction site using objective and patient reported measures of inflammation (skin integrity, erythema, edema and granulation tissue), pain and skin height/numbness to prompt treatment decisions. This addresses the shortcomings of the Holgers scale such as dichotomous subjective responses, not considering long-term wound healing failures such as increased skin height and not encapsulating patient pain [13–15]. Patients qualitative perspectives were assessed using the Surgical Satisfaction Questionnaire (SSQ-8) modified for MIPS and through a semi-structured interview that assessed their experience. The modified SSQ-8 asked patients to use a Likert Scale (1 – very satisfied; 5 – very unsatisfied) to rate their MIPS surgical experience according 8 domains: the result of their surgery, their recovery, satisfaction with abutment length, appearance of

Table 1 The demographic information and operative characteristics from the cohort of MIPS patients followed for a minimum of 12 months

Age	Sen	Previous Diagnosis	Follow-up Duration	Surgery	Admission	Anesthesia	Site
74	F	Psoriasis and Left Mastoid cavity	30 months	MIPS	Day Case	Local	Main OR
58	M	Chronic Suppurative Otitis Media - Previous mastoidectomy	30 months	MIPS	Day Case	General	Main OR
57	F	Chronic Suppurative Otitis Media	28 months	MIPS + Mastoid obliteration	Admitted	General	Main OR
58	M	Chronic Suppurative Otitis Media	24 months	MIPS	Day Case	Local	Main OR
28	F	Chronic Suppurative Otitis Media	23 months	MIPS + Mastoid obliteration	Day Case	General	Main OR
55	M	Chronic Suppurative Otitis Media	20 months	MIPS + Mastoid obliteration	Admitted	General	Main OR
55	M	Chronic Suppurative Otitis Media	18 months	MIPS and Left Tympanoplasty	Admitted	General	Main OR
52	F	Chronic Suppurative Otitis Media	14 months	MIPS + Blind Sac closure	Admitted	General	Main OR
30	M	Chronic Suppurative Otitis Media Tympanomastoidecomy	20 months	MIPS	Day Case	Local	Minor Procedures
65	F	CSOM preexisting mastoid cavity	20 months	MIPS	Day Case	Local	Minor Procedures
41	M	Right Microtia	19 months	MIPS	Day Case	Local	Minor Procedures
74	M	CSOM	17 months	MIPS	Day Case	Local	Minor Procedures

screw, the follow-up they received, overall satisfaction and how likely they would be to recommend MIPS to others who require BAHD. Both the IPS scale and modified SSQ-8 were administered at the patient's most recent follow-up visit.

Statistical analysis

Data from all three observers' IPS scores were analyzed independently and were averaged. Only descriptive analysis was used since this is a small sample evaluation.

Box and whisker plots of survey data were used to present responses.

Results

The mean (SD) soft tissue status score averages using the IPS Scale were low for inflammation 0.1 (0.1), pain 0.1 (0.1), skin height 0.2 (0.1) and total IPS score 0.4 (0.3) indicating minimal soft tissue changes. There was good inter-rater reliability with these scores. Table 3 shows the summarized IPS results. Digital photographs

Table 2 Technical information relating to the MIPS surgery for each of the 12 patients. For each procedure 50 N.cm of torque was obtained. * *Topical application of ciprofloxacin/dexamethasone drops (Ciprodex ®) around abutment*

Sound Processor	Abutment (and change if applicable)	Implant	Length of Surgery (mins)	Skin thickness (mm)	Number of turns	Adjunctive Measures
Left Ponto Plus power	Ponto 9 mm -- > 12 mm	4 mm Ponto BHX	8.2	4.5	S	Abutment lengthened
Left BAHA S	Ponto 12 mm	4 mm Ponto BHX	9.S	7	4.5	Ciprodex* drops 'local toilet'*
Left BAHA 5	Ponto 12 mm	4 mm Ponto BHX	4	6	S	Stay suture applied interiorly
Right Ponto Plus power	Ponto 9 mm	4 mm Wide Ponto	9.6	5	4.5	None
Left BAHA S	Ponto 12 mm -- > 9 mm	4 mm Wide Ponto	8	S	4.5	Abutment shortened Ciprodex* 'local toilet'*
Right BAHA S	Ponto 12 mm	4 mm Wide Ponto	S.2	6	3.25	None
Right BAHA S	Ponto 12 mm	4 mm Ponto BHX	6	S	4.5	Direct trauma to implant, close examination - no apparent harm
Left BAHA S	Ponto 12 mm	4 mm Ponto BHX	4.2	6	5	Slight skin redundancy superiorly at implant site
Right Baha 5	Ponto 12 mm	4 mm Ponto BHX	7	7	4.5	None
Right Ponto Plus	Ponto 12 mm	4 mm Ponto BHX	8	6	4.25	None
Right Baha 5	Ponto 12 mm - > 9 mm	4 mm Ponto BHX	7	S	4.5	Abutment shortened
Right Ponto Plus	Ponto 9 mm	4 mm Ponto BHX	4.5	4	4.5	None

Table 3 A summary of the IPS-scale soft tissue status for patients at their most recent follow-up where they were seen by 3 independent raters

	Inflammation			Pain			Skin Height			Total Score		
Rater	1	2	3	1	2	3	1	2	3	1	2	3
Score	0.3	0.1	0.0	0.2	0.0	0.0	0.3	0.1	0,2	0.8	0.2	0.2
Average	01			0.1			0.2			0.4		

corroborated these findings. Figure 1 shows a sample of such images.

There were few minor complications as can be seen by the soft tissue score. The most common intervention in the early post-operative period was the prescription of topical antimicrobial drops on an 'as required' basis should the patient experience redness or irritation. Later complications noted included 3 patients with abutment length changes, the requirement of stay sutures inferiorly and skin redundancy superiorly. Most importantly, there were no failures to osseointegrate and no fixtures had been lost in this cohort at the time of last follow-up.

In terms of survey data, median (M) and Interquartile Range (IQR) from the MIPS modified SSQ-8 were: result of surgery 1 (1), recovery 1 (1, 2), abutment length satisfaction 1.5 (1, 2), appearance of screw 2 (1, 2), follow-up received 1 (1, 2), overall satisfaction 1 (1, 2), and recommendation of MIPS to others who would benefit 1 (1). Figure 2 presents a graphic summary of modified SSQ-8 survey data.

The patient experiences with MIPS were overwhelmingly positive. All patients reported speedy recoveries, often getting back to routine activities the next day. The surgical experience was felt to be minimized, with patient's reporting they received high quality care. Issues reported

included getting used to having a foreign object on their head and initial maintenance of the implant site. Some patients reported wearing their devices with a degree of selectivity, only using them in more challenging listening environments. A segment from a semi-structured patient interview is included below:

"I had a screw failure with my previous bone conduction surgery. It was a much better experience with MIPS when I was awake. There was virtually no recovery afterwards – I went shopping 1 hour later. This was compared to my previous surgery with lots of bleeding, bandages and overnight admission. I wear my device all the time."

Discussion

As clinicians, we sense a responsibility to carefully assess and evaluate new developments in patient treatment to ensure that the best quality of care continues to be delivered. The MIPS technique is different from the traditional open approach with which most surgeons are familiar, in a number of ways. Visual access to the bony skull is limited to the narrow tract maintained by the cannula.

A steady hand to stabilize the cannula position and fine tactile feedback are needed to confirm that each pass of the drill is aligned with the original 3 mm test hole. Confirmation that the fixture/abutment assembly has also engaged the countersunk hole once the cannula is removed also demands tactile recognition. The assistance of an experienced second pair of hands cannot be over emphasized. Unlike the

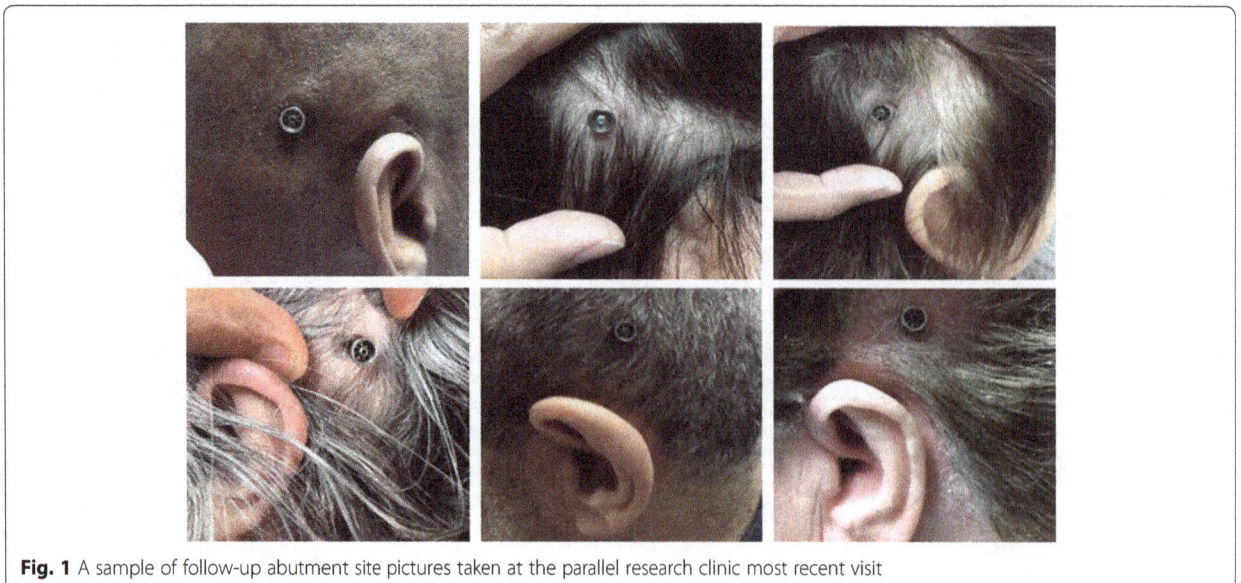

Fig. 1 A sample of follow-up abutment site pictures taken at the parallel research clinic most recent visit

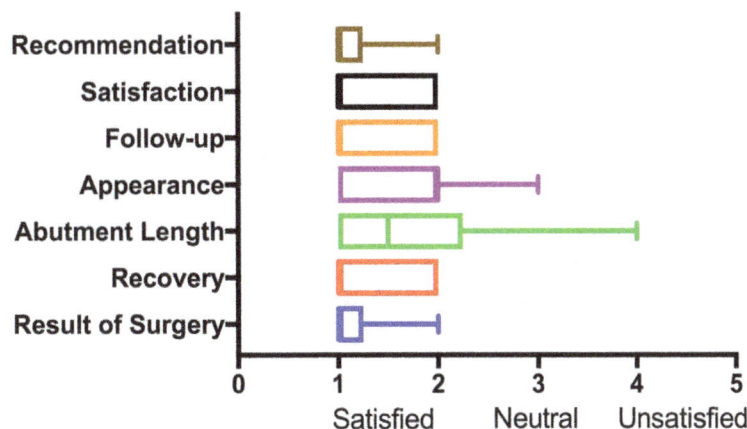

Fig. 2 A box and whisker plot showing survey results from the modified surgical questionnaire for MIPS at latest follow-up

traditional open approach, it is impossible to do this procedure alone. The operating surgeon must maintain the cannula in a stable position for the short duration of the case. The assistant is responsible for the swift loading of drill bits, the application of saline irrigation to the operative site and ultimately attaching the fixture/abutment assembly to the handpiece.

The drills are also very different from what went before. It is intuitive that prolonged drilling, failure to irrigate sufficiently with saline and malalignment of drilling trajectory could all result in fixture failure. As the cannula can only hold a small volume of saline irrigant, this should be cold and not from the warming cabinet. Drilling time should also be as short as possible to prevent heating. Constant refilling of the cannula between stages and removal of bone dust also seems intuitive. At the very end of the procedure, excessive leverage should be avoided when uncoupling the connection to handpiece instrument from the secured abutment. This maneuver risks disturbing even the most perfect of placements and is particularly risky given the increased length of abutments needed when soft tissues are not reduced.

While keen to adopt this simplified approach, we were equally keen to discover whether such changes were possible without compromise to patient care. After performing a round dozen cases, a self-imposed moratorium was observed until sufficient reassurance had been obtained to justify an ongoing change in practice.

Our study has demonstrated that it is possible to maintain secure fixture/abutment placement with the MIPS procedure. With a minimum follow-up of 1 year, skin complications were low, consistent with other invetigators [4]. Implants were stable, and it is reassuring to us that no fixtures were lost in this highly-scrutinized cohort. We have previously shown that this change in practice comes with benefits of cost efficiency and better resource allocation [2].

Here we show additional value in proven patient satisfaction with the MIPS procedure in addition to the well documented improvements in quality of life for BAHD users [16, 17].

It is likely that both training and case selection will have some bearing on surgical outcome. Repeated practice of the surgical steps in a training model prior to real-time surgery would seem to be a prudent prerequisite to successful fixture placement even for those who consider themselves to be experienced surgeons with the traditional system. It is humbling to acknowledge the natural learning curve of any new procedure no matter how simple it may seem. The consequences of failure are significant to the patient.

As the MIPS procedure is performed without soft tissue reduction, longer abutments are used with the same 4 mm fixture of purchase on the skull. Simple rotational physics dictates that increasing the distance from the fulcrum reduces the load necessary to exert a displacing force. This principle is explained by Archimedes' Law of the Lever:

Torque (N.m) = Force (N) x distance (m) from fulcrum

The thicker the scalp, the longer is the required abutment. We note that all our cohort received an abutment of 12 mm or 9 mm. No cases required the longer 14 mm abutment which still relies on just 4 mm of skull purchase. As other centers report their results, it will be interesting to see whether the 14 mm abutments are as stable as we have found the 9 mm and 12 mm abutments to be. If this is not the case, some discretion in patient selection may be appropriate.

A limitation of this study relates to the modified SSQ-8 use for MIPS. Although the SSQ-8 has been independently validated for urogynecological surgeries, the adapted form used for this study has not been studied in the context of otologic surgeries. The survey data was congruent with the interview results, with both methods suggesting encouraging experiences with MIPS. This at least provided the reassurances we were seeking from a quality assurance point of view.

The study's strengths include a long follow-up period for what is still a relatively new technique to North America. With a minimum of 1 year follow-up we anticipated adequate capture of both short and long-term complications. The study also allowed for a robust evaluation of MIPS since objective surgical and subjective patient factors were assessed. The sample size ($N = 12$) for the semi-structured interview was adequate to achieve thematic saturation [18]. The patients will continue to be followed and watched closely to ensure ongoing stability.

Conclusion

As one of the first North American adopters of the MIPS procedure, we thought it diligent to perform a quality assurance project using our own original prospective cohort. Our findings conclude both device stability and patient satisfaction with no loss of fixtures.

Consequently, we have adopted MIPS as our procedure of choice for the placement of all percutaneous BAHDs.

Abbreviations

BAHD: Bone Anchored Hearing Devices; BCHI: Bone Conduction Hearing Implants; HCP: Healthcare Providers; IPS: Inflammation Pain Skin height; MIPS: Minimally Invasive Ponto Surgery; OR: Operating Room; SSQ: Surgical Satisfaction Questionnaire

Acknowledgements

The authors gratefully acknowledge the assistance of the following individuals who were instrumental in helping coordinate and evaluate MIPS patient's in follow-up parallel research clinics:
Carla Roberts (Administrative Assistant, Victoria General Hospital, Halifax).
Mamoona Khalid-Raja (Otology Fellow, Dalhousie University).

Funding

None.

Authors' contributions

YS was responsible for the preparation of the manuscript, coordinating the research clinics to conduct follow-up of the MIPS cohort. YS also completed the literature review, liaised with necessary hospital departments and analyzed the data. NJ prepared and edited of the manuscript, and was the primary surgeon as Otology Fellow for some of the MIPS cases. DPM was the lead surgeon for all MIPS cases, contributed to and edited the manuscript and developed the discussion.

Author's information

YS is a third-year medical student at Dalhousie University. NJ was an Otology Fellow at Dalhousie University and is currently a consulting ENT surgeon and senior clinical lecturer at both Sydney and Macquarie Universities, Sydney, Australia. DPM is a Consultant in Adult and Paediatric Otology/Neurotology at the Queen Elizabeth II Health Science Centre in Halifax Nova Scotia and is an Associate Professor at Dalhousie University.

Competing interests

DPM has participated in scientific meetings, MIPS prototype development and workshops arranged by Oticon Medical where travel and accommodation costs were provided. YS and NJ have none to declare.

Author details

[1]Faculty of Medicine, Dalhousie University, Halifax, NS, Canada. [2]Division of Otolaryngology – Head and Neck Surgery, Dalhousie University, Halifax, NS, Canada. [3]Discipline of Surgery, Sydney Medical School, University of Sydney, Sydney, Australia. [4]Department of Otolaryngology – Head and Neck Surgery, Faculty of Medicine and Health Sciences, Macquarie University, Sydney, Australia. [5]QEII Health Science Center - VG Site Otolaryngology, 5820 University Ave - Rm 3037, Halifax, NS B3H 2Y9, Canada.

References

1. Hultcrantz M. Outcome of the bone-anchored hearing aid procedure without skin thinning: a prospective clinical trial. Otol Neurotol. 2011; 32:1134–9.
2. Sardiwalla Y, Jufas N, Morris DP. Direct cost comparison of minimally invasive punch technique versus traditional approaches for percutaneous bone anchored hearing devices. J Otolaryngol - Head Neck Surg. 2017;46:4–9.
3. Johansson M, Holmberg M, Hultcrantz PM. Bone anchored hearing implant surgery with tissue preservation – a systematic literature review. Oticon Med Rev. 2015. https://www.oticonmedical.com/-/media/medical/main/files/for-professionals/bahs/surgical-materials/papers/eng/literature-review---tissue-preservation---english---m52107.pdf?la=en.
4. Johansson ML, et al. Short-term results from seventy-six patients receiving a bone-anchored hearing implant installed with a novel minimally invasive surgery technique. Clin Otolaryngol. 2017;42:1043–8.
5. Bonilla A, Magri C, Juan E. Findings from the experience with the punch technique for auditory osseointegrated implants: a retrospective single center comparative study. Acta Otorrinolaringol Esp. 2017;68:309–16.
6. Bennett, A., Banigo, A., Lovegrove, D. & Wood, M. Comparison of non soft tissue reduction techniques for BAHA insertion: open approach vs. MIPS in OSSEO (2017).
7. Johansson M, Holmberg M. Design and clinical evaluation of MIPS – a new perspective on tissue preservation. Oticon Med. 2014:1–12. https://doi.org/10.13140/RG.2.1.3624.7762.
8. Calon, T. G. A. et al. Minimally invasive Ponto surgery compared to the linear incision technique without soft tissue reduction for bone conduction hearing implants: study protocol for a randomized controlled trial. Trials 17, 540 (2016).
9. Calon ÄTGA, et al. Minimally invasive Ponto surgery versus the linear incision technique with soft tissue preservation for bone conduction hearing Implants : a multicenter randomized controlled trial. Otol. Neurotol. 2018;39:882–93.
10. Reyes RA, Tjellstrom A, Granstrom G. Evaluation of implant losses and skin reactions around extraoral bone-anchored implants: a 0-to 8-year follow-up. Otolaryngol Neck Surg. 2000;122:272–6.
11. Tjellstrom A, Granstrom G. Long-term follow-up with the bone-anchored hearing aid: a review of the first 100 patients between 1977 and 1985. Ear Nose Throat J. 1994;73:112–4.
12. D'Eredità R, Caroncini M, Saetti R. The new baha implant: a prospective osseointegration study. Otolaryngol - Head Neck Surg (United States). 2012; 146(979–983).
13. Kruyt IJ, Nelissen RC, Johansson ML, Mylanus EAM, Hol MKS. The IPS-scale: a new soft tissue assessment scale for percutaneous and transcutaneous implants for bone conduction devices. Clin Otolaryngol. 2017;42:1410–3.
14. Holgers KM, Tjellstrom A, Bjursten LM, Erlandsson BE. Soft tissue reactions around percutaneous implants: a clinical study of soft tissue conditions around skin-penetrating titanium implants for bone-anchored hearing aids. Am J Otol. 1988;9:56–9.
15. Wazen JJ, et al. Successes and complications of the Baha system. Otol Neurotol. 2008;29:1115–9.
16. Hol MKS, et al. The bone-anchored hearing aid: quality-of-life assessment. Arch Otolaryngol Head Neck Sur. 2004;130:394–9.
17. AruArunachalan PS, Kilby D, Meikle D, Davison T, Johnson I. Bone-anchored hearing aid: quality of life assess by Glasgow benefit inventory. Clin Otolaryngol Allied Sci. 2000;25:570 6.

Permissions

The contributors of this book come from diverse backgrounds, making this book a truly international effort. This book will bring forth new frontiers with its revolutionizing research information and detailed analysis of the nascent developments around the world.

We would like to thank all the contributing authors for lending their expertise to make the book truly unique. They have played a crucial role in the development of this book. Without their invaluable contributions this book wouldn't have been possible. They have made vital efforts to compile up to date information on the varied aspects of this subject to make this book a valuable addition to the collection of many professionals and students.

This book was conceptualized with the vision of imparting up-to-date information and advanced data in this field. To ensure the same, a matchless editorial board was set up. Every individual on the board went through rigorous rounds of assessment to prove their worth. After which they invested a large part of their time researching and compiling the most relevant data for our readers.

The editorial board has been involved in producing this book since its inception. They have spent rigorous hours researching and exploring the diverse topics which have resulted in the successful publishing of this book. They have passed on their knowledge of decades through this book. To expedite this challenging task, the publisher supported the team at every step. A small team of assistant editors was also appointed to further simplify the editing procedure and attain best results for the readers.

Apart from the editorial board, the designing team has also invested a significant amount of their time in understanding the subject and creating the most relevant covers. They scrutinized every image to scout for the most suitable representation of the subject and create an appropriate cover for the book.

The publishing team has been an ardent support to the editorial, designing and production team. Their endless efforts to recruit the best for this project, has resulted in the accomplishment of this book. They are a veteran in the field of academics and their pool of knowledge is as vast as their experience in printing. Their expertise and guidance has proved useful at every step. Their uncompromising quality standards have made this book an exceptional effort. Their encouragement from time to time has been an inspiration for everyone.

The publisher and the editorial board hope that this book will prove to be a valuable piece of knowledge for researchers, students, practitioners and scholars across the globe.

List of Contributors

Scott Kohlert, Laurie McLean and Kristian Macdonald
Department of Otolaryngology, The Ottawa Hospital, 501 Smyth Rd, Ottawa, ON K1H 8L6, Canada
University of Ottawa, Ottawa, ON, Canada

Laura Zuccaro
University of Ottawa, Ottawa, ON, Canada

John E. Iyaniwura
Biomedical Engineering Graduate Program, Western University, 1151 Richmond Street, London, ON N6A 3K7, Canada

Hanif M. Ladak
Biomedical Engineering Graduate Program, Western University, 1151 Richmond Street, London, ON N6A 3K7, Canada
Department of Otolaryngology-Head and Neck Surgery, Western University, London, ON, Canada
Department of Medical Biophysics, Western University, London, ON, Canada
Department of Electrical and Computer Engineering, Western University, London, ON, Canada

Sumit K. Agrawal
Biomedical Engineering Graduate Program, Western University, 1151 Richmond Street, London, ON N6A 3K7, Canada
Department of Otolaryngology-Head and Neck Surgery, Western University, London, ON, Canada
Department of Electrical and Computer Engineering, Western University, London, ON, Canada
London Health Science Centre, Room B1-333, University Hospital, 339 Windermere Rd., London, ON, Canada

Mai Elfarnawany
Department of Otolaryngology-Head and Neck Surgery, Western University, London, ON, Canada

Kevin Martell and Harold Yeehau Lau
Division of Radiation Oncology, Tom Baker Cancer Centre, Calgary, AB, Canada
Department of Oncology, University of Calgary, 1331 29 Street Northwest, Calgary, AB T2N 4 N2, Canada

Joanna Mackenzie
Edinburgh Cancer Centre, Western General Hospital, Edinburgh, Scotland, UK

Warren Kerney
Calgary Zone, Alberta Health Services, Calgary, AB, Canada

Sarah Chorfi and Neil Verma
Faculty of Medicine, McGill University Health Centre, Montreal Children's Hospital, McGill University, Room A02.3015, 1001 Boulevard Decarie, Montreal, QC H4A 3J1, Canada

Joseph S. Schwartz
Department of Otolaryngology-Head and Neck Surgery, McGill University, Montreal, Canada

Lily H. P. Nguyen
Department of Otolaryngology-Head and Neck Surgery, McGill University, Montreal, Canada
Centre for Medical Education, McGill University, Montreal, Canada

Meredith Young
Centre for Medical Education, McGill University, Montreal, Canada
Department of Medicine, McGill University, Montreal, Canada

Lawrence Joseph
Department of Epidemiology and Biostatistics, McGill University, Montreal, Canada

Ilyes Berania, Mohamed Awad, Issam Saliba and Jean-Jacques Dufour
Division of Otolaryngology - Head and Neck Surgery, Université de Montréal, Centre Hospitalier de l'Université de Montréal (CHUM) – Hôpital Notre-Dame, 1560 Sherbrooke Street, Montreal, QC H2L 4M1, Canada

Marc-Elie Nader
Division of Otolaryngology - Head and Neck Surgery, Université de Montréal, Centre Hospitalier de l'Université de Montréal (CHUM) – Hôpital Notre-Dame, 1560 Sherbrooke Street, Montreal, QC H2L 4M1, Canada
Department of Head and Neck Surgery, Unit 1445, The University of Texas MD Anderson Cancer Center, 1515 Holcombe Blvd, Houston, TX 77030, USA

Matthew S. Harris
Department of Otolaryngology – Head and Neck Surgery, Schulich School of Medicine and Dentistry, Western University, London, ON, Canada

Brian W. Rotenberg, Kathryn Roth and Leigh J. Sowerby
Department of Otolaryngology – Head and Neck Surgery, Schulich School of Medicine and Dentistry, Western University, London, ON, Canada

St. Joseph's Healthcare, Western University, 268 Grosvenor Street, London, ON N6A 4 V2, Canada

Hedyeh Ziai
Faculty of Medicine, University of Ottawa, Ottawa, ON, Canada

James P. Bonaparte
Department of Otolaryngology–Head and Neck Surgery, University of Ottawa, 1919 Riverside Drive, Suite 309, Ottawa, ON K1H 7W9, Canada

Woon Won Kim
Department of General Surgery, Haeundae Paik Hospital, Inje University College of Medicine, Busan, Republic of Korea

Tae Kwun Ha
Department of General Surgery, Busan Paik Hospital, Inje University College of Medicine, 75, Bokji-ro, Busanjin-gu, 614-735 Busan, Republic of Korea

Sung Kwon Bae
Department of Medical Management, Kosin University, Busan, Republic of Korea

Jianhua Peng, He Li, Jun Chen, Xianming Wu, and Xiaoyun Chen
Department of Otolaryngology, the First Affiliated Hospital of Wenzhou Medical University, Wenzhou, Zhejiang 325000, China

Tao Jiang
Institute of Translation Medicine, the First Affiliated Hospital of Wenzhou Medical University, Wenzhou, Zhejiang 325000, China

Jason J. Xu, Caitlin McMullen, Han Zhang, Antoine Eskander, Ralph Gilbert, Jonathan Irish, Patrick Gullane, Dale Brown, John R. de Almeida and David P. Goldstein
Department of Otolaryngology—Head and Neck Surgery, University Health Network, University of Toronto, Toronto, Ontario, Canada

Eugene Yu
Department of Medical Imaging, University Health Network, University of Toronto, Toronto, Ontario, Canada

Jesse Pasternak and Lorne Rotstein
Department of Surgery, Division of General Surgery, University Health Network, University of Toronto, Toronto, Ontario, Canada

Jim Brierley and Richard Tsang
Department of Radiation Oncology, University Health Network, University of Toronto, Toronto, Ontario, Canada

Anna M. Sawka
Department of Medicine, Division of Endocrinology, University Health Network University of Toronto, Toronto, Ontario, Canada

Christopher M. Yao, Hedyeh Ziai, Gordon Tsang, Andrea Copeland, Dale Brown, Jonathan C. Irish, Ralph W. Gilbert, David P. Goldstein, Patrick J. Gullane and John R. de Almeida
Department of Otolaryngology-Head and Neck Surgery/Surgical Oncology, Princess Margaret Cancer Centre, University Health Network, 610 University Avenue, 3-955, Toronto, ON M5G 2 M9, Canada

Alex Hopkins, Vincent L. Biron, Hadi Seikaly and David W. J. Côté
Department of Surgery, Division of Otolaryngology-Head and Neck Surgery, University of Alberta, Edmonton, AB, Canada

Adrian Mendez
Department of Surgery, Division of Otolaryngology-Head and Neck Surgery, University of Alberta, Edmonton, AB, Canada
E4 Walter C Mackenzie Centre, 8440-112 Street NW, Edmonton, AB T6G 2B7, Canada

Lin Fu Zhu
Faculty of Medicine and Dentistry, University of Alberta, Edmonton, AB, Canada

Caroline C. Jeffery and Allan Ho
Division of Otolaryngology-Head and Neck Surgery, University of Alberta, Hospital, 8440 112 Street, Edmonton, AB T6G 2B7, Canada
Faculty of Medicine and Dentistry, University of Alberta, Hospital, 8440 112 Street, Edmonton, AB T6G 2B7, Canada

Cameron Shillington and Colin Andrews
Faculty of Medicine and Dentistry, University of Alberta, Hospital, 8440 112 Street, Edmonton, AB T6G 2B7, Canada

Kazunori Kubota, Sachio Takeno, Takayuki Taruya, Atsushi Sasaki, Takashi Ishino and Katsuhiro Hirakawa
Department of Otolaryngology, Head and Neck Surgery, Division of Clinical Medical Science, Programs for Applied Biomedicine, Graduate School of Biomedical Sciences, Hiroshima University, 1-2-3 Kasumi, Minami-ku, Hiroshima 734-8551, Japan

Ingo Todt, Gloria Grupe, Andreas Stratmann, Arne Ernst and Philipp Mittmann
Department of Otolaryngology, Head and Neck Surgery, Unfallkrankenhaus Berlin, Warenerstr.7, 12683 Berlin, Germany

Grit Rademacher and Sven Mutze
Department of Radiology, Unfallkrankenhaus Berlin, Berlin, Germany

Kristian I. Macdonald and Shaun J. Kilty
MD FRCSC, Department of Otolaryngology – Head and Neck Surgery, University of Ottawa, Ottawa, ON, Canada

Carl van Walraven
MD MSc FRCPC, Department of Medicine, Ottawa Hospital Research Institute, University of Ottawa, Ottawa, ON, Canada

P. Horwich, M. H. Rigby, C. MacKay, J.Melong, B.Williams, R. Hart, J. Trites and S. M. Taylor
Department of Surgery, Division of Otolaryngology–Head and Neck Surgery, Queen Elizabeth II Health Science Centre and Dalhousie University, 3rd Floor Dickson Building, VG Site, 5820 University Avenue, Halifax, NS B3H 2Y9, Canada

M. Bullock
Department of Pathology, Division of Anatomical Pathology, Queen Elizabeth II Health Science Centre and Dalhousie University, Halifax, NS, Canada

Alexandra E. Quimby
Department of Otolaryngology-Head and Neck Surgery, University of Ottawa, S3, 501 Smyth Road, Ottawa, ON K1H 8L6, Canada

Edmund S. H. Kwok
Department of Emergency Medicine, University of Ottawa, 501 Smyth Rd, Ottawa, ON K1H 8L6, Canada

Daniel Lelli
Department of Medicine, Division of Neurology, University of Ottawa, 501 Smyth Rd, Ottawa, ON K1H 8L6, Canada

Peter Johns
Department of Emergency Medicine, University of Ottawa, 501 Smyth Rd, Ottawa, ON K1H 8L6, Canada

Darren Tse
Department of Otolaryngology-Head and Neck Surgery, University of Ottawa, 501 Smyth Rd, Ottawa, ON K1H 8L6, Canada

A. E. Quimby and S.Kohlert
Department of Otolaryngology - Head and Neck Surgery, University of Ottawa, 501 Smyth Rd, Module S, Room M2566, Ottawa, ON K1H 8L6, Canada

L. Caulley
Bringham and Women's Hospital, Department of Neuroendocrinology, 75 Francis St, Boston, MA 02115, USA

M. Bromwich
Division of Otolaryngology – Head and Neck Surgery, Children's Hospital of Eastern Ontario, 401 Smyth Rd, Ottawa, ON K1H 8L1, Canada

Ying-Chieh Hsu
Department of Otorhinolaryngology, Cathay General Hospital, 280 Ren-Ai Rd. Sec. 4, Taipei, Taiwan

Tzu-Chin Huang
Department of Otorhinolaryngology, Cathay General Hospital, 280 Ren-Ai Rd. Sec. 4, Taipei, Taiwan. Department of Otorhinolaryngology, Hsinchu Cathay General Hospital, Hsinchu, Taiwan.

Chin-Lung Kuo
Department of Otolaryngology, Taoyuan Armed Forces General Hospital, Taoyuan, Taiwan, Republic of China

M. Elise Graham
Division of Otolaryngology – Head and Neck Surgery, Western University and London Health Sciences Centre, 5010, 800 Commissioners Road E, London, Ontario, Canada

Brian D. Westerberg, Jane Lea, Rochelle Galleto and Hannah Foggin
Division of Otolaryngology – Head and Neck Surgery, University of British Columbia, Vancouver, BC, Canada

Paul Hong
IWK Health Center and Division of Otolaryngology–Head and Neck Surgery, Dalhousie University, Halifax, NS, Canada

Simon Walling and Andrea L. O. Hebb
Division of Neurosurgery, Dalhousie University, Halifax, NS, Canada

David P. Morris Emily Papsin and Maeve Mulroy
Division of Otolaryngology, Head and Neck Surgery, Dalhousie University, Halifax, NS, Canada

Manohar Bance
Division of Otolaryngology, Head and Neck Surgery, Dalhousie University, Halifax, NS, Canada University of Cambridge, Cambridge, UK

Melody J. Xu
Department of Radiation Oncology, University of California San Francisco, San Francisco, CA, USA

Sue S. Yom
Department of Radiation Oncology, University of California San Francisco, San Francisco, CA, USA Division of Head and Neck Oncologic Surgery, Department of Otolaryngology-Head and Neck Surgery, University of California San Francisco, San Francisco, CA, USA

Tara J. Wu
Department of Head and Neck Surgery, University of California Los Angeles, Los Angeles, CA, USA

Annemieke van Zante
Department of Pathology, University of California San Francisco, San Francisco, CA, USA

Ivan H. El-Sayed, William R.Ryan and Patrick K. Ha
Division of Head and Neck Oncologic Surgery, Department of Otolaryngology-Head and Neck Surgery, University of California San Francisco, San Francisco, CA, USA

Alain P. Algazi
Department of Medicine, University of California San Francisco, San Francisco, CA, USA

Brent A. Chang, Kimberly Luu, Robert M.McKenzie and Donald W. Anderson
Division of Otolaryngology – Head and Neck Surgery, University of British Columbia, Vancouver, BC, Canada

Oleksandr Butskiy
Division of Otolaryngology – Head and Neck Surgery, University of British Columbia, Vancouver, BC, Canada
Gordon and Leslie Diamond Health Care Centre, 4th. Fl. 4299B-2775 Laurel Street, Vancouver, BC V5Z 1M9, Canada

Clifford Scott Brown, Ralph Abi-Hachem and David Woojin Jang
Division of Head and Neck Surgery and Communication Sciences, Department of Surgery, Duke University Medical Center, DUMC 3805, Durham, NC 27710, USA

Lisa Jin and Daphne Lu
Faculty of Medicine, University of British Columbia, 317-2194 Health Sciences Mall, Vancouver, BC V6T 1Z3, Canada

Neil K. Chadha and Frederick K.Kozak
Faculty of Medicine, University of British Columbia, 317-2194 Health Sciences Mall, Vancouver, BC V6T 1Z3, Canada
Division of Pediatric Otolaryngology-Head and Neck Surgery, BC Children's Hospital, 4480 Oak St, Vancouver, BC V6H 3N1, Canada

Paula Téllez and Julie Pauwels
Division of Pediatric Otolaryngology-Head and Neck Surgery, BC Children's Hospital, 4480 Oak St, Vancouver, BC V6H 3N1, Canada

Ruth Chia
Department of Audiology, BC Children's Hospital, 4480 Oak St, Vancouver, BC V6H 3N1, Canada

Simon Dobson
Sidra Medical and Research Centre, Doha, Qatar

Hazim Al Eid
Department of Surgery, Division of Otolaryngology King Fahad Specialist Hospital, Dammam, Kingdom of Saudi Arabia

Vincent Wu
School of Medicine, Faculty of Health Sciences, Queen's University, 80 Barrie St, Kingston, ON K7L 3J8, Canada

Stephen F. Hall
Department of Otolaryngology – Head and Neck Surgery, Queen's Cancer Research Institute, Queen's University, 10 Stuart St, Level 2, Kingston, ON K7L 3N6, Canada

Margaret Aron
Division of Otolaryngology-Head and Neck Surgery, Université de Sherbrooke, Sherbrooke, QC, Canada
Centre Hospitalier Université de Sherbrooke, Service d'Otorhinolaryngoloie et Chirurgie Cervicofaciale, Site Hôtel-Dieu, 580 rue Bowen Sud, Sherbrooke, QC J1G 2E8, Canada

Thomas G. Landry
Division Otolaryngology-Head and Neck Surgery, Nova Scotia Health Authority, Dalhousie University, Halifax, NS, Canada

Manohar Bance
Division Otolaryngology-Head and Neck Surgery, Nova Scotia Health Authority, Dalhousie University, Halifax, NS, Canada

David Forner, Liane B. Johnson, Matthew H. Rigby, Jonathan R. Trites, Mark S. Taylor and Robert D. Hart
Division of Otolaryngology – Head and Neck Surgery, Department of Surgery, Dalhousie University, 5820 University Ave. 3rd Floor Dickson Bldg, Halifax, NS B3H 2Y9, Canada

Timothy Wallace
Division of Otolaryngology – Head and Neck Surgery, Department of Surgery, Dalhousie University, 5820 University Ave. 3rd Floor Dickson Bldg, Halifax, NS B3H 2Y9, Canada
Division of Otolaryngology – Head and Neck Surgery, Department of Surgery, Cumberland Regional Health Care Center, Amherst, NS, Canada

Christopher J. Chin
Division of Otolaryngology – Head and Neck Surgery, Department of Surgery, Dalhousie University, 5820 University Ave. 3rd Floor Dickson Bldg, Halifax, NS B3H 2Y9, Canada

Division of Otolaryngology – Head and Neck Surgery, Department of Surgery, Saint John Regional Hospital, Saint John, NB, Canada

Martin Bullock and Daniel Manders
Department of Pathology, Dalhousie University, Halifax, NS, Canada

Kimberly Luu and Arif Janjua
Division of Otolaryngology – Head and Neck Surgery, University of British Columbia, Gordon and Leslie Diamond Health Care Centre, DHCC, Vancouver General Hospital, 4th. Floor Rm. 4299B 2775 Laurel Street, Vancouver, BC V5Z 1M9, Canada

Jason Sutherland and Giuping Liu
UBC Centre for Health Services and Policy Research, Vancouver Campus, 201-2206 East Mall, Vancouver, BC V6T 1Z3, Canada

Trafford Crump
University of Calgary, 2500 University Dr. NW, Calgary, AB T2N 1N4, Canada

Ashley Hinther
Department of Surgery, Section of Otolaryngology-Head and Neck Surgery, Cumming School of Medicine, University of Calgary, HRIC 2A02, 3280 Hospital Dr NW, Calgary, AB T2N 4Z6, Canada

Shamir P. Chandarana, T. Wayne Matthews and Joseph C. Dort
Department of Surgery, Section of Otolaryngology-Head and Neck Surgery, Cumming School of Medicine, University of Calgary, HRIC 2A02, 3280 Hospital Dr NW, Calgary, AB T2N 4Z6, Canada
Ohlson Research Initiative, Arnie Charbonneau Cancer Institute, Cumming School of Medicine, University of Calgary, Calgary, AB, Canada

Steven C. Nakoneshny
Ohlson Research Initiative, Arnie Charbonneau Cancer Institute, Cumming School of Medicine, University of Calgary, Calgary, AB, Canada

Sena Turkdogan
McGill University Health Center, Montreal, QC, Canada

Véronique-Isabelle Forest and Michael P. Hier
Department of Otolaryngology-Head and Neck Surgery, Sir Mortimer B. Davis-Jewish General Hospital, Montreal, Canada

Richard J. Payne
Department of Otolaryngology-Head and Neck Surgery, Sir Mortimer B. Davis-Jewish General Hospital, Montreal, Canada

Department of Otolaryngology-Head and Neck Surgery, McGill University Health Centre, Montreal, Canada

Michael Tamilia
Department of Endocrinology and Metabolism, Sir Mortimer B. Davis-Jewish General Hospital, Montreal, Canada

Anca Florea
Department of Pathology, Sir Mortimer B. Davis-Jewish General Hospital, Montreal, Canada

Francisco Lee, Kristine A. Smith and J. Douglas Bosch
Section of Otolaryngology – Head and Neck Surgery, Department of Surgery, Cumming School of Medicine, University of Calgary, HRIC 2A02, 3280 Hospital Dr NW, Calgary, AB T2N 4Z6, Canada

Steven C. Nakoneshny
Ohlson Research Initiative, Arnie Charbonneau Cancer Institute, Cumming School of Medicine, University of Calgary, Calgary, Alberta, Canada

Yaeesh Sardiwalla
Faculty of Medicine, Dalhousie University, Halifax, NS, Canada

David P. Morris
Faculty of Medicine, Dalhousie University, Halifax, NS, Canada
Division of Otolaryngology – Head and Neck Surgery, Dalhousie University, Halifax, NS, Canada
QEII Health Science Center - VG Site Otolaryngology, 5820 University Ave - Rm 3037, Halifax, NS B3H 2Y9, Canada

Nicholas Jufas
Division of Otolaryngology – Head and Neck Surgery, Dalhousie University, Halifax, NS, Canada
Discipline of Surgery, Sydney Medical School, University of Sydney, Sydney, Australia
Department of Otolaryngology – Head and Neck Surgery, Faculty of Medicine and Health Sciences, Macquarie University, Sydney, Australia

Index